# Neuroanatomy

## Basic and clinical

*For David and Betty Dickens*

# Neuroanatomy

## Basic and clinical

*Second Edition*

# M. J. T. FitzGerald MD, PhD, DSc, MRIA

Professor and Chairman, Department of Anatomy, University College, Galway, Ireland; formerly
Associate Professor at the Department of Biological Structure, University of Washington School
of Medicine, Seattle; and Lecturer in Anatomy at the Department of Anatomy,
St Thomas's Hospital Medical School, London

## Baillière Tindall

LONDON   PHILADELPHIA   TORONTO   SYDNEY   TOKYO

This book is printed on acid-free paper

*Baillière Tindall*
W. B. Saunders

24–28 Oval Road
London, NW1 7DX

The Curtis Center
Independence Square West
Philadelphia, PA 19106-3399, USA

55 Horner Avenue
Toronto, Ontario, M8Z 4X6, Canada

Harcourt Brace Jovanovich Group (Australia) Pty Ltd
30–52 Smidmore Street
Marrickville,
NSW 2204, Australia

Harcourt Brace Jovanovich Japan Inc.
Ichibancho Central Building, 22-1 Ichibancho
Chiyoda-ku, Tokyo 102, Japan

First published 1985
Reprinted 1985 and 1990
Second edition 1992

Typeset by Paston Press, Loddon, Norfolk
Printed in Great Britain by Butler and Tanner Ltd, Frome, Somerset

A catalogue record for this book is available from the British Library

ISBN 0-7020-1432-X

# Contents

# Acknowledgements

First, I would like to thank my wife. As well as being a doctor and a professional histologist, Maeve has been at pains to read the text and illustrations, with many reminders that the book should be written to inform students rather than to impress colleagues. As a result, I believe students will find the text very readable, although some 'heavy going' is unavoidable in later chapters owing to the nature of the material.

For constructive comments on the first edition, I thank Professor M. Berry, Guy's Hospital Medical School, London; Professor J. P. Fraher, University College, Cork; Professor Dr med. Hans-Joachim Kretschmann, University of Hannover Medical School; and Dr B. L. Munger, Hershey Medical Center, Pennsylvania State University. Many points made by students, in Galway and elsewhere, were also taken into account.

For comments on preliminary drafts of the present main text, I again thank Professors Berry and Fraher, and I thank Professor J. S. G. Miller, University of Newcastle upon Tyne. Dr J. M. O'Donnell, Department of Pharmacology, University College, Galway helped me with the chapter on the autonomic nervous system; and Dr Simone Backhauss, Anatomisches Institut der Heinrich Heine Universität, Düsseldorf, made suggestions for the chapter on the skin. The clinical panels were checked by Professor Hugh Staunton of The Richmond Institute for Neurology and Neurosurgery, Dublin; by Dr J. D'Alton, Neurological Services P.C., Franklin Street, Framingham, Massachusetts; and by Dr J. Moran, Consultant Neurologist, University College Hospital, Galway. I should emphasize that any errors that may have persisted in the text or illustrations are entirely my own responsibility.

Ms Barbara Keane, UCHG, provided opportunities to observe and discuss the work of physical therapists in neurorehabilitation.

Photographs of gross and sectional anatomy were provided through the good offices of Dr T. H. Williams, College of Medicine, University of Iowa and the J. B. Lippincott Company, Pennsylvania. Several series of MR images were provided by Professor Paul Finn, Department of Radiology, New Deaconess Hospital, Boston. Carotid angiograms were provided by Dr J. Toland, Department of Radiology, Beaumont Hospital, Dublin and by Professor J. F. Toole, The Bowman Gray School of Medicine, Winston-Salem, North Carolina. Sources for other illustrations are acknowledged in the text.

I am also glad to acknowledge the secretarial assistance of Ms Mary O'Donnell, and photographic assistance by Mr John Furey.

My publishing colleagues at Baillière Tindall have been most supportive. Associate Editor Dr Steven Handley has looked after my every need with courteous efficiency. The illustrators appointed by the Publishers, Marks Creative Consultants, besides giving a professional rendition of my drawings, added numerous imaginative touches; I believe readers will agree that the collaborative effort has been worthwhile.

# Preface

In addition to being updated, the material for the second edition has been modified in several respects. The text has been significantly shortened by removal of material of little clinical relevance. It has also been simplified, to make it more accessible to undergraduates; the first edition seems to have appealed mainly to residents/registrars in clinical neurology. A chapter on embryology has been inserted in order to explain the basic relationships of parts in the adult brain, and two chapters on gross anatomy have been introduced to explain the appearance of 'slices' of the living brain derived from MRI (magnetic resonance imaging).

Permission to use some photographs for this edition has, I believe, been used to good effect. The photographs range across gross anatomy, sectional anatomy of the cerebral hemispheres and brain stem, MRI appearances, angiography, and clinical conditions. Color has also been introduced where advantageous, and my final line drawings have been rendered by professionals.

During the course of preparing an invited report on undergraduate medical anatomy teaching,[1] I have been impressed by the perception by educationalists of the need to present the basic and applied aspects of any topic *together* if learning is to be effective. The following quotations should suffice to make the point. 'The successful retrieval of information at some time in the future is promoted when the retrieval cues are encoded together with the information.'[2] 'The closer the resemblance between the situation in which something is learned and the situation in which it is applied, the better the performance.'[3] '[There is] an apparent lack of utility of basic science information in the clinical reasoning process when the basic science information is provided out of context of the clinical problem.'[4] With these strictures in mind, I have interspersed clinical comments within the general text. I have also shifted the more formal descriptions of clinical disorders from the rump of various chapters into 'clinical panels' placed alongside the relevant basic material.

Because of the perceived importance of problem-solving in medical education (as distinct from rote learning),[5] I have included four sets of neuroanatomical diagnostic problems.

In the first chapter of his book, *The Effective Clinical Neurologist*,[6] Dr Louis Caplan (Tufts University School of Medicine, Boston) asks: 'Is the neurologist's compulsion with anatomy reasonable and justified?' His affirmative answer stresses the value of ascertaining the probable site of a lesion before any of the newer technologies are brought to bear. The present book aims to serve this purpose by explaining the clinical consequences of lesions at many different levels of the nervous system.

I should appreciate receiving comments from students and from colleagues, about ways in which the present edition might be improved—without being made longer. The third edition of a textbook is often the best!

*Turlough FitzGerald*

## REFERENCES

1 FitzGerald, M. J. T. (1992) Undergraduate medical anatomy teaching. *Journal of Anatomy* **180**: 203–209.
2 Tulving, E. and Thompson, D. M. (1973) Encoding specificity and retrieval processes in episodic memory. *Psychological Review* **80**: 352–373.
3 Schmidt, H. G. (1983) Problem-based learning: rationale and description. *Medical Education* **17**: 11–16.
4 Patel, V. L., Groen, G. J. and Scott, H. M. (1988) Biomedical knowledge in explanations of clinical problems by medical students. *Medical Education* **22**: 398–406.
5 Walton, H. J. (1989) Editorial. *Medical Education* **23**: 219–220.
6 Caplan, L. R. (1990) *The Effective Clinical Neurologist*. Cambridge: Blackwell.

# 1

# Embryology

The objective of this chapter is to provide a basis for understanding the arrangement of major parts in the adult nervous system.

For descriptive purposes, the human embryo is in the prone (face down) position. The terms *dorsal* and *ventral* correspond to the adult *anterior* and *posterior*. The terms *rostral* and *caudal* correspond to *superior* and *inferior*.

## SPINAL CORD

### Neurulation (Figure 1.1)

The entire nervous system originates from the **neural plate**, an ectodermal thickening in the floor of the amniotic sac. During the third week after fertilization the plate forms paired **neural folds,** which unite to create the **neural tube** and **neural canal**. Union of the folds commences in the future neck region of the embryo and proceeds rostrally and caudally from there. The open ends of the tube, the **neuropores,** are closed off before the end of the fourth week. The process of formation of the neural tube from the ectoderm is known as **neurulation.**

Cells at the edge of each neural fold escape from the line of union and form the **neural crest** alongside the tube. Cell types derived from the neural crest include spinal and autonomic ganglion cells and the Schwann cells of peripheral nerves.

### Spinal nerves (Figure 1.2)

The dorsal part of the neural tube is called the **alar plate**; the ventral part is the **basal plate.** Neurons developing in the alar plate are predominantly sensory in function and receive *dorsal nerve roots* growing in from the spinal ganglia. Neurons in the basal plate are predominantly motor and give rise to *ventral nerve roots*. At appropriate levels of the spinal cord the ventral roots also contain autonomic fibers. The dorsal and ventral roots unite to form the *spinal nerves*, which emerge from the vertebral canal in the interval between the neural arches being formed by the mesenchymal vertebrae.

The cells of the spinal (dorsal root) ganglia are initially bipolar. They become unipolar by the coalescence of their two processes at one side of the parent cells.

## BRAIN

### Brain vesicles (Figure 1.3)

Rostrally, the closed neural tube expands in the form of three **brain vesicles: the prosencephalon** or forebrain, the **mesencephalon** or midbrain, and the **rhombencephalon** or hindbrain.

The alar plate of the prosencephalon expands on each side to form the **telencephalon,** or cerebral hemispheres. The basal plate remains in place here, as the **diencephalon.** Finally, an *optic outgrowth* from the diencephalon is the forerunner of the retina and optic nerve.

*The diencephalon, mesencephalon and rhombencephalon constitute the embryonic brainstem.*

The brainstem buckles as development proceeds. As a result, the mesencephalon is carried to the summit of the brain. The rhombencephalon folds upon itself, causing the alar plates to flare and creating the rhomboid (diamond-shaped) **fourth ventricle** of the brain. The rostral part of the rhombencephalon gives rise to the **pons** and **cere-**

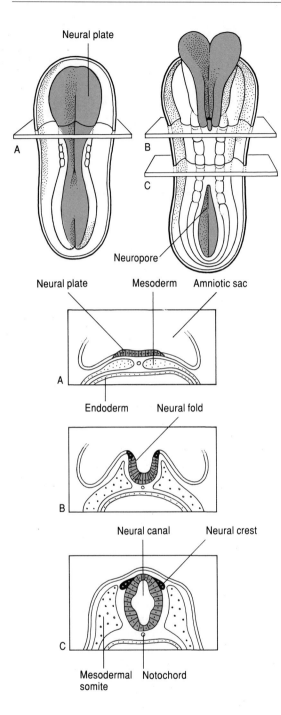

**Figure 1.1.** Cross-section *A* is from a 3-somite (20-day) embryo. Cross-sections *B* and *C* are from an 8-somite (22-day) embryo.

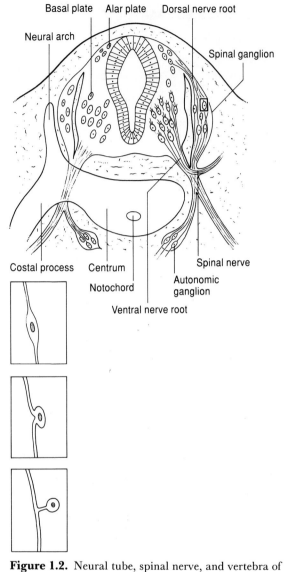

**Figure 1.2.** Neural tube, spinal nerve, and vertebra of an embryo at 8 weeks. Inset shows transformation of a spinal ganglion cell from bipolar to unipolar form.

**bellum**. The caudal part gives rise to the **medulla oblongata** (*Table 1.1*).

## Ventricular system and choroid plexuses

The neural canal dilates within the cerebral hemispheres, forming the **lateral ventricles**; these communicate with the **third ventricle** within the

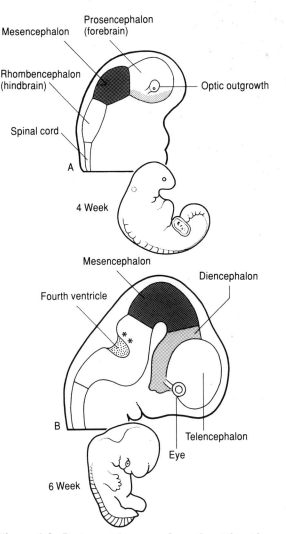

**Figure 1.3.** Brain vesicles, seen from the right side. Mesencephalon shaded, diencephalon stippled. Asterisks indicate the site of initial development of the cerebellum.

**Table 1.1** Some derivatives of the brain vesicles

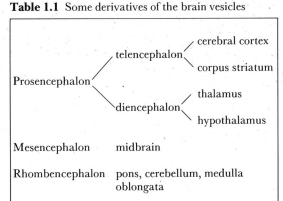

| Prosencephalon | telencephalon | cerebral cortex |
| | | corpus striatum |
| | diencephalon | thalamus |
| | | hypothalamus |
| Mesencephalon | midbrain | |
| Rhombencephalon | pons, cerebellum, medulla oblongata | |

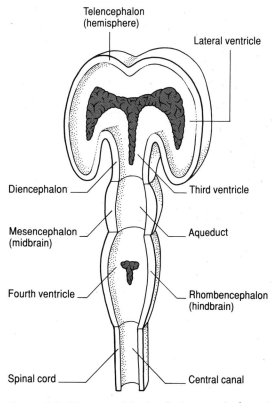

**Figure 1.4.** Diagram of the developing ventricular system. Choroid plexuses are shown in red.

diencephalon. The third and fourth ventricles communicate through the **aqueduct** of the midbrain (*Figure 1.4*).

The thin roofs of the forebrain and hindbrain are invaginated by tufts of capillaries which form the **choroid plexuses** of the four ventricles. The choroid plexuses secrete *cerebrospinal fluid* which flows through the ventricular system. The fluid leaves the fourth ventricle through three apertures in its roof (*Figure 1.5*).

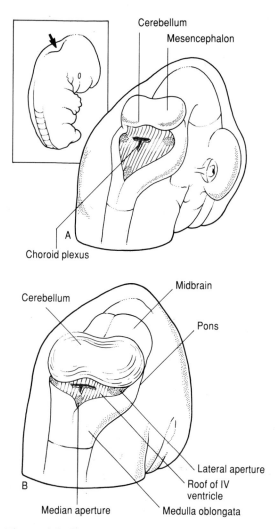

**Figure 1.5.** Dorsal views of the developing hindbrain (see arrow in inset). (A) At 6 weeks, initial development of the cerebellum occurs under cover of the thin roof of the fourth ventricle. (B) At 10 weeks, the ventricle is being covered over by the cerebellum.

### Cranial nerves

*Figure 1.6* illustrates the state of development of the cranial nerves during the sixth week after fertilization. The *olfactory nerve* (I) forms from bipolar neurons developing in the epithelium lining the olfactory pit. The *optic nerve* (II) is growing centrally from the retina. The *oculomotor* (III) and *trochlear* (IV) *nerves* arise from the mid-

brain, and the *abducens* (VI) arises from the pons; all three will supply extrinsic muscles of the eye.

The three divisions of the *trigeminal* (V) *nerve* will be sensory to the skin of the face and scalp, to the mucous membranes of the oro-nasal cavity, and to the teeth. A *motor root* will supply the muscles of mastication (chewing).

The *facial* (VII) *nerve* will supply the muscles of facial expression. The *vestibulocochlear* (VIII) *nerve* will supply the organs of hearing and balance, which develop from the otocyst.

The *glossopharyngeal* (IX) *nerve* is composite. Most of its fibers will be sensory to the oropharynx. The *vagus* (X) *nerve* is also composite; it contains a large sensory element for the supply of the mucous membranes of the digestive system, and a large motor (parasympathetic) element for the supply of the heart and gastrointestinal tract.

The *cranial accessory* (XIc) *nerve* will be distributed by the vagus to the muscles of the larynx and pharynx. The *spinal accessory* (XIs) *nerve* will supply the sternomastoid and trapezius muscles. The *hypoglossal* (XII) *nerve* will supply the muscles of the tongue.

### Cerebral hemispheres

In the telencephalon, mitotic activity takes place in the *ventricular zone*, just outside the lateral ventricle. Daughter cells migrate to the outer surface of the expanding hemisphere and form the *cerebral cortex.*

Expansion of the cerebral hemispheres is not uniform. A region on the lateral surface, the **insula**, is relatively quiescent and forms a pivot around which the expanding hemisphere rotates. **Frontal, parietal, occipital** and **temporal lobes** can be identified at 14 weeks' gestational age (*Figure 1.7*).

On the medial surface of the hemisphere, a patch of cerebral cortex, the **hippocampus**, belongs to a fifth, **limbic lobe** of the brain. The hippocampus is drawn into the temporal lobe, leaving in its wake a strand of fibers called the **fornix.** Within the concavity of this arc is the **choroid fissure**, through which the choroid plexus invaginates into the lateral ventricle (*Figure 1.8*).

The **anterior commissure** develops as a connection linking olfactory (smell) regions of the left and right sides. Above this, a much larger commissure, the **corpus callosum** links matching areas of

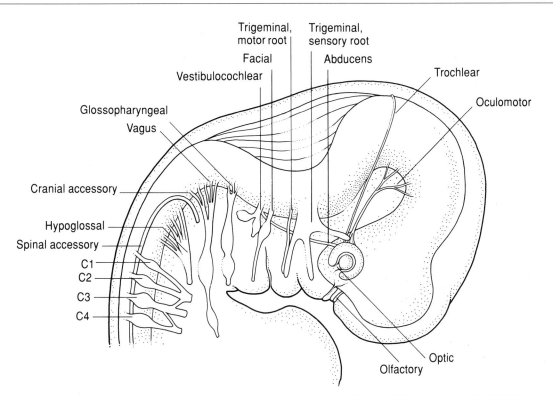

**Figure 1.6.** Cranial nerves of an embryo early in the 6th week. (Adapted from Bossy *et al.*, 1990.)

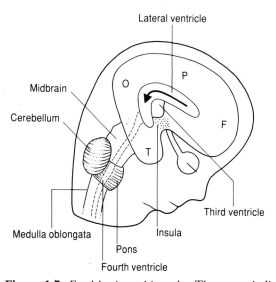

**Figure 1.7.** Fetal brain at 14 weeks. The arrow indicates the C-shaped growth of the hemisphere around the insula. F, P, O, T, frontal, parietal, occipital, temporal lobes.

the cerebral cortex of the two sides. It extends backward above the fornix.

Coronal sections of the telencephalon reveal a mass of gray matter in the base of each hemisphere which is the forerunner of the **corpus striatum.** Beside the third ventricle the diencephalon gives rise to the **thalamus** and **hypothalamus** (*Figure 1.9*).

The expanding cerebral hemispheres come into contact with the diencephalon and they fuse with it (see 'site of fusion' in *Figure 1.9A*). One consequence is that the term 'brainstem' is restricted thereafter to the remaining, free parts: midbrain, pons, and medulla oblongata. A second consequence is that the cerebral cortex is able to project fibers direct to the brainstem. Together with fibers projecting from thalamus to cortex, they split the corpus striatum into **caudate** and **lentiform nuclei** (*Figure 1.9B*).

By the 28th week of development, several *sulci* (fissures) have appeared on the surface of the brain, notably the *lateral, central, and calcarine* sulci (*Figure 1.10*).

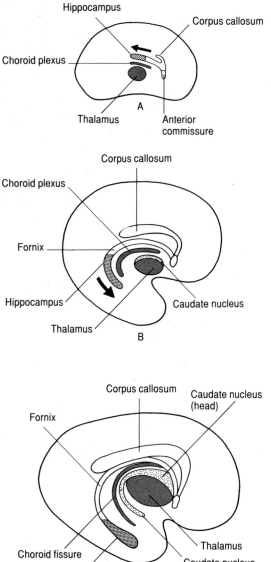

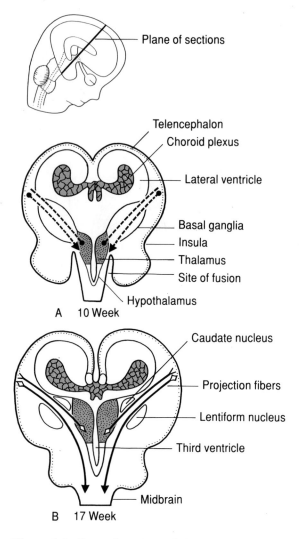

**Figure 1.8.** Medial aspect of developing left hemisphere. The hippocampus, initially dorsal to the thalamus, migrates into the temporal lobe (arrows in A and B), leaving the fornix in its wake. The concavity of the arch so formed contains the choroid fissure (the line of insertion of the choroid plexus into the lateral ventricle) and the tail of the caudate nucleus.

**Figure 1.9.** Coronal sections of the developing cerebrum. The corpus striatum is cleft by fibers projecting to and from the cerebral cortex. See text for other details.

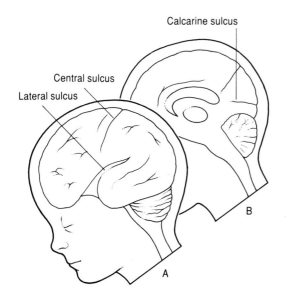

**Figure 1.10.** Three major cortical sulci in a fetus of 28 weeks. (A) Lateral surface of hemisphere; (B) medial surface of hemisphere.

## REFERENCES

Bossy, J., O'Rahilly, R. and Muller, F. (1990) Ontogenese du systeme nerveux. In *Anatomie Clinique: Neuroanatomie* (Bossy, J., ed.), pp. 357–388. Paris: Springer-Verlag.

Lemire, R.J., Loeser, J.D., Leech, R.W. and Alvord, E.C. (1975) *Normal and Abnormal Development of the Nervous System.* Hagerstown: Harper & Row.

O'Rahilly, R. and Gardner, E. (1979) The initial development of the human brain. *Acta Anat.* **104:** 123–133.

O'Rahilly, R. and Muller, F. (1987) The developmental anatomy and histology of the human central nervous system. In *Handbook of Clinical Neurology, Vol. 6, Malformations* (Myrianthopoulos, N.C., ed.), pp. 1–17. Amsterdam: Elsevier.

Sadler, T.W. (1990) *Langman's Medical Embryology*, 6th edn. Baltimore: Williams & Wilkins.

# 2

# Cerebral topography

**CHAPTER SUMMARY**

Surface features
Lobes
Diencephalon
Internal anatomy of the cerebrum
Thalamus, caudate and lentiform nuclei
Internal capsule
Lateral and third ventricles

The following account of cerebral gross anatomy is intended to provide the student with baseline information required for interpretation of brain scans.

The advent of nuclear magnetic resonance imaging (MRI) of the living brain has made it possible to define the more discrete types of brain lesions—notably tumors and hematomas—with great accuracy. An understanding of the gross anatomy, as seen in different planes of section, is quite fundamental to the interpretation of computer-produced 'slices' of the brain.

## SURFACE FEATURES

### Lobes

The surfaces of the two cerebral hemispheres are furrowed by **sulci,** the intervening ridges being called **gyri**. Most of the cerebral cortex is concealed from view in the walls of the sulci. Although the patterns of the various sulci vary from brain to brain, some are sufficiently constant to serve as descriptive landmarks.

The deepest sulci are the **lateral sulcus** *(Sylvian fissure)* and the **central sulcus** *(Rolandic fissure)* *(Figure 2.1A)*. These two serve to divide the hemisphere into four **lobes,** with the aid of two imaginary lines: one line extends back from the lateral sulcus; the other reaches from the upper end of the **parieto-occipital sulcus** *(Figure 2.1B)* to a blunt *pre-occipital notch* at the lower border of the hemisphere. The lobes are called **frontal, parietal, occipital and temporal**.

The blunt tips of the frontal, occipital and temporal lobes are the respective **poles** of the brain.

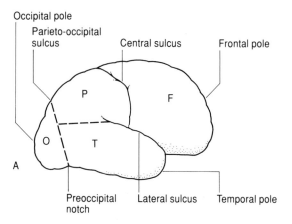

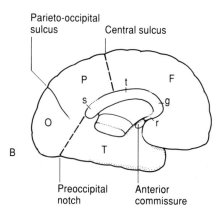

**Figure 2.1.** Boundaries of the frontal (F), parietal (L), occipital (O), and temporal (T) lobes. s, Splenium; t, trunk; g, genu; r, rostrum of corpus callosum.

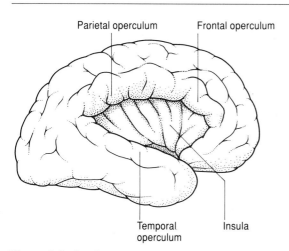

**Figure 2.2.** Insula, seen upon retraction of the opercula.

The lips **(opercula)** of the lateral sulcus can be pulled apart to expose the **insula** (*Figure 2.2*). The insula was mentioned in Chapter 1 as being relatively quiescent during prenatal expansion of the telencephalon.

The medial surface of the hemisphere is exposed by cutting the **corpus callosum,** a massive band of white matter connecting matching areas of the cortex of the two hemispheres. The corpus callosum consists of a main part or *trunk*, a posterior end or *splenium*, an anterior end or *genu* ('knee'), and a narrow *rostrum* reaching from the genu to the **anterior commissure** (*Figure 2.1B*). The frontal lobe lies anterior to a line drawn from the upper end of the central sulcus to the trunk of the corpus callosum (*Figure 2.1B*). The parietal lobe lies behind this line, and it is separated from the occipital lobe by the parieto-occipital sulcus. The temporal lobe lies in front of a line drawn from the preoccipital notch to the splenium.

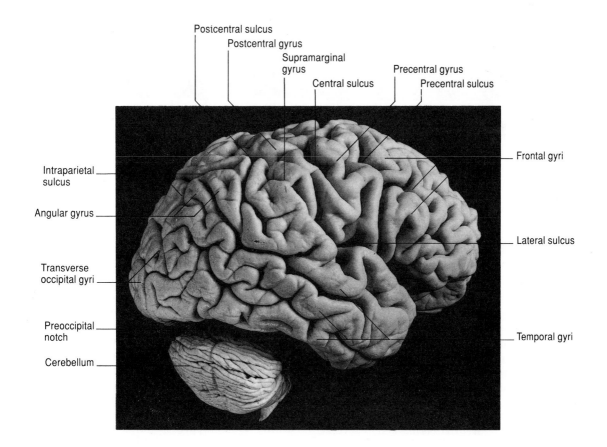

**Figure 2.3.** Lateral view of right cerebral hemisphere. (Photograph reproduced from Gluhbegovic and Williams (1980) with kind permission of the authors and of J.B. Lippincott, Inc.)

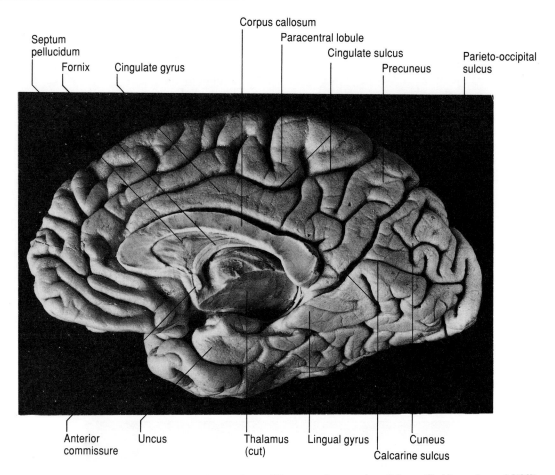

Septum
pellucidum
Fornix    Cingulate gyrus
Corpus callosum
Paracentral lobule
Cingulate sulcus
Precuneus
Parieto-occipital
sulcus

Anterior            Uncus            Thalamus      Lingual gyrus            Cuneus
commissure                          (cut)                      Calcarine sulcus

**Figure 2.4.** Medial view of right cerebral hemisphere. (Photograph reproduced from Gluhbegovic and Williams (1980) with kind permission of the authors and of J.B. Lippincott, Inc.)

*Figures 2.3* to *2.6* should be consulted along with the following description of surface features of the lobes of the brain.

### Frontal lobe

The lateral surface of the frontal lobe contains the **precentral gyrus** bounded in front by the precentral sulcus. Further forward, **superior, middle,** and **inferior frontal gyri** are separated by superior and inferior frontal sulci. On the medial surface, the superior frontal gyrus is separated from the **cingulate gyrus** by the cingulate sulcus. The inferior or orbital surface is marked by several **orbital gyri**. In contact with this surface are the **olfactory bulb** and **olfactory tract.**

### Parietal lobe

The anterior part of the parietal lobe contains the **postcentral gyrus** bounded behind by the postcentral sulcus. The posterior parietal lobe is divided into **superior** and **inferior parietal lobules** by an intra-parietal sulcus. The inferior parietal lobule shows a **supramarginal gyrus,** capping the upturned end of the lateral sulcus, and an **angular gyrus** capping the superior temporal sulcus. The medial surface contains the posterior part of the **paracentral lobule** and, behind this, the **precuneus**. The paracentral lobule (partly contained in the frontal lobe) is so called because of its relationship to the central sulcus.

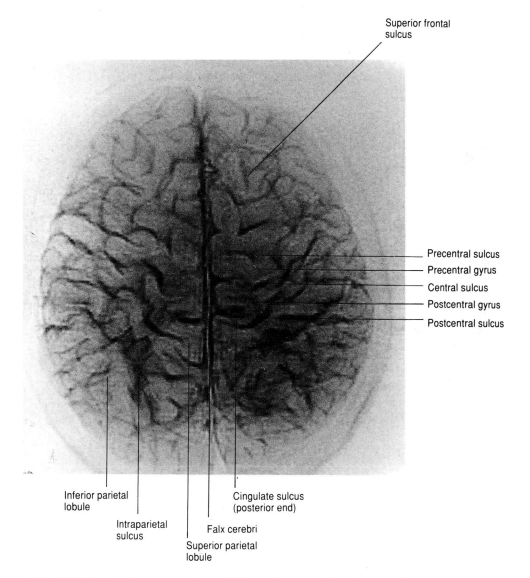

Superior frontal sulcus

Precentral sulcus
Precentral gyrus
Central sulcus
Postcentral gyrus
Postcentral sulcus

Inferior parietal lobule

Intraparietal sulcus

Superior parietal lobule

Falx cerebri

Cingulate sulcus (posterior end)

**Figure 2.5.** 'Thick slice' surface anatomy brain MR scan from a healthy volunteer. (Reproduced from *Neuroradiology* (1990) **32:** 439–448 with kind permission of Professor K. Katada and of the Publishers.)

## Occipital lobe

The lateral surface of the occipital lobe is marked by several **lateral occipital gyri.** The medial surface contains the **cuneus** ('wedge') between the parieto-occipital sulcus and the important **calcarine sulcus**. The inferior surface shows three gyri and three sulci. The **lateral** and **medial occipito-temporal gyri** are separated by the occipito-temporal sulcus. The **lingual gyrus** lies between

the collateral sulcus and the anterior end of the calcarine sulcus.

## Temporal lobe

The lateral surface of the temporal lobe displays **superior, middle,** and **inferior temporal gyri** separated by superior and inferior temporal sulci. The inferior surface shows the anterior parts of the occipitotemporal gyri. The lingual gyrus continues

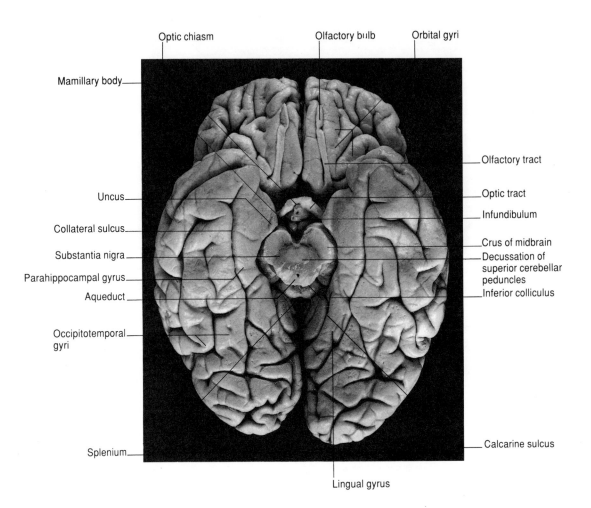

Optic chiasm   Olfactory bulb   Orbital gyri

Mamillary body

Olfactory tract

Uncus

Optic tract

Infundibulum

Collateral sulcus

Crus of midbrain

Substantia nigra

Decussation of
superior cerebellar
peduncles

Parahippocampal gyrus

Aqueduct

Inferior colliculus

Occipitotemporal
gyri

Splenium

Calcarine sulcus

Lingual gyrus

**Figure 2.6.** Cerebrum, viewed from below. (Photograph reproduced from Gluhbegovic and Williams (1980) with kind permission of the authors and of J.B. Lippincott, Inc.)

forward as the **parahippocampal gyrus** which ends in a blunt medial projection, the **uncus**. As will be seen later in views of the sectioned brain, the parahippocampal gyrus underlies a rolled-in part of the cortex, the **hippocampus**.

### Limbic lobe

A fifth, **limbic lobe** of the brain surrounds the medial margin of the hemisphere. Surface contributors to the limbic lobe include the cingulate and parahippocampal gyri. It is more usual to

speak of the *limbic system*, which includes the hippocampus, fornix, amygdala and other elements.

### Diencephalon (Figure 2.7)

The largest components of the diencephalon are the **thalamus** and the **hypothalamus.** These nuclear groups form the side walls of the third ventricle. Between them is a shallow *hypothalamic sulcus*, which represents the rostral limit of the embryonic sulcus limitans. The hypothalamus forms the floor of the third ventricle as well.

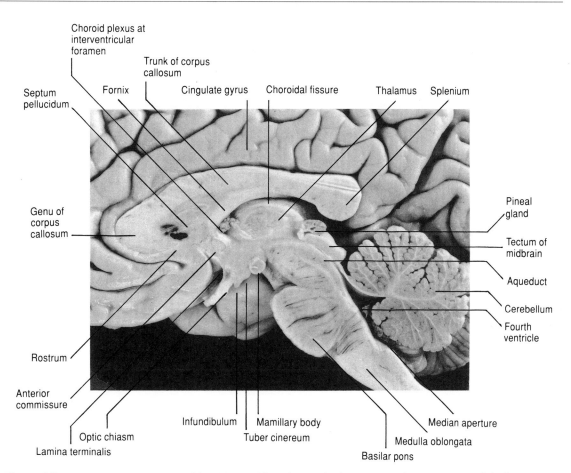

**Figure 2.7.** Median sagittal section of fixed brain. Note that in the living state, the orientation of the brainstem is more vertical (cf. *Figure 2.8*). (Photograph reproduced from Gluhbegovic and Williams (1980) by kind permission of the authors and of J.B. Lippincott, Inc.)

The MRI picture in *Figure 2.8* should be examined in conjunction with *Figures 2.4* and *2.7*.

## INTERNAL ANATOMY OF THE CEREBRUM

The arrangement of the following structures will now be described: thalamus, caudate and lentiform nuclei, internal capsule; hippocampus and fornix; association and commissural fibers; lateral and third ventricles.

### Thalamus, caudate and lentiform nuclei, internal capsule

The two thalami face one another across the slot-like third ventricle. More often than not, they kiss, creating an *interthalamic adhesion* (*Figure 2.9*).

In *Figure 2.10* the thalamus, caudate nucleus, internal capsule, lentiform nucleus and internal capsule are assembled piecemeal. In contact with the upper surface of the thalamus are the *head* and *body* of the **caudate nucleus**. The *tail* of the caudate nucleus passes forward below the thalamus, but not in contact with it.

The thalamus is separated from the lentiform nucleus by the **internal capsule**, which is a common site for a *stroke* resulting from local arterial hemorrhage. The internal capsule contains fibers running from thalamus to cortex and from cortex to thalamus, brainstem and spinal cord. In the interval between cortex and internal capsule, these ascending and descending fibers form the **corona radiata**. Below the internal capsule, the *crus* of the

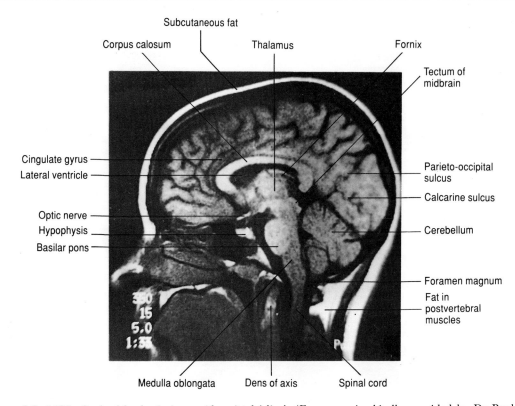

Subcutaneous fat

Corpus calosum    Thalamus    Fornix

Tectum of midbrain

Cingulate gyrus
Lateral ventricle

Parieto-occipital sulcus

Calcarine sulcus

Optic nerve
Hypophysis
Basilar pons

Cerebellum

Foramen magnum
Fat in postvertebral muscles

Medulla oblongata    Dens of axis    Spinal cord

**Figure 2.8.** MRI of a healthy brain in a mid-sagittal 'slice'. (From a series kindly provided by Dr Paul Finn, Department of Radiology, New Deaconess Hospital, Boston.) (*Note:* Lipid-rich tissues are especially enhanced, e.g., CNS myelin, subcutaneous fat, lipid in muscle and bone marrow.)

midbrain receives descending fibers continuing into the brainstem.

The lens-shaped **lentiform nucleus** is composed of two parts, **putamen** and **globus pallidus.** The putamen and caudate nucleus are of similar structure and their anterior ends are fused. Behind this they are linked by strands of gray matter which traverse the internal capsule: hence the term **corpus striatum** (or, simply, *striatum*) used to include the putamen and caudate nucleus. The term *pallidum* refers to the globus pallidus.

The caudate and lentiform nuclei belong to the **basal ganglia**, a term originally applied to a half-dozen masses of gray matter located near the base of the hemisphere. In current usage the term designates four nuclei known to be involved in motor control: the caudate and lentiform nuclei, the subthalamic nucleus in the diencephalon, and the substantia nigra in the midbrain (*Table 2.1*).

**Table 2.1** Nomenclature of basal ganglia*

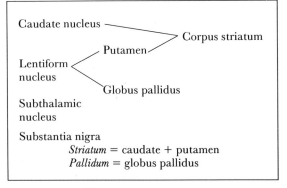

Caudate nucleus
Corpus striatum
Putamen
Lentiform nucleus
Globus pallidus
Subthalamic nucleus
Substantia nigra
    *Striatum* = caudate + putamen
    *Pallidum* = globus pallidus

*Further details in Chapter 24*

In horizontal section, the internal capsule has a dog-leg shape (see photograph of a fixed-brain

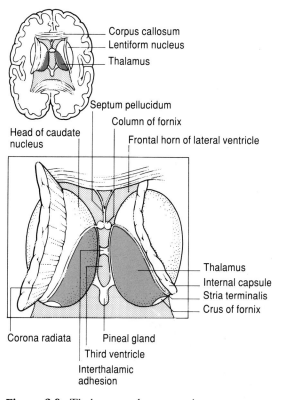

**Figure 2.9.** Thalamus and corpus striatum, seen upon removal of the trunk of the corpus callosum and the body of the fornix.

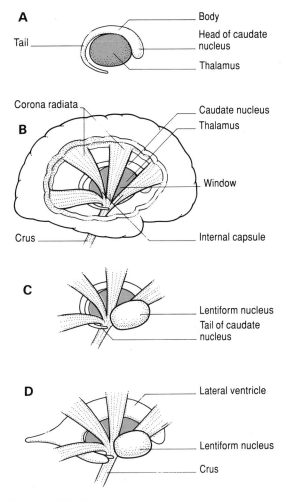

**Figure 2.10.** Diagrammatic reconstruction of corpus striatum and related structures (right side, lateral view). (A) Caudate nucleus and thalamus. (B) Addition of projections from cerebral cortex to brainstem. Three windows (W) have been made in the corona radiata. (C) Addition of lentiform nucleus. (D) Addition of lateral ventricle.

section in *Figure 2.11*, and living-brain MR 'slice' in *Figure 2.12*). The internal capsule has four named parts in horizontal sections:

1. *Anterior limb*, between the lentiform nucleus and the head of the caudate nucleus;
2. *Genu*;
3. *Posterior limb*, between the lentiform nucleus and the thalamus;
4. *Retrolentiform part*, behind the lentiform nucleus and lateral to the thalamus.

The position of the **corticospinal tract** in the posterior limb of the internal capsule is indicated in *Figure 2.11*. It is also called the *pyramidal tract*. (A *tract* is a bundle of fibers serving a common function.) The corticospinal tract originates mainly from the *motor cortex* within the precentral gyrus. It descends through the corona radiata, internal capsule, and crus of midbrain and con-

tinues to the lower end of the brainstem before crossing to the opposite side of the spinal cord.

From a clinical standpoint, *the corticospinal tract is the most important pathway in the entire CNS*, for two reasons. First, it mediates voluntary movements of all kinds, and interruption of the tract by disease leads to motor weakness (called *paresis*) or motor *paralysis*. Secondly, it extends the entire vertical

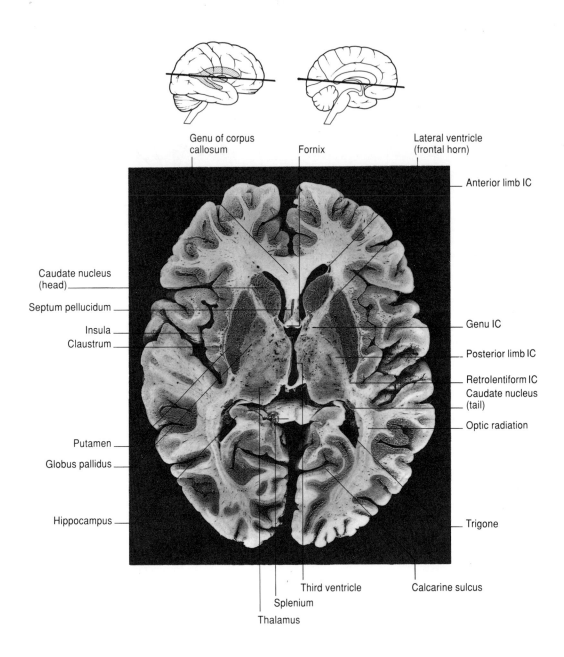

**Figure 2.11.** Horizontal section of fixed brain in the plane indicated at top. IC, internal capsule. (Photograph reproduced from Gluhbegovic and Williams (1980) with kind permission of the authors and of J.B. Lippincott, Inc.)

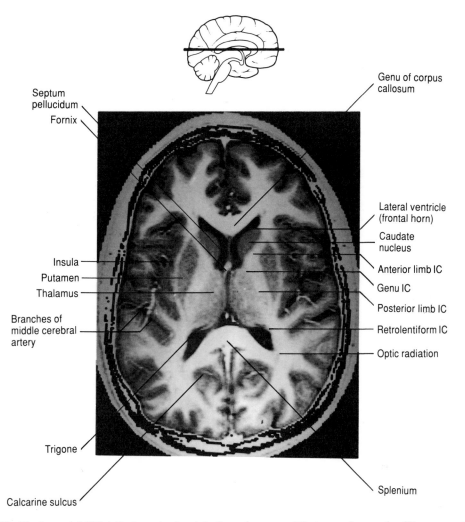

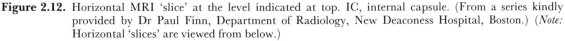

**Figure 2.12.** Horizontal MRI 'slice' at the level indicated at top. IC, internal capsule. (From a series kindly provided by Dr Paul Finn, Department of Radiology, New Deaconess Hospital, Boston.) (*Note:* Horizontal 'slices' are viewed from below.)

length of the CNS, rendering it vulnerable to disease or trauma in the cerebral hemisphere or brainstem on one side, and to spinal cord disease or trauma on the other side.

A coronal section through the anterior limb is represented in *Figure 2.13*; a corresponding MR image is shown in *Figure 2.14*. A coronal section through the posterior limb from a fixed brain is shown in *Figure 2.15*; a corresponding MR 'slice' is shown in *Figure 2.16*.

Lateral to the lentiform nucleus are the *external capsule, claustrum,* and *extreme capsule.*

### *Hippocampus and fornix*

The **hippocampus** is first seen in embryonic life above the thalamus (Chapter 1). The bulk of it retains a high position in lower mammals, including rodents. In primates it retreats into the temporal lobe as this develops, leaving a tract of white matter, the **fornix,** in its wake. The mature hippocampus stretches the full length of the floor of the inferior (temporal) horn of the lateral ventricle (*Figure 2.17*). The mature fornix comprises a *body,* beneath the trunk of the corpus callosum, a *crus*

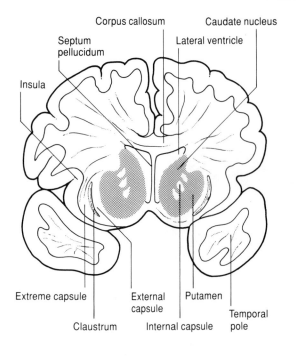

which enters it from each hippocampus, and two *pillars (columns)* which leave it to enter the diencephalon. Intimately related to the crus and body is the *choroid fissure*, through which the choroid plexus is inserted into the lateral ventricle.

### Association and commissural fibers

Fibers leaving the cerebral cortex fall into three groups:

- *Association fibers* pass from one part of a single hemisphere to another
- *Commissural fibers* link matching areas of the two hemispheres

**Figure 2.13.** Drawing of a coronal section through the anterior limb of the internal capsule (cf. *Figure 3.14*).

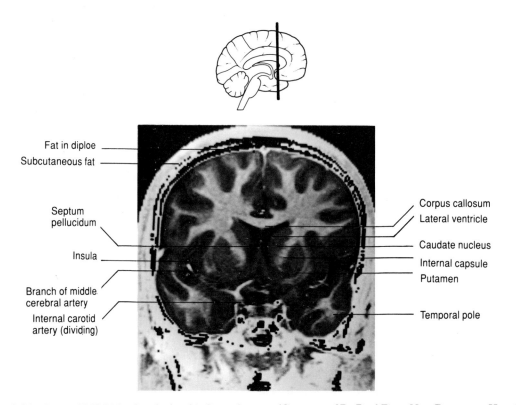

**Figure 2.14.** Coronal MRI 'slice' at the level indicated at top. (Courtesy of Dr Paul Finn, New Deaconess Hospital, Boston.) *(Note:* Coronal 'slices' are viewed from the front.)

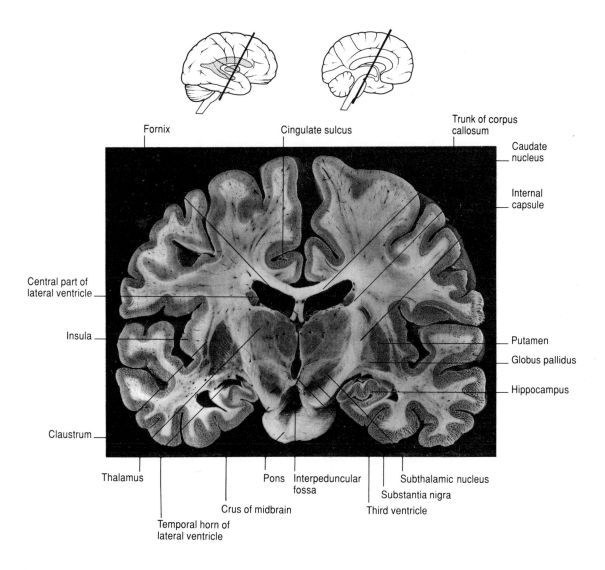

**Figure 2.15.** Coronal section of fixed brain at the level indicated at top. (Photograph reproduced from Gluhbegovic and Williams (1980) with kind permission of the authors and of J.B. Lippincott, Inc.)

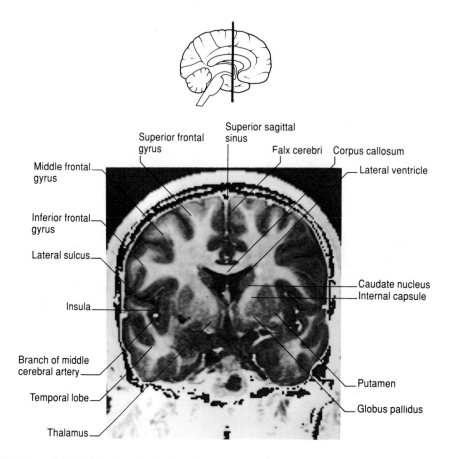

**Figure 2.16.** Coronal MRI 'slice' at the level indicated at top. (From a series kindly provided by Dr Paul Finn, Department of Radiology, New Deaconess Hospital, Boston.)

- *Projection fibers* run to subcortical nuclei in the cerebral hemisphere, brainstem, and spinal cord.

### Association fibers *(Figure 2.18)*

*Short* association fibers pass from one gyrus to another within a lobe. *Long* association fibers link one lobe with another. Bundles of long association fibers include:

- The *superior longitudinal fasciculus,* linking the frontal and occipital lobes
- The *inferior longitudinal fasciculus,* linking the occipital and temporal lobes
- The *arcuate fasciculus,* linking the frontal lobe with the occipitotemporal cortex
- The *uncinate fasciculus,* linking the frontal and anterior temporal lobes

- The *cingulum,* underlying the cortex of the cingulate gyrus.

### Cerebral commissures

CORPUS CALLOSUM (*FIGURE 2.19*)
The corpus callosum is much the largest of the *commissures* linking matching areas of the left and right cerebral cortex. From the trunk, some fibers pass laterally and upward, intersecting the corona radiata. Other fibers pass laterally and then bend downward as the **tapetum** to reach the lower parts of the temporal and occipital lobes. Fibers traveling to the medial wall of the occipital lobe emerge from the splenium on each side and form the **occipital** (major) **forceps.** The **frontal** (minor) **forceps** emerges from each side of the genu to reach the medial wall of the frontal lobe.

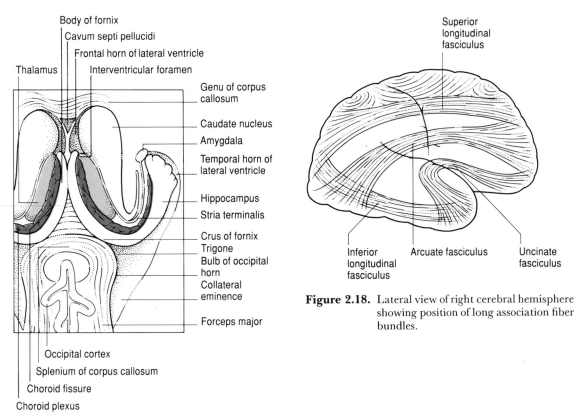

**Figure 2.17.** Continuity of structures in central part and temporal horn of lateral ventricle. *Note:* Amygdala, stria terminalis and tail of caudate nucleus occupy the roof of the temporal horn.

**Figure 2.18.** Lateral view of right cerebral hemisphere showing position of long association fiber bundles.

MINOR COMMISSURES (*FIGURE 2.20*)

The **anterior commissure** interconnects the anterior parts of the temporal lobes, as well as the two olfactory tracts.

The **posterior commissure** and the **habenular commissure** lie directly in front of the pineal gland.

The **commissure of the fornix** contains some fibers traveling from one hippocampus to the other by way of the two crura.

### Lateral and third ventricles

The **lateral ventricle** consists of a *central part*, within the parietal lobe, and *frontal* (anterior),

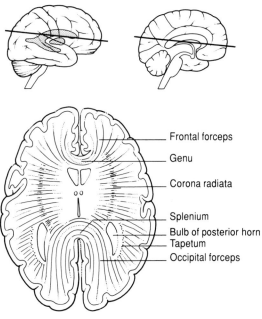

**Figure 2.19.** Horizontal section through genu and splenium of corpus callosum. Fibers passing laterally from the trunk intersect the corona radiata.

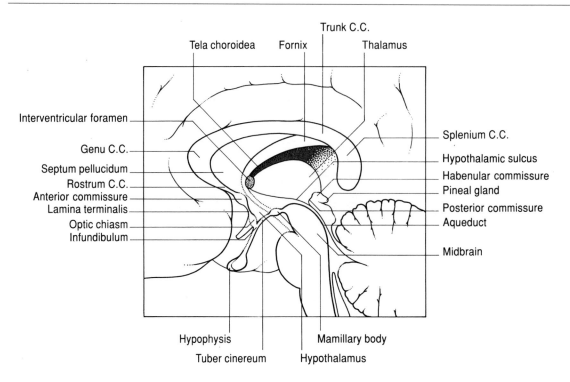

**Figure 2.20.** Sagittal section of diencephalon and surroundings. C.C., corpus callosum.

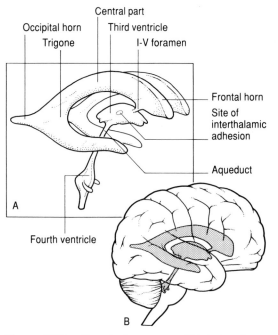

**Figure 2.21.** Ventricular system. (A) isolated cast; (B) ventricular system *in situ*.

*occipital* (posterior) and *temporal* (inferior) *horns* (*Figure 2.21*). The anterior limit of the central part is the *interventricular foramen*, located between thalamus and anterior pillar of the fornix, through which it communicates with the third ventricle (*Figure 2.20*). The central part joins the occipital and temporal horns at the *(collateral) trigone* (*Figure 2.22*).

Relationships of the lateral ventricle are listed below.

*Frontal horn*: lies between head of caudate nucleus and septum pellucidum. Its other boundaries are formed by the corpus callosum: trunk above, genu in front, rostrum below.

*Central part*: lies below the trunk of the corpus callosum and above the thalamus and anterior part of the body of the fornix. Medially is the septum pellucidum, which tapers away posteriorly where the fornix rises to meet the corpus callosum. The septum pellucidum is formed of the thinned out walls of the two cerebral hemispheres. Its bilateral origin may be indicated by a central cavity *(cavum)*.

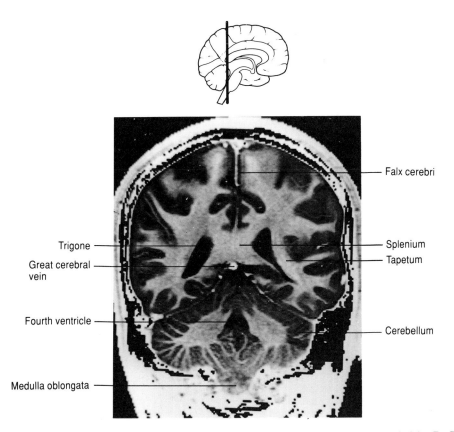

Falx cerebri

Trigone

Great cerebral vein

Splenium

Tapetum

Fourth ventricle

Cerebellum

Medulla oblongata

**Figure 2.22.** Coronal MRI 'slice' at the level indicated at top. (From a series kindly provided by Dr Paul Finn, Department of Radiology, New Deaconess Hospital, Boston.)

*Occipital horn:* roof and lateral wall formed by the tapetum of the corpus callosum. On the medial side, the forceps major forms the *bulb of the posterior horn* and, below this, the calcarine sulcus creates a second bulge, the *calcar avis.*

*Temporal horn:* in the roof are the tail of the caudate nucleus and, at the anterior end, the **amygdala** (*Figure 2.17*), a nucleus belonging to the limbic system. The hippocampus and its associated structures occupy the full length of the floor. Outside these is the *collateral eminence,* created by the collateral sulcus.

The **third ventricle** is the cavity of the diencephalon. Its boundaries are shown in *Figure 2.20.* A *choroid plexus* hangs from its roof, which is formed of a double layer of pia mater called the *tela choroidea.* Above this are the fornix and corpus callosum. In each side wall are the thalamus and hypothala-mus. The anterior wall is formed by the anterior commissure, the lamina terminalis, and the optic chiasm. In the floor are the infundibulum, the tuber cinereum, the mamillary bodies (also spelt 'mammillary'), and the upper end of the midbrain. The pineal gland and related commissures form the posterior wall. The pineal is often calcified, and the habenular commissure is sometimes, even as early as the second decade of life, thereby becoming detectable even on plain radiographs of the skull. The pineal is sometimes displaced to one side by a tumor, hematoma or other space-occupying lesion within the cranial cavity.

## REFERENCES

DeArmond, S.J., Fusco, M.M. and Dewey, M.M. (1976) *Structure of the Human Brain: a Photographic Atlas,* 2nd edn. Oxford: Oxford University Press.

Gluhbegovic, N. and Williams, T.H. (1980) *The Human Brain: a Photographic Guide*. New York: Harper & Row.

Kretschmann, H-J. and Weinrich, W. (1992) *Clinical Neuroanatomy and Neuroimaging*. Stuttgart: Georg Thieme.

Ludwig, E. and Klingler, J. (1956) *Atlas Cerebri Humani*. Boston: Little Brown & Co.

Niewenhuys, R., Voogd, J. and van Huijzen, C. (1988) *The Human Central Nervous System: a Synopsis and Atlas*, 3rd edn. New York: Springer-Verlag.

Roberts, M., Hanaway, J. and Morest, D.K. (1987) *Atlas of the Human Brain in Section*, 2nd edn. Philadelphia: Lea & Febiger.

# 3

# Midbrain, hindbrain, spinal cord

This chapter describes the surface features of the brainstem, cerebellum, and spinal cord. Salient features of transverse sections are also described.

The midbrain connects the diencephalon to the hindbrain. As explained in Chapter 1, the hindbrain is made up of the pons, medulla oblongata, and cerebellum. The medulla oblongata joins the spinal cord within the foramen magnum of the skull.

## BRAINSTEM

### Ventral view (Figures 3.1, 3.2)

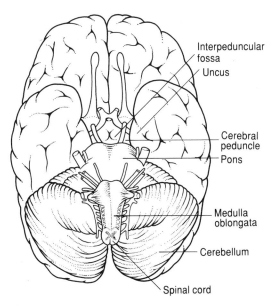

**Figure 3.1.** Ventral view of the brainstem, *in situ*.

## Midbrain

The ventral surface of the midbrain shows two massive **cerebral peduncles** bordering the **interpeduncular fossa**. The **optic tracts** wind around the midbrain at its junction with the diencephalon. On the lateral side is the uncus of the temporal lobe. The **oculomotor nerve** (III) emerges from the medial surface of the peduncle. The **trochlear**

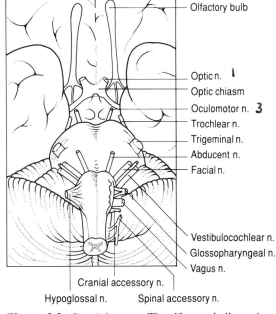

**Figure 3.2.** Cranial nerves. The olfactory bulb receives the olfactory nerve from the nose.

nerve (IV) can be seen between the peduncle and the uncus.

## Pons

The bulk of the pons is composed of *transverse fibers* which raise numerous surface ridges. On each side, the pons is marked off from the **middle cerebellar peduncle** by the attachment of the **trigeminal nerve** (V). The middle cerebellar peduncle plunges into the hemisphere of the cerebellum.

At the lower border of the pons are the attachments of the **abducens** (VI), **facial** (VII), and **vestibulocochlear** (VIII) **nerves.**

## Medulla oblongata

The **pyramids** are alongside the **anterior median fissure.** Just above the spinomedullary junction, the fissure is invaded by the **decussation of the pyramids**, where fibers of the two pyramids intersect while crossing the midline. Lateral to the pyramid is the **olive**, and behind the olive is the **inferior cerebellar peduncle**. Attached between pyramid and olive is the **hypoglossal nerve** (XII). Attached between olive and inferior cerebellar peduncle are the **glossopharyngeal, vagus, and cranial accessory nerves** (IX, X, XIc). The **spinal accessory nerve** (XIs) arises from the spinal cord and runs up through the foramen magnum to join the cranial accessory.

## Dorsal view *(Figure 3.3)*

The roof or **tectum** of the midbrain is composed of four **colliculi**. The **superior colliculi** belong to the visual system and the **inferior colliculi** belong to the auditory system. The **trochlear nerve** (IV) emerges below the inferior colliculus on each side.

The diamond-shaped **fourth ventricle** lies behind the pons and upper medulla oblongata, under cover of the cerebellum. The upper half of the diamond is bounded by the **superior cerebellar peduncles** which are attached to the midbrain. The lower half is bounded by the **inferior cerebellar peduncles,** which are attached to the medulla oblongata. The middle cerebellar peduncles enter from the pons and overlap the other two.

Below the fourth ventricle, the medulla oblon-

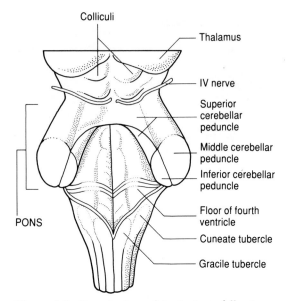

**Figure 3.3.** Dorsal view of brainstem, following removal of the cerebellum.

gata shows a pair of **gracile tubercles** flanked by a pair of **cuneate tubercles.**

## Sectional views

### Sagittal section *(Figure 3.4A)*

In the midbrain, the central canal of the embryonic neural tube is represented by the **aqueduct.** Behind the pons and upper medulla oblongata, it is represented by the fourth ventricle, which is tent shaped in this view. The central canal resumes at mid-medullary level; it is continuous with the central canal of the spinal cord, although movement of cerebrospinal fluid into the cord canal is negligible.

The intermediate region of the brainstem is called the **tegmentum.** Ventral to this in the pons is the **basilar region.** Ventral to it in the medulla oblongata are the pyramids.

### Transverse sections

The tegmentum of the entire brainstem is permeated by an important network of neurons, the **reticular formation.** The tegmentum also contains *ascending sensory pathways* carrying general sensory information from the trunk and limbs. *Motor pathways* to cell groups in the brainstem and

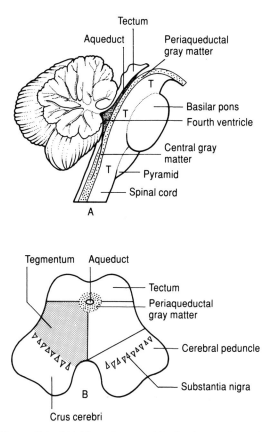

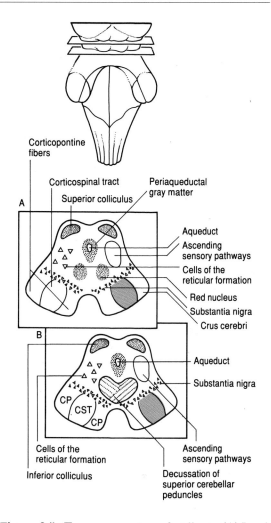

**Figure 3.4.** (A) Named parts of the brainstem in sagittal section; (B) named parts of the midbrain. (T), tegmentum.

**Figure 3.5.** Transverse sections of midbrain. (A) Level of superior colliculi; (B) level of inferior colliculi.

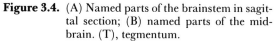

spinal cord are placed more ventrally: they occupy the crura of the midbrain, the basilar pons, and the pyramids of the medulla oblongata. The largest motor pathways are corticopontine, to the pons, and corticospinal, to the spinal cord.

*Note:* In this introductory account the positions of the cranial nerve nuclei are not included. (For these, see Chapter 14.) In the tegmentum, the reticular formation is shown on one side and ascending sensory pathways on the other side. In life, both exist bilaterally.

### MIDBRAIN

The midbrain comprises the tectum, the tegmentum, and the crus cerebri (*Figure 3.4B*). The central gray matter surrounds the aqueduct; it is called the *periaqueductal gray matter.*

The most ventral structure in the tegmentum is **the substantia nigra.** The crus contains motor pathways descending from the cerebral cortex to

the brainstem and spinal cord. The lateral part of the tegmentum contains sensory pathways ascending to the thalamus. The *cerebral peduncle* of gross anatomy includes the ventral part of the tegmentum.

The **red nucleus** occupies the tegmentum on each side at the level of the superior colliculi (*Figure 3.5A*). The **decussation of the superior cerebellar peduncles** straddles the midline at the level of the inferior colliculi (*Figure 3.5B*).

### PONS

The cavity of the fourth ventricle is bordered laterally by the superior cerebellar peduncles and

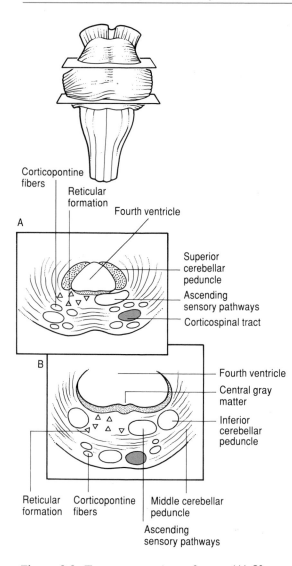

**Figure 3.6.** Transverse sections of pons. (A) Upper; (B) lower.

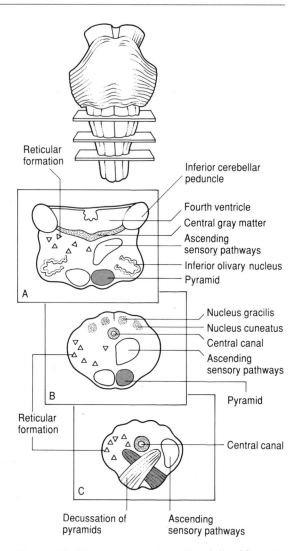

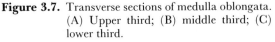

**Figure 3.7.** Transverse sections of medulla oblongata. (A) Upper third; (B) middle third; (C) lower third.

by the inferior cerebellar peduncles below (*Figure 3.6*). Ventral to it is the central gray matter. The tegmentum contains ascending sensory pathways as well as elements of the reticular formation. The basilar region contains descending motor pathways, also millions of transverse fibers which enter the middle cerebellar peduncle.

### Medulla oblongata

The medulla oblongata shows distinctive features at three different levels. The upper third shows the wrinkled **inferior olivary nucleus**, which creates the olive of gross anatomy (*Figure 3.7A*). The middle third shows the **gracile and cuneate nuclei,** which create the gracile and cuneate tubercles (*Figure 3.7B*). (The gracile and cuneate nuclei are also called the *posterior column nuclei* because they receive massive inputs from the posterior white columns of the spinal cord.) The lower third of the medulla shows the decussation of the pyramids (*Figure 3.7C*).

The tegmentum contains ascending sensory pathways and elements of the reticular formation.

## CEREBELLUM

The cerebellum is made up of two **hemispheres** connected by the **vermis** in the midline (*Figure 3.8*). The vermis is distinct only on the under surface, where it occupies the floor of a deep groove, the **vallecula**. The hemispheres show numerous deep **fissures**, with **folia** between (*Figure 3.9A*). About 80% of the **cortex** (surface gray matter) is hidden from view on the surfaces of the folia.

The oldest part of the cerebellum (present even in fishes) is the flocculonodular lobe consisting of the **nodule** of the vermis and the **flocculus** in the hemisphere on each side. More recent is the **anterior lobe** which is bounded posteriorly by the **fissura prima** and contains the **pyramid** and the **uvula**. Most recent is the **posterior lobe**. A prominent feature of the posterior lobe is the **tonsil**. The tonsil lies directly above the foramen magnum of the skull; if the intracranial pressure is raised (for example by a brain tumor), one or both tonsils may descend into the foramen and pose a

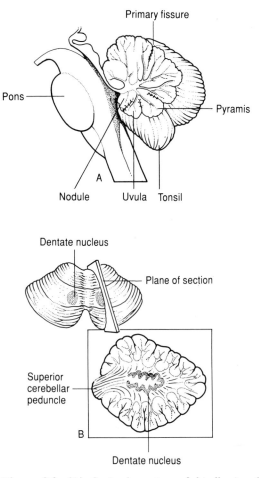

**Figure 3.9.** (A) Sagittal section of hindbrain; (B) oblique section of cerebellum.

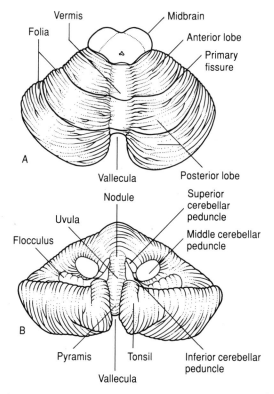

**Figure 3.8.** Cerebellum. (A) Viewed from above; (B) viewed from the position of the pons.

threat to life by compressing the medulla oblongata.

The white matter contains several **central nuclei**. The largest of these is the **dentate nucleus** (*Figure 3.9B*).

## SPINAL CORD

### General features

The spinal cord occupies the upper half of the vertebral canal. Thirty-one pairs of spinal nerves are attached to it, by means of dorsal and ventral nerve roots (*Figure 3.10A*). The cord shows **cervical** and **lumbar enlargements** which accommo-

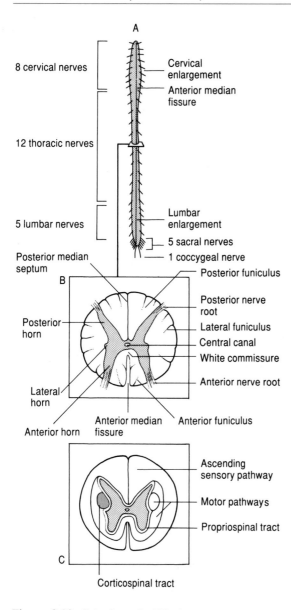

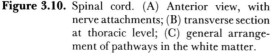

**Figure 3.10.** Spinal cord. (A) Anterior view, with nerve attachments; (B) transverse section at thoracic level; (C) general arrangement of pathways in the white matter.

date nerve cells supplying the upper and lower limbs.

### Internal anatomy

In transverse sections, the cord shows butterfly-shaped gray matter surrounded by three columns or **funiculi** of white matter: an **anterior funiculus** in the interval between the **anterior median fissure** and the emerging anterior nerve roots; a **lateral funiculus** between the anterior and posterior nerve roots; and a **posterior funiculus** between the posterior roots and the **posterior median septum** (*Figure 3.10B*). The gray matter consists of central gray matter surrounding a minute central canal, and **anterior** and **posterior gray horns.** At the levels of attachment of the twelve thoracic and upper two or three lumbar nerve roots a **lateral gray horn** is present as well.

Axons pass from one side of the spinal cord to the other in the **gray commissures**, and in the **white commissure** deep to the anterior median fissure.

### Location of pathways (*Figure 3.10C*)

Adjacent to the central gray matter is the **propriospinal tract**, containing fibers linking one level of the cord with another. Outside this are motor pathways descending from the brain. Outermost are sensory pathways ascending to the brainstem and thalamus.

### REFERENCES

See list for Chapter 2.

CHAPTER SUMMARY

Cranial meninges
Spinal meninges
Circulation of cerebrospinal fluid
*CLINICAL PANELS*
Extradural/subdural hematomas · Hydrocephalus

# 4

# Meninges

**The meninges perform an engineering feat in suspending the brain and spinal cord in a protective fluid jacket which is renewed three times a day. The integrity of the system can be breached by physical injury, by infections or tumors, or by deterioration with advancing age.**

The meninges surround the central nervous system and suspend it in the protective jacket provided by the cerebrospinal fluid. The meninges comprise the tough **dura mater** or *pachymeninx* (Greek, thick membrane), and the *leptomeninges* (Greek, slender membranes) consisting of the **arachnoid mater** and **pia mater**. Between the arachnoid and the pia is the **subarachnoid space** filled with cerebrospinal fluid.

## Cranial meninges

### Dura mater *(Figure 4.1)*

The terminology used to describe the cranial dura mater varies among different authors. It seems best to regard it as a single, tough layer of fibrous tissue which is fused with the inner periosteum of the skull except where it is reflected into the interior of the vault or is stretched across the skull base. Wherever it separates from the periosteum, the intervening space contains venous sinuses.

Two great dural folds extend into the cranial cavity and help to stabilize the brain. These are the **falx cerebri** and the **tentorium cerebelli.**

The falx cerebri occupies the longitudinal fissure between the cerebral hemispheres. Its attached border extends from the crista galli of the ethmoid bone to the upper surface of the tentorium cerebelli. Along the vault of the skull it encloses the **superior sagittal sinus.** Its free border contains the **inferior sagittal sinus** which unites with the great cerebral vein to form the **straight sinus** *(Figure 4.2)*. The straight sinus travels along the line of attachment of falx to tentorium and meets the superior sagittal sinus at the **confluence of the sinuses.**

The tentorium cerebelli arches like a tent above the posterior cranial fossa, being lifted up by the falx cerebri in the midline. The attached margin of the tentorium encloses the **transverse sinuses** on the inner surface of the occipital bone and the **superior petrosal sinuses** along the upper border of the petrous temporal bone. The attached margin reaches to the posterior clinoid processes of the sphenoid bone. Most of the blood from the superior sagittal sinus enters the right transverse sinus *(Figure 4.3)*.

The free margin of the tentorium is U-shaped. The tips of the U are attached to the anterior clinoid processes. Just behind this, the two limbs of the U are linked by a sheet of dura, the **diaphragma sellae**, which is pierced by the pituitary stalk. Laterally, the dura falls away into the middle cranial fossae from the limbs of the U, creating the **cavernous sinus** on each side. Behind the sphenoid bone, the concavity of the U encloses the midbrain.

The cavernous sinus receives blood from the orbit via the ophthalmic veins *(Figure 4.2)*. The superior petrosal sinus joins the transverse sinus at its junction with the **sigmoid sinus.** The sigmoid sinus descends along the occipital bone and discharges into the bulb of the internal jugular vein. The bulb receives the **inferior petrosal sinus** which descends along the edge of the occipital bone.

The tentorium cerebelli divides the cranial cavity into a *supratentorial compartment* containing the forebrain and an *infratentorial compartment* containing the hindbrain.

### Innervation of the cranial dura mater

The dura mater lining the supratentorial compartment of the cranial cavity receives sensory inner-

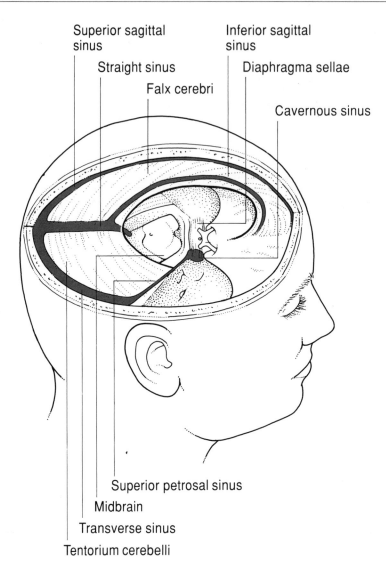

Superior sagittal sinus

Inferior sagittal sinus

Straight sinus

Diaphragma sellae

Falx cerebri

Cavernous sinus

Superior petrosal sinus

Midbrain

Transverse sinus

Tentorium cerebelli

**Figure 4.1.** Dural reflections and venous sinuses. The midbrain occupies the tentorial notch.

vation from the trigeminal nerve. Stretching or inflammation of the supratentorial dura gives rise to frontal or parietal headache.

The dura mater lining the infratentorial compartment is supplied by branches of the upper cervical spinal nerves. Occipital and posterior neck pains accompany disturbance of the infratentorial dura. Acute meningitis involving the posterior cranial fossa is associated with *neck rigidity* and often with *head retraction* brought about by reflex contraction of the posterior nuchal muscles, which are supplied by cervical nerves.

**Meningeal arteries**

Embedded in the inner periosteum of the skull are several *meningeal arteries* whose main function is to supply the diploe (bone marrow). Much the largest is the middle meningeal artery, which ramifies over the inner surface of the temporal and parietal

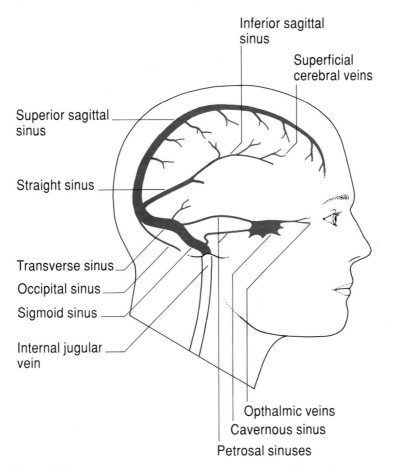

**Figure 4.2.** Side view of intracranial venous sinuses and their tributaries.

bones. Tearing of this artery, with its accompanying vein, is the usual source of an *extradural hematoma* (Panel 4.1).

### Arachnoid mater *(Figure 4.4)*

The arachnoid (Greek, spidery) is a thin, fibrocellular layer in direct contact with the dura mater. The outermost cells of the arachnoid are bonded to one another by tight junctions which seal the subarachnoid space. Innumerable *arachnoid trabeculae* cross the space to reach the pia mater.

### Pia mater *(Figure 4.4)*

The pia mater invests the brain closely, following its contours and lining the various sulci. Like the arachnoid, it is fibrocellular. The cellular component of the pia is external and is permeable to cerebrospinal fluid. The fibrous component occupies a narrow *subpial space* which is continuous with *perivascular spaces* around cerebral blood vessels penetrating the brain surface.

*Note:* Although the subarachnoid and subpial spaces are proven, there is no sign of any 'subdural space' in properly fixed material. Such a space can be created, however, by leakage of blood into the cellular layer of the dura mater following a tear of a cerebral vein at its point of anchorage to the fibrous layer. (See subdural hematoma in Panel 4.1.)

### Subarachnoid cisterns *(Figure 4.5)*

Along the base of the brain and the sides of the brainstem, pools of cerebrospinal fluid occupy

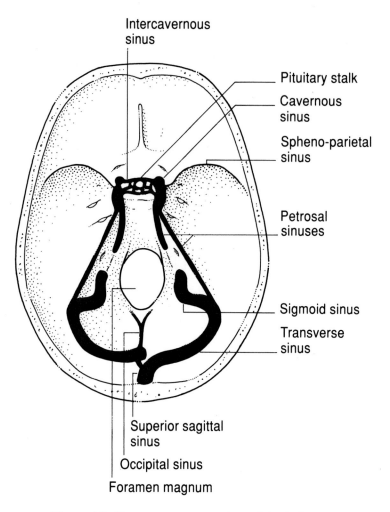

Intercavernous sinus

Pituitary stalk

Cavernous sinus

Spheno-parietal sinus

Petrosal sinuses

Sigmoid sinus

Transverse sinus

Superior sagittal sinus

Occipital sinus

Foramen magnum

**Figure 4.3.** Venous sinuses on the base of the skull.

subarachnoid cisterns. The largest of these is the **cisterna magna**, in the interval between the cerebellum and the medulla oblongata. More rostrally are the **cisterna pontis** ventral to the pons, the **interpeduncular cistern** between the cerebral peduncles, and the **cisterna ambiens** at the side of the midbrain (*Figure 4.6*).

### Sheath of the optic nerve (*Figure 4.7*)

The optic nerve is composed of CNS white matter, and it has a complete meningeal investment. The central vessels of the retina pierce the meninges to enter it. Any sustained elevation of intracranial pressure will be transmitted to the subarachnoid space surrounding the nerve. The *central vein* will be compressed, resulting in swelling of the retinal tributaries of the vein and edema of the optic papilla, where the optic nerve begins. The condition is known as *papilledema* (*Figure 4.8*). It can be recognized on inspection of the retina with an ophthalmoscope.

### *Spinal meninges* (Figure 4.9)

The spinal dural sac is like a test tube, attached to the rim of the foramen magnum and reaching down to the level of the second sacral vertebra. The outer surface of the tube is adherent to the posterior longitudinal ligament of the vertebrae in the midline; elsewhere it is surrounded by fat containing an epidural (internal vertebral) plexus of veins (Chapter 10).

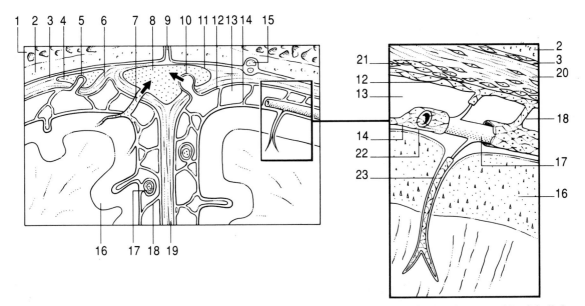

**Figure 4.4.** Coronal section of the superior sagittal sinus and related structures. 1, Diploe; 2, inner table of skull; 3, periosteum; 4, venous lacuna; 5, arachnoid granulation; 6, dura mater; 7, superficial cerebral vein; 8, superior sagittal sinus; 9, sagittal suture; 10, arachnoid granulation; 11, vascular endothelium; 12, arachnoid mater; 13, subarachnoid space; 14, pia mater; 15, meningeal vessels; 16, cerebral cortex; 17, cerebral artery; 18, arachnoid trabecula; 19, falx cerebri; 20, fibrous layer of dura mater; 21, cellular layer of dura mater; 22, subpial space; 23, perivascular space.

## CLINICAL PANEL 4.1 • EXTRADURAL/SUBDURAL HEMATOMAS

An *extradural (epidural) hematoma* is typically caused by a blow to the side of the head severe enough to cause a fracture with associated tearing of the anterior or posterior branch of the middle meningeal artery. Following the initial *concussion* of the brain, with loss of consciousness, there may be a *lucid interval* of several hours. Onset of increasing headache and drowsiness signals cerebral *compression* produced by expansion of the hematoma. Coma and death will supervene unless the hematoma is drained though a burr-hole drilled close to the fracture line.

*Subdural hematomas* are caused by rupture of superficial cerebral veins in transit from the brain to an intracranial venous sinus.

An *acute* subdural hematoma most often follows severe head injury in children. It must always be suspected where a child remains unconscious after a head injury. *Child battering* is a possible explanation if this situation arises in the home.

A *subacute* subdural hematoma may follow head injury at any age. Symptoms and signs of raised intracranial pressure (described in Chapter 6) develop up to 3 weeks after the injury.

*Chronic* subdural hematomas occur in older people, where the transit veins have become brittle and made taut by shrinkage of the aging brain. Head injury may be mild or even absent. A significant number of these patients are alcoholics with reduced blood clotting. Presenting symptoms are variable and include personality changes, headaches, and epileptic seizures.

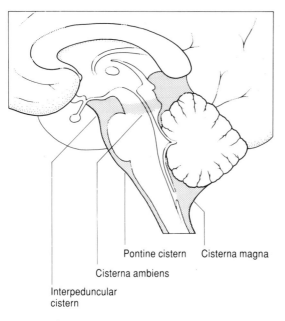

The internal surface of the dura is lined with arachnoid mater. The pia mater lines the surface of the spinal cord and is attached to the dura mater at regular intervals by the serrated **ligamentum denticulatum**.

Because the spinal cord reaches only to first or second lumbar vertebral level, a large **lumbar cistern** is created, containing the free-floating roots of the sacral and lower lumbar spinal nerves (see Chapter 11). The lumbar cistern may be tapped to procure samples of cerebrospinal fluid for analysis ('lumbar puncture' or 'spinal tap').

### Circulation of cerebrospinal fluid

The principal source of the cerebrospinal fluid is the secretion of the choroid plexuses into the ventricles of the brain. From the lateral ventricles the CSF enters the third through the interventricu-

Pontine cistern    Cisterna magna

Cisterna ambiens

Interpeduncular
cistern

**Figure 4.5.** Subarachnoid cisterns.

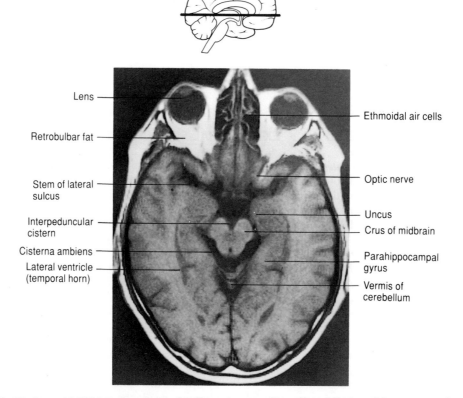

Lens

Retrobulbar fat

Stem of lateral
sulcus

Interpeduncular
cistern

Cisterna ambiens

Lateral ventricle
(temporal horn)

Ethmoidal air cells

Optic nerve

Uncus

Crus of midbrain

Parahippocampal
gyrus

Vermis of
cerebellum

**Figure 4.6.** Horizontal MRI 'slice' at the level indicated at top. Note the proximity of the uncus to the crus of the midbrain (cf. *uncal herniation* in Chapter 5). (From a series kindly provided by Dr Paul Finn, Department of Radiology, New Deaconess Hospital, Boston.)

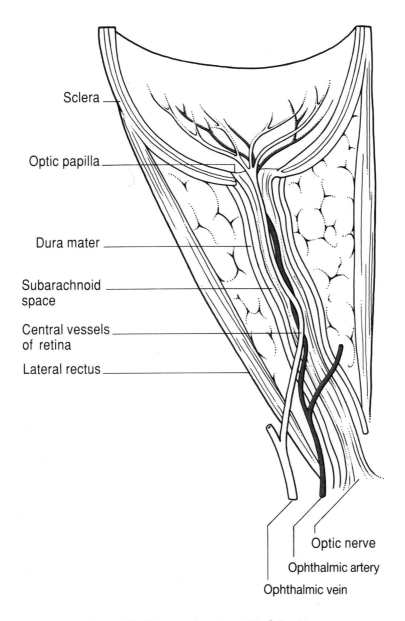

Sclera

Optic papilla

Dura mater

Subarachnoid space

Central vessels of retina

Lateral rectus

Optic nerve

Ophthalmic artery

Ophthalmic vein

**Figure 4.7.** Horizontal section of the left orbit.

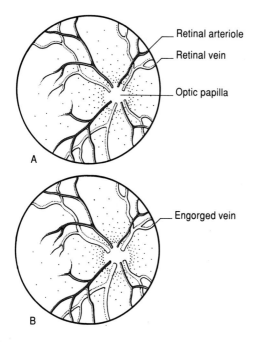

**Figure 4.8.** (A) Normal fundus oculi; (B) Papilledema (the optic papilla is swollen).

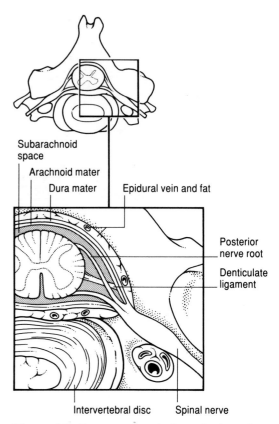

**Figure 4.9.** Contents of cervical vertebral canal.

---

### CLINICAL PANEL 4.2 • HYDROCEPHALUS

*Hydrocephalus* (Greek, water in the head) denotes accumulation of cerebrospinal fluid (CSF) in the ventricular system. With the exception of overproduction of CSF by a rare papilloma of the choroid plexus, hydrocephalus results from obstruction of the normal CSF circulation, with consequent dilatation of the ventricles. The term is *not* used to describe the accumulation of fluid in the ventricles and subarachnoid space in association with senile atrophy of the brain.

In the great majority of cases, hydrocephalus is caused by obstruction of the outlets from the fourth ventricle into the subarachnoid space. A major cause of outlet obstruction in *infancy* is the *Arnold–Chiari malformation*, in which the cerebellum is partly extruded into the vertebral canal during fetal life because the posterior cranial fossa is underdeveloped. In untreated cases the child's head may become as large as a football and the cerebral hemispheres paper thin. The condition is nearly always associated with *spina bifida* (Chapter 10). Early treatment is essential to prevent severe brain damage. The obstruction can be bypassed by means of a catheter having one end inserted into a lateral ventricle and the other inserted into the internal jugular vein.

A major cause of outlet ostruction in *adults* is displacement of the cerebellum into the foramen magnum by a space-occupying lesion such as a tumor or hematoma (see Chapter 5).

*Meningitis* can cause hydrocephalus at any age. The development of leptomeningeal adhesions may compromise CSF circulation at the level of the ventricular outlets, the tentorial notch, and/or the arachnoid granulations.

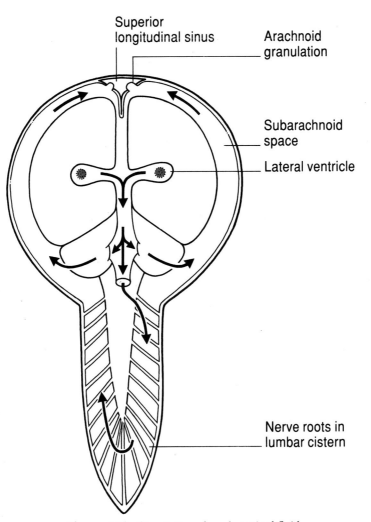

**Figure 4.10.** Circulation of cerebrospinal fluid.

lar foramen. It descends to the fourth through the aqueduct, and gains the subarachnoid space through the median and lateral apertures. (Flow within the central canal of the spinal cord is negligible.)

Within the subarachnoid space, some of the CSF descends through the foramen magnum, reaching the lumbar cistern in about 12 hours. A small amount is absorbed into spinal segmental veins; the rest returns to the cranial subarachnoid space.

From the subarachnoid space at the base of the brain, the CSF ascends through the tentorial notch and bathes the surface of the cerebral hemispheres before being returned to the blood through the **arachnoid granulations** (*Figure 4.4*). The arachnoid granulations are pinhead pouches of arachnoid mater projecting through the dural wall of the major venous sinuses—especially the superior sagittal sinus and the small venous **lacunae** that open into it. CSF is transported across the arachnoid epithelium in giant vacuoles.

About 300 ml of CSF are secreted by the choroid plexuses every 24 hours. Another 200 ml are produced from other sources, as described in Chapter 26. Blockage of flow through the ventricular system or cranial subarachnoid space will cause back-up within the ventricular system: a state of *hydrocephalus* (Panel 4.2).

## REFERENCES

Alskne, J.F. and Lovings, E.T. (1972) Functional ultrastructure of the arachnoid villus. *Arch. Neurol.* **27:** 371–377.

Hutchings, M. and Weller, R.O. (1986) Anatomical relationships of the pia mater to cerebral blood vessels in man. *J. Neurosurg.* **65:** 316–325.

Nicholas, D.S. and Weller, R.O. (1988) The fine anatomy of the human spinal meninges. *J. Neurosurg.* **69:** 276–282.

Prockop, L.D. and Shah, C.P. (1989) Hydrocephalus. In *Merritt's Textbook of Neurology*, 8th edn (Rowland, L.P., ed.). Philadelphia: Lea & Febiger.

<table>
<tr><td>

**CHAPTER SUMMARY**

Neurons
Synapses
Neuroglial cells of the CNS
*CLINICAL PANELS*
Clinical relevance of neuronal transport ·
  Gliomas · Multiple sclerosis

</td></tr>
</table>

# 5

# Neurons and neuroglia

**A knowledge of microscopic anatomy is essential for an understanding of normal and abnormal neurological function. This chapter deals with the histology of the central nervous system; the next chapter deals with peripheral nerves.**

Nerve cells, or **neurons**, are the structural and functional units of the nervous system. They generate and conduct electrical changes in the form of nerve impulses. They communicate chemically with other neurons at points of contact called **synapses.**

**Neuroglia** (literally, 'nerve glue') is the connective tissue of the nervous system. Neuroglial cells outnumber neurons by about ten to one. They have important nutritive and supportive functions.

## NEURONS

Billions of neurons form a shell, or **cortex,** on the surface of the cerebral and cerebellar hemispheres. **Nuclei** are aggregates of neurons buried within the white matter.

In the central nervous system, almost all neurons are multipolar, their cell bodies or **somas** having multiple poles or angles. At every pole but one, a **dendrite** emerges and divides repeatedly (*Figure 5.1*). On some neurons the shafts of the dendrites are smooth. On others the shafts show numerous short **spines.** The dendrites receive synaptic contacts from other neurons, both on the spines and on the shaft surface.

The remaining pole of the soma gives rise to the **axon**, which conducts nerve impulses. Most axons give off **collateral** branches. **Terminal** branches synapse upon target neurons.

Most synaptic contacts between neurons are either **axodendritic** or **axosomatic**. Axodendritic

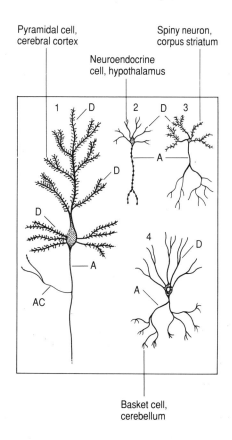

**Figure 5.1.** Profiles of neurons from the brain. 1, Pyramidal cell, cerebral cortex; 2, neuroendocrine cell, hypothalamus; 3, spiny neuron, corpus striatum; 4, basket cell, cerebellum. Neurons 1 and 3 show dendritic spines. A, axon; AC, axon collateral; D, dendrite.

synapses are usually excitatory in their effect upon target neurons, whereas most axosomatic synapses have an inhibitory effect.

### Internal structure of neurons (Figures 5.2 and 5.3)

All parts of neurons are permeated by three skeletal elements, **microtubules, neurofilaments,** and **microfilaments.** The soma contains the nucleus and the cytoplasm or **perikaryon** (Greek, around the nucleus). The perikaryon contains clumps of granular endoplasmic reticulum known as *Nissl bodies*; also Golgi complexes, free ribosomes, mitochondria, and smooth endoplasmic reticulum (SER).

### Intracellular transport

Turnover of membranous and skeletal material takes place in all cells. In neurons, fresh components are continuously synthesized in the soma and moved into the axon and dendrites by a process of *anterograde transport*. At the same time, worn out materials are returned to the soma by *retrograde transport*, for degradation in lysosomes (see also *target recognition*, later).

Anterograde transport is of two kinds, rapid and slow. Included in *rapid* transport (at a speed of 300–400 mm per day) are free elements such as synaptic vesicles, transmitter substances (or their precursor molecules), and mitochondria. Also included are lipid and protein molecules (including receptor proteins) for insertion into the plasma membrane. *Slow* anterograde transport has long

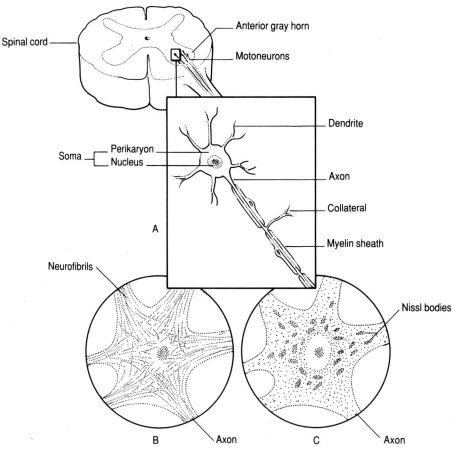

**Figure 5.2.** Motoneuron from the anterior gray horn of the spinal cord. (A) General features; (B) neurofibrils (matted neurofilaments) seen after staining with silver salts; (C) Nissl bodies (clumps of granular endoplasmic reticulum) seen after staining with a cationic dye such as thionin.

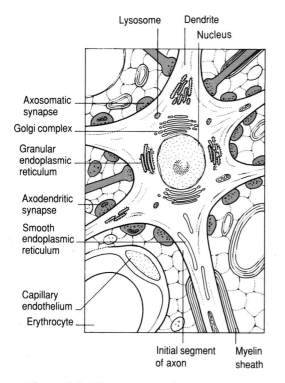

Lysosome   Dendrite
Nucleus

Axosomatic
synapse

Golgi complex

Granular
endoplasmic
reticulum

Axodendritic
synapse

Smooth
endoplasmic
reticulum

Capillary
endothelium

Erythrocyte

Initial segment   Myelin
of axon           sheath

**Figure 5.3.** Ultrastructure of a motoneuron.

been thought to consist of bulk movement of cytoplasm along with the three skeletal elements contained within it. However, the view is gaining ground that the skeletal elements and the smooth endoplasmic reticulum are largely stationary. Microtubules do appear to move along when observed in living axons, but this effect may be achieved by addition of rapidly transported structural protein molecules to their distal ends while their proximal ends are being dismantled. Neurofilaments become largely stationary in the more distal parts of axons.

Retrograde transport of worn out mitochondria, SER and plasma membrane (including receptors therein) is fairly rapid (150–200 mm per day). In addition to its function in waste disposal, retrograde transport is involved in *target cell recognition*. At synaptic contacts, axons constantly 'nibble' the plasma membrane of target neurons by means of endocytotic vesicular uptake, the vesicles being brought to the soma and incorporated into Golgi complexes there. Uptake of target cell 'marker' molecules is important for cell recognition during development. It may also be necessary for viability later on because adult neurons

shrink and may even die if their axons are severed proximal to their first branches.

TRANSPORT MECHANISMS

Microtubules are the supporting structures for neuronal transport. Microtubule-associated proteins, in the form of ATPases, propel organelles and molecules along the outer surface of the microtubules. Distinct ATPases are used for orthograde and retrograde work.

Neurofilaments do not seem to be involved in the transport mechanism. They are rather evenly spaced, having side-arms that keep them apart and provide skeletal stability by attachment to proteins beneath the axolemmal membrane. Neurofilament numbers are in direct proportion to axonal diameter and the filaments may in truth *determine* axonal diameter.

Some points of clinical relevance are highlighted in Panel 5.1.

## SYNAPSES

### Chemical synapses

Synapses are the points of contact between neurons. Conventional synapses are *chemical*, depending for their effect on the release of a transmitter substance. The typical chemical synapse comprises a **presynaptic** membrane, a **synaptic cleft,** and a **postsynaptic membrane** (*Figure 5.4*). The presynaptic membrane belongs to the terminal bouton, the postsynaptic membrane to the target neuron. Transmitter substance is released from the bouton by exocytosis, traverses the narrow synaptic cleft and activates receptors in the postsynaptic membrane. Underlying the postsynaptic membrane is a **subsynaptic web,** in which numerous biochemical changes are initiated by receptor activation.

The bouton contains **synaptic vesicles** loaded with transmitter substance, together with numerous mitochondria and sacs of SER. Following conventional methods of fixation *presynaptic dense projections* are visible, and microtubules seem to guide the synaptic vesicles to *active zones* in the intervals between the projections.

Transmitter-loaded synaptic vesicles have three possible sources, as shown in *Figure 5.5*:

1. Some vesicles are formed and loaded in the Golgi apparatus and shipped to the synaptic boutons by rapid transport.

## CLINICAL PANEL 5.1 ● CLINICAL RELEVANCE OF NEURONAL TRANSPORT

TETANUS

Wounds contaminated by soil or street dust may contain ***Clostridium tetani***. The toxin produced by this organism binds to the plasma membrane of nerve endings, is taken up by endocytosis and carried to the spinal cord by retrograde transport. Other neurons upstream take in the toxin by endocytosis—notably Renshaw cells (Chapter 13) which normally exert a braking action upon motoneurons through the release of an inhibitory transmitter substance, glycine. Tetanus toxin prevents the release of glycine. As a result, motoneurons go out of control, particularly those supplying the muscles of the face, jaws and spine. These muscles exhibit prolonged, agonizing spasms. About half of the patients who show these classical signs of tetanus die of exhaustion within a few days. Tetanus is entirely preventable by appropriate and timely immunization.

VIRUSES AND TOXIC METALS

Retrograde axonal transport has been blamed for the passage of viruses from the nasopharynx to the CNS; also for the uptake of toxic metals such as lead and aluminium. Viruses, in particular, may be spread widely through the brain by means of retrograde transneuronal uptake.

PERIPHERAL NEUROPATHIES

Defective *anterograde* transport seems to be involved in certain 'dying back' neuropathies in which the distal parts of the longer peripheral nerves undergo progressive atrophy.

2. Some transmitter precursors and requisite enzymes are shipped to the boutons individually, before being taken into vesicles budded from terminal sacs of SER.

3. Some transmitter molecules are retrieved from the synaptic cleft by endocytosis and returned to the synaptic vesicular pool.

### *Receptor activation*

Transmitter molecules cross the synaptic cleft and activate receptor proteins which straddle the postsynaptic membrane (*Figure 5.5*). The activated receptors initiate ionic events that either raise or lower the postsynaptic membrane potential (depending upon the receptor type). The voltage change passes over the soma in a decremental wave called *electrotonus*, and alters the resting potential of the first part or *initial segment* of the axon. (See physiology texts for details of the ionic events.) If excitatory postsynaptic potentials are dominant, the initial segment will be depolarized to threshold and generate a burst of action potentials.

### Lock and key analogy for drug therapy

The receptor may be likened to a lock, the transmitter being the key that operates it. The transmitter output of certain neurons may falter as a consequence of age or disease, and a duplicate key can often be provided in the form of a drug which mimics the action of the transmitter. Such a drug is called an *agonist*. On the other hand, excessive production of a transmitter may be countered by a

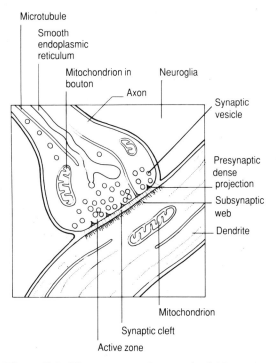

**Figure 5.4.** Ultrastructure of an axodendritic synapse following conventional tissue fixation.

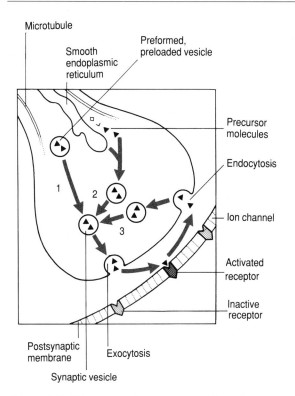

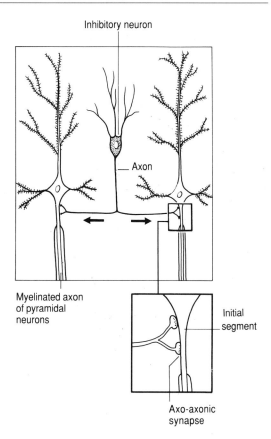

**Figure 5.5.** Diagram to show origin and fate of synaptic vesicles, and transmitter–receptor binding. For numbers, see text.

**Figure 5.6.** Axo-axonic synapses in the cerebral cortex. Arrows indicate direction of impulse conduction.

*receptor blocker*—the equivalent of a dummy key which will occupy the lock without activating it.

### Less common chemical synapses

Two varieties of *axo-axonic* synapses are recognized. In both cases the boutons belong to inhibitory neurons. One variety occurs on the initial segment of the axon, where it exercises a powerful veto on impulse generation (*Figure 5.6*). In the second kind, the boutons are applied to excitatory boutons of other neurons, and they inhibit transmitter release. The effect is called *presynaptic inhibition*, any conventional contact being *postsynaptic* in this context (*Figure 5.7*).

*Dendrodendritic* (D-D) synapses occur between dendritic spines of contiguous spiny neurons and alter the electrotonus of the target neuron rather than generating nerve impulses. In *one-way* D-D synapses, one of the two spines contains synaptic vesicles. In reciprocal synapses, both do. Excitatory D-D synapses are shown in *Figure 5.8*. Inhibitory D-D synapses are numerous in relay nuclei of the thalamus (Chapter 21).

Somatodendritic and somatosomatic synapses have also been identified, but they are scarce.

### Electrical synapses

Electrical synapses consist of gap junctions (nexuses) between dendrites or somas of contiguous neurons. They permit electrotonic changes to pass from one neuron to another. Their function seems to be to ensure synchronous activity of neurons having a common action. An example is the *inspiratory center* in the medulla oblongata, where all of the cells exhibit synchronous discharge during inspiration.

### NEUROGLIAL CELLS OF THE CNS

Four different types of neuroglial cell are found in the CNS, as follows.

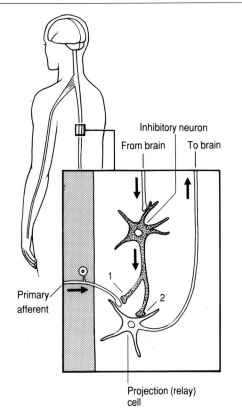

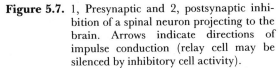

**Figure 5.7.** 1, Presynaptic and 2, postsynaptic inhibition of a spinal neuron projecting to the brain. Arrows indicate directions of impulse conduction (relay cell may be silenced by inhibitory cell activity).

**Figure 5.8.** Dendrodendritic excitation. The dendrites belong to three separate neurons. On the right is a reciprocal synapse. Arrows indicate direction of electrotonic waves.

## Astrocytes *(Figure 5.9)*

**Astrocytes** are bushy cells with dozens of fine radiating processes. The cytoplasm contains abundant intermediate filaments. This confers a degree of rigidity on these cells which helps to support the brain as a whole. Glycogen granules, which are also abundant, provide an immediate source of glucose for the neurons.

Some astrocyte processes form **glial limiting membranes** on the inner (ventricular) and outer (pial) surfaces of the brain. Other astrocyte processes are wrapped around capillaries and help to maintain the specialized structure of capillary endothelium in the CNS (Chapter 26). Still other processes invest synaptic contacts between neurons.

As well as maintaining the capillary endothelium, three further functions of astrocytes may be mentioned. They are engaged in mopping up $K^+$ ions during periods of intense neuronal activity; in recycling certain neurotransmitter substances following release (notably the excitatory transmitter, glutamate); and in phagocytosis of decaying synaptic boutons.

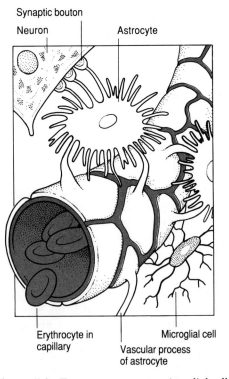

**Figure 5.9.** Two astrocytes, one microglial cell.

## CLINICAL PANEL 5.2 • GLIOMAS

Brain tumors most commonly originate from neuroglial cells, especially astrocytes.

*General* symptoms produced by brain tumors are those of *raised intracranial pressure.* They include headache, drowsiness, and vomiting. Radiological investigation may reveal displacement of midline structures to the opposite side. Tumors below the tentorium (usually cerebellar) are likely to block the exit of cerebrospinal fluid from the fourth ventricle, in which case ballooning of the ventricular system will add to the intracranial pressure.

*Local* symptoms depend upon the position of the tumor. For example, clumsiness of an arm or leg may be caused by a cerebellar tumor on the same side; and motor weakness of an arm or leg may be caused by a cerebral tumor on the opposite side.

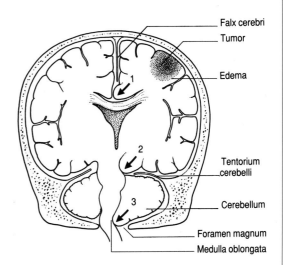

**Figure CP 5.2.1.** Brain herniations. For numbers, see text.

### Progression

Expansion of a tumor may cause one or more *brain hernias* to develop, as shown in *Figure CP 5.2.1:*

(1) *Subfalcal herniation* (in the interval between falx cerebri and corpus callosum) seldom causes specific symptoms.

(2) *Uncal herniation* is the term used to denote displacement of the uncus of the temporal lobe into the tentorial notch. Compression of the ipsilateral crus cerebri by the uncus may give rise to contralateral motor weakness. Alternatively, compression of the *contralateral* crus against the sharp edge of the tentorium cerebelli may cause *ipsilateral* motor weakness.

(3) *Pressure coning*: a cone of cerebellar tissue (the tonsil) may descend into the foramen magnum, squeezing the medulla oblongata and causing death from respiratory/cardiovascular failure by inactivation of *vital centers* in the reticular formation (Chapter 18).

---

Unlike neurons, whose multiplication has ceased around the time of birth, astrocytes can multiply at any time. As part of the healing process following CNS injury, proliferation of astrocytes and their processes results in dense glial scar tissue *(gliosis)*. More importantly, spontaneous local proliferation of astrocytes may give rise to a brain tumor (Panel 5.2).

### *Oligodendrocytes* (Figure 5.10)

**Oligodendrocytes** are responsible for wrapping myelin sheaths around axons in the white matter. In the gray matter they form **satellite cells** which seem to participate in ion exchange with neurons.

### Myelination

Myelination commences during the middle period of gestation, and continues well into the second decade. A single oligodendrocyte lays myelin on upwards of three dozen axons by means of a spiraling process whereby the inner and outer faces of the plasma membrane form the alternating *major* and *minor dense lines* seen in transverse sections of the myelin sheath. Some cytoplasm remains in *paranodal pockets* at the ends of each myelin segment. In the intervals between the glial wrappings the axon is exposed, at *nodes*.

Myelination greatly increases the speed of impulse conduction because the depolarization process jumps from node to node (see Chapter 6).

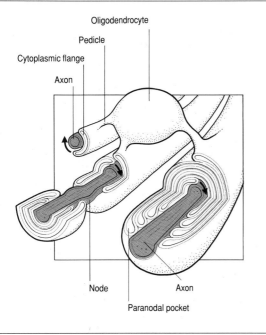

During myelination, K⁺ ion channels are deleted from the underlying axolemma. For this reason, demyelinating diseases such as multiple sclerosis (Panel 5.3) are accompanied by failure of impulse conduction.

Unmyelinated axons abound in the gray matter. They are fine (0.2 $\mu$m in diameter or less) and not individually ensheathed.

### Microglia (Figure 5.9)

**Microglia** develop from monocytes entering from the circulation during fetal life. They are the chief phagocytes of the CNS.

**Figure 5.10.** Myelination in the CNS. Arrows indicate movement of the growing edge of the cytoplasmic flange of the oligodendrocyte.

---

### CLINICAL PANEL 5.3 • MULTIPLE SCLEROSIS

Multiple sclerosis (MS) is the commonest neurological disorder of young adults in the temperate latitudes north and south of the equator. It is more prevalent in women, with a female:male ratio of 3:2. The peak age of onset is around 30 years, the range being 15 to 45.

MS is a *primary demyelinating disease*: the initial feature is the development of plaques (patches) of demyelination in the white matter while the axons remain intact. The denuded axons are unable to conduct impulses because K⁺ channels are normally deleted from the axolemmal membrane when myelin sheaths are initially laid down. Impulse conduction in neighboring myelinated fibers is also compromised by edema (inflammatory exudate). Over time, the plaques are progressively replaced by glial scar tissue and the trapped axons degenerate as well. Old plaques feel firm (sclerotic) in postmortem slices of the brain.

Common locations of early plaques are the cervical spinal cord, upper brainstem, optic nerve, and periventricular white matter including that of the cerebellum. MS is not a systems disease: it is not anatomically selective, and a plaque may involve parts of adjacent motor and sensory pathways. Curiously, the symptoms do not correlate well with the sites of plaques detected by means of MRI scans.

Presenting symptoms can be correlated with lesion sites, as follows:

*Motor weakness,* usually in one or both legs, signifies a lesion involving the corticospinal tract.

*Clumsiness* in reaching and grasping usually accompanies a lesion in the cerebellar white matter.

*Numbness/tingling,* often spreading up from the legs to the trunk, may be caused by a lesion in the posterior white matter of the spinal cord.

*Diplopia* (double vision) may be produced by a plaque within the pons or midbrain affecting the function of one of the ocular motor nerves.

A *scotoma* (patch of blindness in the visual field of one eye) is produced by a plaque within the optic nerve.

*Urinary retention* (failure of the bladder to empty) can be caused by interruption of the central autonomic pathway descending from the brainstem to the lower part of the cord.

The usual course of the disease is one of *remissions and relapses,* with an overall slow progression and development of multiple disabilities.

## *Ependyma*

**Ependymal cells** line the ventricular system of the brain. Cilia on their free surface help the propulsion of cerebrospinal fluid through the ventricles.

## REFERENCES

Morell, P. and Quarles, R.H. (1989) Formation, structure, and biochemistry of myelin. In *Basic Neurochemistry: Molecular, Cellular, and Medical Aspects*, 4th edn (Siegel, G.J. *et al.*, eds), pp.109–138. New York: Raven Press.

Raine, C.S. (1989) Neurocellular anatomy. In *Basic Neurochemistry: Molecular, Cellular, and Medical Aspects*, 4th edn (Siegel, G.J. *et al.*, eds), pp. 3–33. New York: Raven Press.

Sano, Y. (1989) Morphological aspects of neurons as secretory cells. *Arch. Histol. Cytol.* **52:** 107–112.

Vallee, R.B. (1991) Mechanisms of fast and slow axonal transport. *Ann. Rev. Neurosci.* **14:** 59–92.

Vernadakis, A. (1988) Neuron-glia interrelations. *Int. Rev. Neurobiol.* **30:** 149–224.

Waxman, S.G. (1987) Molecular neurobiology of the myelinated nerve fiber: ion-channel distributions and their implications for demyelinating diseases. In *Molecular Neurobiology in Neurology and Psychiatry* (Kandel E.R., ed.), pp. 7–37. New York: Raven Press.

Westrum, L.E. and Gray, E.J. (1986) New observations on the substructure of the active zone of brain synapses and motor endplates. *Proc. R. Soc.Lond.* B **229:** 29–38.

# 6

# Peripheral nerves: general features

**CHAPTER SUMMARY**

General features
Microscopic structure of peripheral nerves
Degeneration and regeneration of peripheral
  nerves

This chapter describes the general composition of the cranial and spinal nerves, and their microscopic structure including the process of myelin formation. The events occurring after physical injury to peripheral nerves are outlined, and are compared with those following injury to the CNS.

The peripheral nerves comprise the cranial and spinal nerves linking the brain and spinal cord to the peripheral tissues. The neurons contributing to peripheral nerves are partly contained within the central nervous system. The cells giving rise to the motor *(efferent)* nerves to skeletal muscles occupy the CNS gray matter, and the central processes of peripheral sensory *(afferent)* neurons enter the white matter before making contact with other neurons *(Figure 6.1)*.

The spinal nerves supply *somatic efferent* fibers to the skeletal muscles of the trunk and limbs, and *somatic afferent* fibers to the skin, muscles and joints. They all carry *visceral efferent*, autonomic fibers and some carry *visceral afferent* fibers as well. The cranial nerves are more diverse, and collectively also include *branchial efferent* fibers for the supply of muscles that originated from the branchial arches in embryonic life, and *special sense afferents* serving smell, taste, hearing and balance.

The **spinal nerves** are formed by the union of **anterior** and **posterior nerve roots** at their points of exit from the vertebral canal. The spinal nerve proper is only 1 cm long and occupies an intervertebral foramen. Upon emerging from the foramen it divides into **anterior** and **posterior rami.** Posterior rami supply the erector spinae muscles and the overlying skin. Anterior rami supply the muscles and skin of the side and front of the trunk, including the limbs; they also supply sensory fibers to the parietal pleura and parietal peritoneum.

The cervical, brachial and lumbosacral plexuses are derived from *anterior rami*, which form

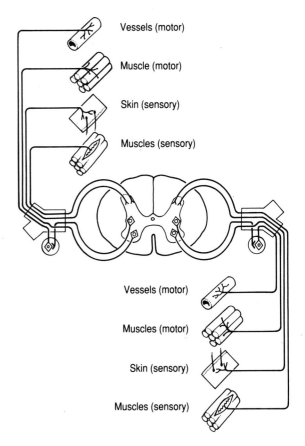

Vessels (motor)

Muscle (motor)

Skin (sensory)

Muscles (sensory)

Vessels (motor)

Muscles (motor)

Skin (sensory)

Muscles (sensory)

**Figure 6.1.** Fiber composition of a thoracic spinal nerve. *Left:* components of a posterior ramus. *Right:* components of an anterior ramus.

the **roots** of the plexuses. The term 'root' therefore has two different meanings, depending on the context.

## MICROSCOPIC STRUCTURE OF PERIPHERAL NERVES

*Figure 6.2* illustrates the structure of a typical peripheral nerve. It is not possible to designate individual nerve fibers as motor or sensory on the basis of structural features alone.

Peripheral nerves are invested with **epineurium,** a loose, vascular connective tissue sheath outside the fascicles (bundles of fibers) that make up the nerve. Nerve fibers are exchanged between fascicles along the course of the nerve.

Each fascicle is covered by **perineurium,** composed of several layers of squamous epithelial cells bonded by tight junctions. Surrounding the individual Schwann cells is a network of reticular collagenous fibers, the **endoneurium.**

Less than half of the nerve fibers are enclosed in myelin sheaths. The remaining, unmyelinated fibers travel in deep gutters along the surface of Schwann cells.

The term 'nerve fiber' is usually used in the context of nerve impulse conduction, where it is equivalent to 'axon'. An anatomical definition is possible for a myelinated fiber: it comprises axon, myelin and neurolemmal sheaths, and endoneurium. A definition is not possible for unmyelinated axons because they share neurolemmal and endoneurial sheaths.

### Myelin formation (Figure 6.3)

**The Schwann cell** is the representative neuroglial cell of the peripheral nervous system. It forms chains of **neurolemmal cells** along the nerves. Modified Schwann cells form **satellite cells** in

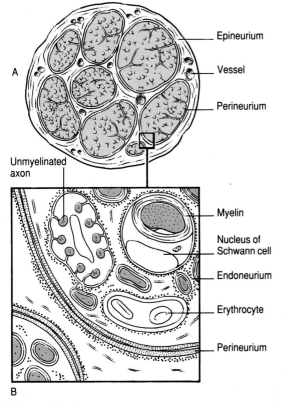

**Figure 6.2.** Transverse section of a nerve trunk. (A) Light microscopy; (B) electron microscopy.

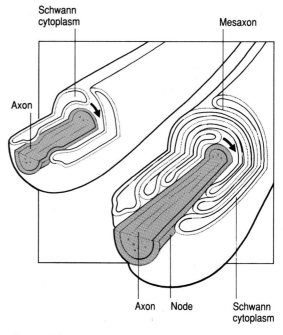

**Figure 6.3.** Myelination in peripheral nervous system. Arrows indicate movement of flange of Schwann cytoplasm.

posterior root ganglia (Chapter 11) and **teloglia** at encapsulated sensory nerve endings (Chapter 8).

If an axon is to be myelinated, it receives the simultaneous attention of a sequence of Schwann cells along its length. Each one encloses the axon completely, creating a 'mesentery' of plasma membrane, the **mesaxon.** The mesaxon is displaced progressively, being rotated around the axon. Successive layers of plasma membrane come into apposition to form the major and minor dense lines (see histology texts for myelin ultrastructure).

*Paranodal pockets* of cytoplasm persist at the ends of the myelin segments, on each side of the *nodes of Ranvier.* (Louis Ranvier discovered them 80 years before CNS nodes were seen in the electron microscope in the early 1960s.) The paranodal pockets may be responsible for maintaining the dense population (about $10^5$) of $Na^+$ channels in the nodal plasma membrane.

## Myelin expedites conduction

Along unmyelinated fibers impulse conduction is *continuous* (uninterrupted). Its maximum speed is 15 m/s (meters per second). Along myelinated fibers excitable membrane is confined to the nodes of Ranvier because myelin is an electrical insulator. Impulse conduction is called *saltatory* ('jumping') because it jumps from node to node. Speed of conduction is much greater along myelinated fibers, with a maximum of 120 m/s. The *number* of impulses that can be conducted by myelinated fibers is also much greater.

The larger the myelinated fiber the more rapid the conduction, because larger fibers have longer internodal segments and the nerve impulses take longer 'strides' between nodes. A 'rule of six' can be used to express the ratio between size and speed: a fiber of 10 $\mu$m external diameter will conduct at 60 m/s, one of 15 $\mu$m at 90 m/s, and so on.

Degeneration

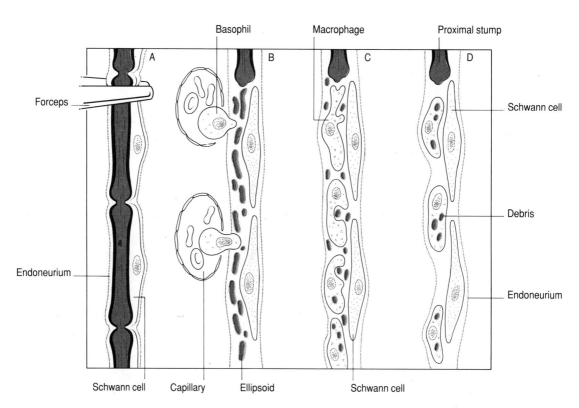

**Figure 6.4.** Events in degeneration of a single myelinated nerve fiber. (A) Intact fiber, showing its four components. The fiber is being pinched at its upper end. (B) The myelin and axon have broken up into 'ellipsoids' and droplets. Monocytes are entering the endoneurial tube from the blood. (C) The droplets are being engulfed by monocytes. (D) Clearance of debris is almost complete. Schwann cells and endoneurium remain intact.

In physiological recordings, peripheral nerve fibers are classified in accordance with conduction velocities and other criteria. Motor fibers are classified into Groups A, B, and C in descending order. Sensory fibers are classified into Types I–IV. In practice, there is some interchange of usages: for example, unmyelinated sensory fibers are usually called C fibers rather than Type IV.

## DEGENERATION AND REGENERATION OF PERIPHERAL NERVES

When nerves are cut or crushed, their axons degenerate distal to the lesion, because axons are pseudopodial outgrowths and depend on their parent cells for survival. In the peripheral nervous system regeneration is vigorous and it is often complete. In the CNS, on the other hand, it is neither vigorous nor complete.

### Wallerian degeneration of peripheral nerves (Waller, 1816–1870)

The principal events in peripheral nerve degeneration are represented in *Figure 6.4* and described in the caption. Following a crush or cut injury to a nerve, the axons and myelin sheaths distal to the cut break up to form 'ellipsoids' during the first 48 hours—mainly because of lysosomal activity by Schwann cells. The debris is cleared by monocytes which enter the damaged endoneurial sheaths from the blood and become macrophages. The end result of degeneration is a shrunken nerve skeleton with intact connective tissue and perineurial sheaths, and a core of intact Schwann cells.

### Regeneration

The principal events are summarized in *Figure 6.5*. Following a clean cut, axons begin to sprout from

Regeneration

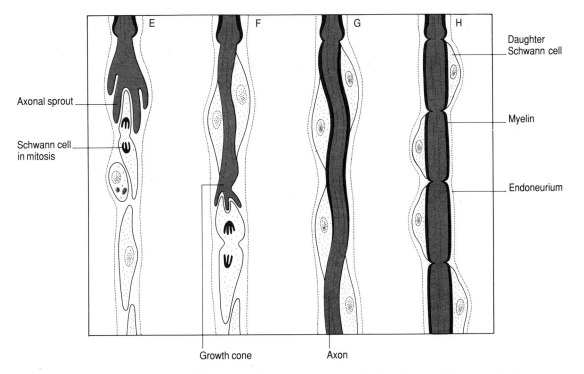

**Figure 6.5.** Events in regeneration. (E) An axonal sprout has entered the distal stump. The sprout is mitogenetic to each Schwann cell it encounters. (F) The growth cone is extending distally along the surface of Schwann cells. (G) Myelination is commencing along the proximal part of the regenerating axon. (H) When regeneration is complete the fiber has a normal appearance but the myelin segments are shorter than the originals.

the face of the proximal stump within a few hours, but in the more common crush or tear injuries seen clinically, the axons die back for 1 cm or more and sprouting may be delayed for a week. Successful regeneration requires that the axons make contact with Schwann cells of the distal stump (or at least with their basement membranes). Failure to make contact leads to production of a *neuroma* consisting of whorls of regenerating axons trapped in scar tissue at the site of the initial injury. Following amputation of a limb, an *amputation neuroma* can be a source of severe pain.

Successful nerve tips exhibit swellings called **growth cones,** from which fine **filopodia** extend along Schwann cell basement membranes. The filopodia develop surface receptors which become anchored temporarily to complimentary molecules in the basement membrane. Filaments of actin within the filopodia become attached to the surface receptors; from these points of anchorage they are able to exert onward traction on the growth cones.

Growth cones are mitogenic to Schwann cells, which complete a single mitotic cycle before wrapping the larger axons with myelin lamellae.

Regeneration proceeds at about 5 mm per day in the larger nerve trunks, slowing down to 2 mm per day in the finer branches. If appropriate endo-neurial tubes have been entered, complete functional recovery is likely. Good recovery depends on accurate alignment of proximal and distal stumps, because sensory axons are quite capable of growing along former motor tubes, and motor sprouts along sensory ones. For this reason the outlook is better following a crush injury (endoneurium preserved) than a cut.

When nerve trunks have been completely severed, it is common practice to wait about 3 weeks before attempting repair. By that time, the connective tissue sheaths will have thickened a little and will be better able to hold suture material than are freshly injured, edematous sheaths. Moreover, the trimming of the nerves required before insertion of sutures creates a second axotomy, on the axons emerging from the proximal stump. In animal experiments, a second axotomy induces a more vigorous and sustained regenerative response.

### Upstream effects of nerve section

- Within a few days of axotomy, Nissl bodies can no longer be identified by cationic dyes in parent cells in the dorsal root ganglia and spinal gray matter (*Figure 6.6*). The phenomenon is known as chromatolysis ('loss of color'). Electron microscopy reveals that the granular endo-

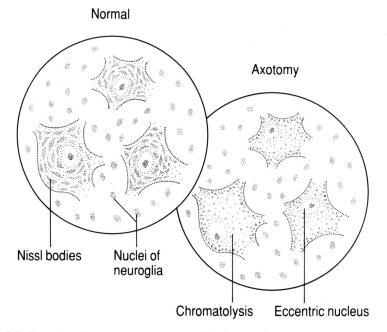

**Figure 6.6.** Reaction of motoneurons to injury (Nissl stain; the axon is below, for each cell).

plasmic reticulum is in fact increased in amount. Instead of being in clumps it is dispersed throughout the perikaryon, with accumulations deep to the plasma membrane.

- The nucleus becomes eccentric due to osmotic changes in the perikaryon.
- Parent motoneurons become isolated from synaptic contacts by the intrusion of neuroglial cells into all of the synaptic clefts.

## Degeneration in the CNS

Following injury to the white matter, distal degeneration occurs after the manner of peripheral nerves. However, clearance of debris by microglial cells and fresh monocytes is much slower. Debris can still be identified after 6 months in the CNS, whereas in peripheral nerves it is virtually cleared in 6 days.

Chromatolysis is unusual in the CNS. Instead, large-scale necrosis (death) of injured neurons is the rule. Neurons that survive may appear wasted, with permanent isolation from synaptic contacts.

### Transneuronal atrophy

CNS neurons have a trophic (sustaining) effect upon one another. If the main input to a group of neurons is destroyed, the group is likely to waste away and die. This is known as *orthograde transneuronal atrophy*. It is comparable to the atrophy that occurs in skeletal muscle when its motor nerve is cut. In some situations *retrograde transneuronal degeneration* takes place, in neurons upstream to those destroyed by the lesion.

### End result of CNS injury

If the lesion has been small, the neuronal debris is ultimately replaced by a glial scar composed of astrocyte processes. A large lesion may result in cystic cavities walled by scar tissue, containing cerebrospinal fluid and hemolyzed blood.

## Regeneration in the CNS

Remarkable degrees of functional recovery are often observed after CNS lesions. However, injured motor and sensory pathways do not reestablish their original connections. They regenerate for a few millimeters at most, and such synapses as develop are upon other neurons close to the site of injury.

One of the most active areas in neurobiological research is the use of *embryonic* nervous tissue to replace neurons that have been lost from injury or disease. The mammalian CNS in general seems to be lacking in *trophic factors* required for successful regeneration. Such factors are evidently present in embryonic neurons because when these are transplanted (with immunological precautions) into adult brain they grow well. This approach is beginning to be applied to patients having restricted areas of brain pathology—notably Parkinson's disease (Chapter 24).

## REFERENCES

Birch, R., Bonney, G., Payan, J., Wynn Parry, C.B. and Iggo, A. (1986) Peripheral nerve injuries. *J. Bone Joint Surg.* **68B**: 2–21.

Gag, F.H. and Fisher, L.J. (1991) Intracerebral grafting: a tool for the neurobiologist. *Neuron* **6**: 1–12.

Goldberg, D.J. and Burmeister, D.W. (1989) Looking into growth cones. *Trends Neurosci.* **12**: 503–506.

Ide, C. and Kato, S. (1990) Peripheral nerve regeneration. *Neurosci. Res. Suppl.* **13**: S157-S164.

McQuarry, I.G. (1988) Cytoskeleton of the regenerating axon. In *Current Issues in Neural Regeneration Research*, pp. 23–32. New York: Alan R. Liss.

O'Reilly, P.M.R. and FitzGerald, M.J.T. (1985) Internodal segments in human laryngeal nerves. *J. Anat.* **140**: 645–650.

Stoll, G., Griffin, J.W., Li, C.Y. and Trapp, R.D. (1989) Wallerian degeneration in the peripheral nervous system: participation of both Schwann cells and macrophages in myelin degradation. *J. Neurocytol.* **18**: 671–683.

Tetzlaff, W., Graeber, M.B. and Kreutzberg, G.W. (1986) Reaction of motoneurons and their microenvironment to axotomy. *Exp. Brain Res. Suppl.* **13**: S3–8.

# 7

# Innervation of muscles and joints

The nerve endings in muscles and joints provide the peripheral equipment which the CNS exploits to brilliant effect in a multitude of motor activities. This chapter describes the functional anatomy of the nerve endings, and some simple reflexes they mediate at spinal cord level.

In gross anatomy, the nerves to skeletal muscles are branches of mixed peripheral nerves. The branches enter the muscles about one-third of the way along their length, at *motor points* (*Figure 7.1*). Motor points have been identified for all major muscle groups, for the purpose of *functional electrical stimulation* by physical therapists, in order to increase muscle power.

Only 60% of the axons in the nerve to a given muscle are motor to the muscle fibers that make up the bulk of the muscle. The rest are sensory in nature although the largest sensory receptors—the neuromuscular spindles—have a motor supply of their own.

## MOTOR INNERVATION OF SKELETAL MUSCLE

The nerve of supply branches within the muscle belly, forming a plexus from which groups of axons emerge to supply the muscle fibers (*Figure 7.1*). The axons supply single **motor end plates** placed about half way along the muscle fibers (*Figure 7.2A*).

A *motor unit* comprises a motor neuron in the spinal cord or brainstem together with the *squad* of muscle fibers it innervates. In large muscles (e.g. the flexors of the hip or knee) each motor unit contains 1000 muscle fibers or more. In small muscles (e.g. the intrinsic muscles of the hand) each unit contains ten muscle fibers or less. Small units contribute to the finely graded contractions used for delicate manipulations.

There are three different types of skeletal muscle fiber. (a) Slow-twitch, oxidative (SO) fibers are small, rich in mitochondria and blood capillaries (hence, they are red). They exert small forces and are fatigue resistant. They are deeply placed and suited to sustained postural activities, including standing. (b) Fast, glycolytic (FG) fibers are large, mitochondria poor, and capillary poor (hence, white). They produce brief, powerful contractions. They predominate in superficial

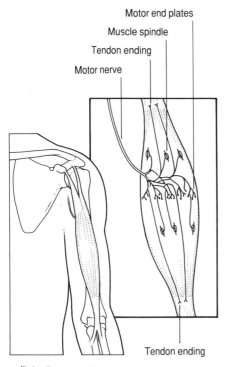

Motor end plates
Muscle spindle
Tendon ending
Motor nerve

Tendon ending

**Figure 7.1.** Pattern of innervation of skeletal muscle.

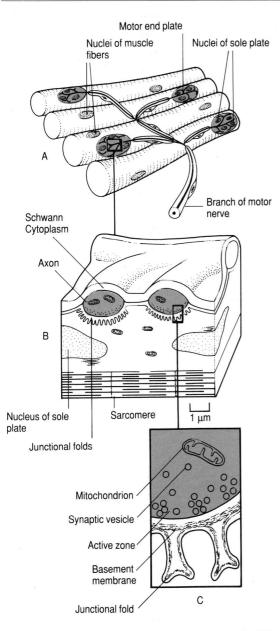

**Figure 7.2.** Motor nerve supply to skeletal muscle. (A) Four motor end plates supplied from a single axon; (B) enlargement from (A); (C) enlargement from (B) showing active zones.

muscles. (c) Intermediate (fast, oxidative–glycolytic, FOG) fibers have properties intermediate between the other two. Every muscle contains all three kinds of fiber, but a given motor unit contains only one kind. The fibers of each unit interdigitate with those of other units.

## Motor end plates

At the *myoneural junction* the axon forms a handful of branchlets which groove the surface of the muscle fiber (*Figure 7.2B*). The underlying sarcolemma is thrown into *junctional folds*. The basement membrane of the muscle fiber traverses the synaptic cleft and lines the folds. The underlying sarcoplasm shows an accumulation of nuclei, mitochondria and ribosomes known as a *sole plate*.

Each axonal branchlet forms an elongated terminal bouton, containing thousands of synaptic vesicles loaded with acetylcholine (ACh). Synaptic transmission takes place at *active zones* facing the crests of the junctional folds (*Figure 7.2C*). ACh is extruded by exocytosis into the synaptic cleft. It diffuses through the basement membrane to reach ACh receptors in the sarcolemma. Activation of the receptors leads to depolarization of the sarcolemma. The depolarization is led into the interior of the muscle fiber by T-tubules. The sarcoplasmic reticulum liberates $Ca^{2+}$ ions which initiate contraction of the sarcomeres (see biochemistry texts for details).

Cholinesterase enzyme is concentrated in the basement membrane, and about 30% of released ACh is hydrolyzed without reaching the postsynaptic membrane. After hydrolysis, the choline moiety is returned to the axoplasm.

## Motor units in old age

The progressive wasting of muscles seen in the elderly is due to loss of motoneurons from the spinal cord and brainstem, and to low-grade peripheral neuropathy arising from vascular disease and often from nutritional deficiency. Electromyographic (EMG) records taken from contracting muscles show *giant motor unit* potentials during the seventh and eighth decades. The extra-large potentials result from takeover of vacated motor end plates of lost motoneurons, by *collateral sprouts* from the axons of adjacent healthy motor units.

The commonest disorder of the myoneural junction is *myasthenia gravis* (Panel 7.1).

---

### CLINICAL PANEL 7.1 • MYASTHENIA GRAVIS

The ACh receptors of skeletal muscle normally undergo turnover, having a half-life (i.e. a 50% loss) of 10 days. New receptors are constantly synthesized in Golgi complexes located around the nuclei of the sole plate and inserted into the sarcolemma of the junctional folds. Old receptors are removed by endocytosis and degraded by lysosomes.

In myasthenia gravis, the immune system produces antibodies to the ACh receptor. The antigen–antibody complex has a half-life of only 2 days, leading to a progressive loss of receptors and of junctional folds. Muscles most affected are those supplied by cranial nerves.

Clinically, myasthenia gravis is characterized by weakness and easy fatigue of the muscles of the orbit, face, and mouth. The limbs are sometimes affected as well. In severe cases, weakness of the muscles of swallowing and respiration may be life-threatening.

Administration of an anticholinesterase drug such as neostigmine can be both diagnostic and therapeutic. By prolonging the binding time of ACh with the remaining receptors, it usually causes prompt improvement in muscle power.

The abnormal antibodies seem to originate in the thymus gland, which is usually hyperplastic in these cases and contains a lymphoid tumor in 10% of patients. Removal of the thymus may be beneficial if symptoms cannot be otherwise controlled.

---

## SENSORY INNERVATION OF SKELETAL MUSCLE

### *Neuromuscular spindles*

Muscle spindles are up to 1 cm in length and vary in number from a dozen to several hundred in different muscles. They are abundant (a) in the antigravity muscles along the vertebral column, femur and tibia; (b) in the muscles of the neck; and (c) in the intrinsic muscles of the hand. All of these muscles are rich in slow, oxidative muscle fibers. Spindles are scarce where FG or FOG fibers predominate.

Muscle spindles contain up to a dozen *intrafusal* muscle fibers (*Figure 7.3*). (Ordinary muscle fibers are *extrafusal* in this context.) The larger intrafusal fibers emerge from the *poles* (ends) of the spindle and are anchored to connective tissue (perimysium). The smaller ones are anchored to the collagenous spindle capsule. At the spindle *equator* (middle), the sarcomeres are replaced almost entirely by nuclei, in the form of 'bags' (in large fibers) or 'chains' (in small fibers).

### Innervation

Spindles have a motor as well as a sensory nerve supply. The motor fibers, called *fusimotor*, are in the A$\gamma$ size range, in contrast to the A$\alpha$ fibers supplying extrafusal muscle. The fusimotor axons divide to supply the striated segments at both ends of the intrafusal muscles (*Figure 7.3*). A single

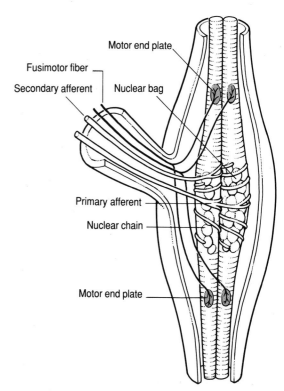

**Figure 7.3.** Representative pattern of innervation of a neuromuscular spindle. One bag muscle fiber and one chain muscle fiber are shown. The primary afferent is supplying both, the secondary afferent is supplying the chain fiber. Fusimotor fibers are supplying the striated segments of both.

*primary* sensory fiber of Type Ia caliber forms *annulospiral* wrappings around the bag/chain segments of the intrafusal muscle fibers. *Secondary* sensory endings are found on one or both sides of the primary; they are supplied by Type II fibers.

## Activation

Muscle spindles are *stretch receptors*. Ion channels in the surface membrane of the sensory terminals are opened by stretch, creating positive electrotonic waves which summate close to the final heminode of the parent sensory fiber. Summation produces a *receptor potential* which will fire off nerve impulses when it reaches threshold.

Muscle spindles may be stretched either *passively* or *actively*.

### PASSIVE STRETCH

Passive stretch of muscle spindles occurs when an entire muscle belly is passively lengthened. For example, in eliciting a tendon reflex such as the *knee jerk*, the spindles in the belly of the muscle are passively stretched when the tendon is struck. The Type Ia and Type II fibers discharge to the spinal cord, where they synapse upon the dendrites of $\alpha$ motoneurons (*Figure 7.4*). ($\alpha$ motoneurons are so called because they give rise to axons of A$\alpha$ diameter.) The response to the *positive feedback* from spindles is a twitch of contraction in the extrafusal muscle fibers. The spindles, because they lie in parallel with the extrafusal muscle, are passively shortened; they are described as being *unloaded*.

Tendon reflexes are *monosynaptic* reflexes. They have a latency (stimulus–response interval) of about 15–25 milliseconds.

In addition to exciting homonymous motoneurons (that is, motoneurons supplying the same muscles), the spindle afferents *inhibit* the $\alpha$ motoneurons supplying the antagonist muscles, through the medium of inhibitory internuncial (interposed) neurons (*Figure 7.4*). This effect is called *reciprocal inhibition*. The inhibitory neurons involved are called *Ia internuncials*.

### INFORMATION CODING

Spindle primary afferents are most active *during* the stretching process. The more rapid the stretch, the more impulses they fire off. They therefore encode the *rate* of stretch.

Spindle secondary afferents are more active than the primaries when a given position is held. The greater the degree of *maintained* stretch, the more impulses they fire off. They therefore encode the *degree* of muscle stretch.

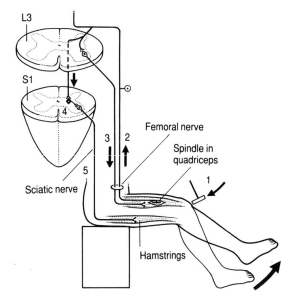

**Figure 7.4.** Patellar reflex, including reciprocal inhibition. Arrows indicate nerve impulses. (1) A tap to the patellar ligament stretches the spindles in quadriceps femoris. (2) Spindles discharge excitatory impulses to the spinal cord. (3) $\alpha$ motoneurons respond by eliciting a twitch in quadriceps, with extension of the knee. (4,5) Ia inhibitory internuncials respond by suppressing any activity in the hamstrings.

### ACTIVE STRETCH

Active stretch is produced by the fusimotor neurons, which elicit contraction of the striated segments of the intrafusal muscle fibers. The connective tissue attachments being relatively fixed, the intrafusal fibers *stretch the spindle equators* by pulling them in the direction of the spindle poles. (This could be called a Christmas-cracker effect.)

During voluntary movements, alpha and gamma motoneurons are *coactivated* by the corticospinal (pyramidal) tract. As a result, the spindles are *not* unloaded by extrafusal muscle contraction. Through ascending connections, the spindle afferents on both sides of the relevant joints are able to keep the brain informed about contractions and relaxations during any given movement.

## Tendon endings

*Golgi tendon organs* are found at muscle–tendon junctions (*Figure 7.5*). A single Ib caliber nerve fiber forms elaborate sprays which intertwine with

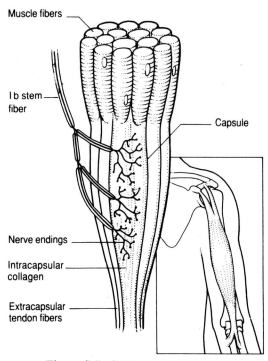

**Figure 7.5.** Golgi tendon organ.

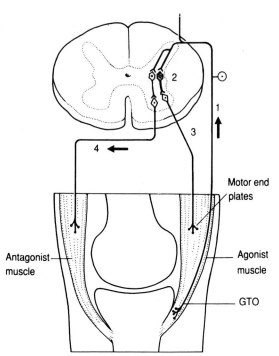

**Figure 7.6.** Reflex effects of Golgi tendon organ (GTO) stimulation. (1) Agonist contraction excites GTO afferent which (2) stimulates inhibitory internuncial synapsing on (3) homonymous motoneuron; and stimulates excitatory internuncial synapsing on (4) antagonist motoneuron.

tendon fiber bundles enclosed within a connective tissue capsule.

A dozen or more muscle fibers insert into the intracapsular tendon fibers, which are *in series* with the muscle fibers. The nerve endings are activated by distortion when tension develops during muscle contraction. Because the rate of impulse discharge along the parent fiber is related to the applied tension, tendon endings signal the *force* of muscle contraction.

The Ib afferents exert *negative feedback* onto the homonymous motoneurons, in contrast to the positive feedback exerted by muscle spindle afferents. The effect is called *autogenetic inhibition*, and the reflex arc is disynaptic because of the interpolation of an inhibitory neuron (*Figure 7.6*). There is an accompanying *reciprocal excitation* of motoneurons supplying antagonist muscles.

### Free nerve endings

Muscles are rich in freely ending nerve fibers, distributed to the intramuscular connective tissue and investing fascial envelopes. They are responsible for pain sensation caused by direct injury or by accumulation of metabolites including lactic acid.

## INNERVATION OF JOINTS

Freely ending unmyelinated nerve fibers are abundant in joint ligaments and capsules, and in the outer parts of intra-articular menisci. They mediate pain when a joint is strained, and they operate an excitatory reflex to protect the capsule. For example, the anterior wrist capsule is supplied by the median and ulnar nerves; if it is suddenly stretched by forced extension, motor fibers in these nerves are reflexly activated and cause wrist flexion.

Animal experiments have shown that when a joint is inflamed, more freely ending nerve fibers are excited than is the case when a healthy joint capsule is stretched. It seems that some nerve endings are *only* stimulated by inflammation.

Encapsulated nerve endings in and around joint capsules include Ruffini endings which signal tension, lamellated endings responsive to pressure, and Pacinian corpuscles responsive to vibration (see Chapter 8).

## REFERENCES

Barker, D. (1974) The morphology of muscle receptors. In *Handbook of Physiology, Vol.III/2, Muscle Receptors* (Hunt, C.D., ed.), pp. 1–191. Berlin: Springer-Verlag.

Binder, M.D. and Stuart, D.G. (1980) Motor-unit muscle receptor interactions: design features of the neuromuscular control system. *Prog. Clin. Neurophysiol.* **8:** 72–98.

Buchthal, F. and Schmalbruch, H. (1980) Motor units of mammalian muscle. *Physiol. Rev.* **60:** 90–125.

Burke, D. and Gandevia, S.C. (1990) Peripheral motor system. In *The Human Nervous System* (Paxinos, G., ed.), pp. 125–148. San Diego: Academic Press.

Salpeter, M.M. (1987) Vertebrate neuromuscular junctions: general morphology, molecular organization, and functional consequences. In *The Vertebrate Neuromuscular Junction* (Salpeter, M.M., ed.), pp. 55–116. New York: Alan R. Liss.

Wyke, B. (1981) The neurology of joints: a review of general principles. *Clin. Rheum. Dis.* **7:** 223–239.

# 8

# Innervation of skin

**CHAPTER SUMMARY**

Sensory units
Nerve endings
*CLINICAL PANELS*
Axon reflex · Peripheral neuropathies

This chapter describes the pattern of cutaneous innervation in hairy and hairless skin. In hairy skin it is stereotyped, conforming to the general mammalian pattern. Sensitivity to touch reaches peak values in the finger pads, which contain a unique pattern of specialized nerve endings designed for the exploration of textured surfaces.

Conscious appreciation of three-dimensional shapes depends upon the integration of cutaneous, muscular, and articular information at the level of the parietal cortex.

From the cutaneous branches of the spinal nerves, innumerable fine twigs enter a *dermal nerve plexus* located in the base of the dermis (*Figure 8.1*). Within the plexus, individual nerve fibers divide and overlap extensively with others before terminating at higher levels of the skin. Because of overlap, the area of anesthesia resulting from injury to a cutaneous nerve (e.g. superficial radial, saphenous) is smaller than its anatomical territory.

## Sensory units; receptive fields

A given stem fiber forms the same kind of nerve ending at all of its terminals. In physiological recordings the stem fiber and its family of endings constitute a *sensory unit*. Together with its parent unipolar nerve cell, the sensory unit is analogous to the motor unit described in Chapter 7.

The territory from which a sensory unit can be excited is its *receptive field*. There is an inverse relationship between the size of receptive fields and sensory acuity. For example, fields measure about 2 cm$^2$ on the arm, 1 cm$^2$ at the wrist, and 5 mm$^2$ on the finger pads.

Sensory units interdigitate so that different *modalities* of sensation can be perceived from a given patch of skin.

## Nerve endings

### Free nerve endings (*Figure 8.2A*)

As they run toward the skin surface, sensory fibers shed their perineurial sheaths and then their myelin sheaths (if any) before branching further in a subepidermal network. The Schwann cell sheaths

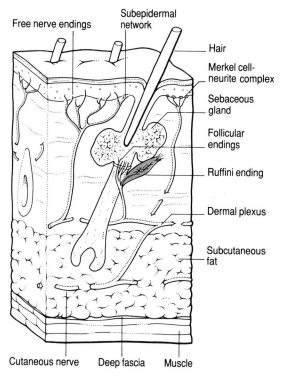

Free nerve endings

Subepidermal network

Hair

Merkel cell-neurite complex

Sebaceous gland

Follicular endings

Ruffini ending

Dermal plexus

Subcutaneous fat

Cutaneous nerve    Deep fascia    Muscle

**Figure 8.1.** Innervation of hairy skin.

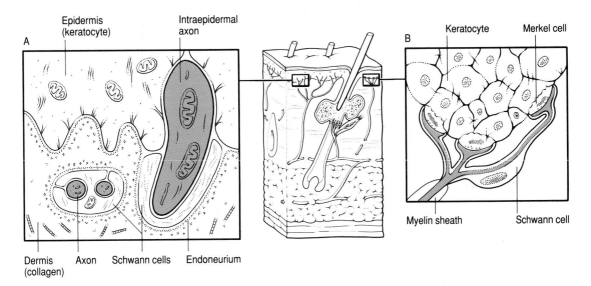

**Figure 8.2.** (A) Unmyelinated axons in dermis (left) and epidermis (right). (B) Merkel cell–neurite complex.

open to permit naked axons to terminate between collagen bundles *(dermal nerve endings)* or within the epidermis *(epidermal nerve endings)*.

FUNCTIONS

Some sensory units with free nerve endings are *thermoreceptive;* they supply either 'warm spots' or 'cold spots' scattered over the skin. Two kinds of *nociceptive* ('painful') units with free endings are also found. One responds to severe mechanical deformation of the skin, such as pinching with a forceps. The parent fibers are finely myelinated (A$\delta$). The other consists of 'polymodal nociceptors'; these are C fiber units responding to mechanical deformation, intense heat (sometimes to intense cold as well), and to irritant chemicals.

C fiber units are responsible for the axon reflex (Panel 8.1).

**Follicular nerve endings** *(Figure 8.1)*

Just below the level of the sebaceous glands, myelinated fibers apply a *palisade* of terminals along the outer root sheath epithelium of the hair follicles. Outside this, a set of *circumferential* terminals encircles the follicle at the same level.

Each follicular unit supplies many follicles and there is much territorial overlap. Follicular units are 'rapidly adapting': they fire when the hairs are being bent, but not when the bent position is held. Rapid adaptation accounts for our being largely

unaware of our clothing except when putting it on or taking it off.

**Merkel cell–neurite complexes** *(Figure 8.2B)*

Expanded nerve terminals are applied to *Merkel cells (tactile menisci)* in the basal epithelium of epidermal pegs and ridges. These *Merkel cell–neurite complexes* are 'slowly adapting' (SA). They discharge continuously in response to sustained pressure (for example, when holding a pen or wearing spectacles), and they are markedly sensitive to the *edges* of objects held in the hand.

**Encapsulated nerve endings**

The capsules of the three nerve endings to be described are composed of an outer coat of connective tissue, a middle coat of perineural epithelium, and an inner coat of modified Schwann cells *(teloglia).* All three are *mechanoreceptors*, responding to mechanical stimulation.

*Meissner's corpuscles* are most numerous in the finger pads, where they lie beside the intermediate ridges of the epidermis *(Figures 8.3 and 8.4A).* In these ovoid receptors, several axons run a zig-zag course among stacks of teloglial lamellae. Meissner's corpuscles are rapidly adapting (RA) receptors. Together with the slowly adapting Merkel cell–neurite complexes, they provide the tools for delicate detective work on textured surfaces

## CLINICAL PANEL 8.1 • NEUROGENIC INFLAMMATION: THE AXON REFLEX

When the skin is stroked with a sharp object, a red line appears in seconds due to capillary dilatation in direct response to the injury. A few minutes later a red *flare* spreads into the surrounding skin, due to arteriolar dilatation, followed by a white *wheal* due to exudation of plasma from the capillaries. These phenomena constitute the *triple response*. The wheal and flare responses are produced by *axon reflexes* in the local sensory cutaneous nerves. The sequence of events is shown by the numbers in *Figure CP 8.1.1*.

1. The noxious stimulus is transduced (converted to nerve impulses) by polymodal nociceptors.

2. As well as transmitting impulses to the CNS in the normal, *orthodromic* direction, the axons send impulses in an *antidromic* direction from points of bifurcation into the neighboring skin. Surprisingly, the nociceptive endings respond to antidromic stimulation by releasing one or more peptide substances, notably *substance P*.

3. Substance P binds with receptors on the walls of arterioles, leading to arteriolar dilatation—the flare response.

4. Substance P also binds with receptors on

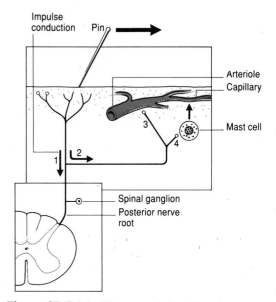

**Figure CP 8.1.1.** The axon reflex. For the numbers, see text.

the surface of mast cells, stimulating them to release *histamine*. The histamine increases capillary permeability and leads to local accumulation of tissue fluid—the wheal response.

---

such as cloth or wood, or on embossed surfaces such as Braille text. Elevations as little as 5 $\mu$m in height can be detected!

*Ruffini endings* are found in both hairy and glabrous skin (*Figures 8.1* and *8.3*). They respond to *drag* (shearing stress) and are slowly adapting (SA) receptors. They are most numerous alongside the fingernails. Their structure resembles that of Golgi tendon organs, having a collagenous core in which one or more axons branch liberally (*Figure 8.4B*).

*Pacinian corpuscles* are the size of grains of rice. They are subcutaneous (*Figure 8.3*). Inside a thin connective sheath are onion-like layers of perineural epithelium containing some blood capillaries. Innermost are several teloglial lamellae surrounding a single central axon which has shed its myelin sheath at its point of entry (*Figure 8.4B*).

Pacinian corpuscles are rapidly adapting (RA) and are especially responsive to *vibration*—particularly to bony vibration. In the limbs, many

Pacinian corpuscles are embedded in the periosteum of the long bones.

The digital receptors are classified as follows by sensory physiologists:

- Merkel cell–neurite complexes = SA I
- Meissner's corpuscles = RA I
- Ruffini endings = SA II
- Pacinian corpuscles = RA II

When three-dimensional objects are being manipulated, out of sight, significant contributions to perceptual evaluation are made by muscle afferents (especially from muscle spindles) and articular afferents from joint capsules. The cutaneous, muscular, and articular afferents relay information independently to the contralateral somatic sensory cortex. The three kinds of information are integrated (brought together at cellular level) in the posterior part of the parietal lobe, which is specialized for *spatial sense*. The tactile dimension of

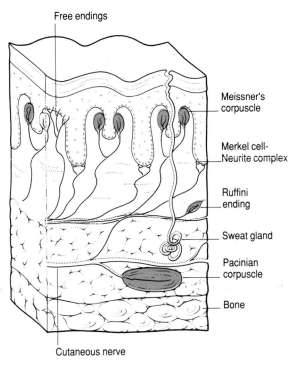

**Figure 8.3.** Innervation of finger pad.

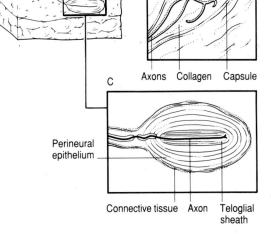

**Figure 8.4.** (A) Meissner's corpuscle; (B) Ruffini ending; (C) Pacinian corpuscle.

spatial sense is called *stereognosis*. In the clinic, this faculty is tested by asking the patient to identify an object such as a key without looking at it.

### Peripheral neuropathies

Panel 8.2 gives a short account of peripheral nerve diseases, with special reference to leprosy.

---

## CLINICAL PANEL 8.2 ● PERIPHERAL NEUROPATHIES: LEPROSY

Diseases of peripheral nerves *(peripheral neuropathies)* have a wide variety of causes which include inherited and acquired metabolic disorders, nutritional deficiencies, reaction to drugs, and infections. The most common peripheral neuropathy in demographic terms is *leprosy*. Leprosy is prevalent in India and central Africa and is endemic in pockets elsewhere including the Gulf Coast region of the United States.

The leprosy bacillus enters the skin through minor abrasions. It travels proximally within the perineurium of the cutaneous nerves and kills off the Schwann cells. Loss of myelin seg-

ments ('segmental demyelination') blocks impulse conduction in the larger nerve fibers. Later, the inflammatory response to the bacillus compresses all of the axons, leading to Wallerian degeneration of entire nerves and gross thickening of the connective tissue sheaths. Patches of anesthetic skin develop on the fingers, toes, nose and ears. The protective function of skin sensation is lost and the affected parts suffer injury and loss of tissue. *Motor paralyses* occur later on, as a consequence of invasion of mixed nerve trunks proximal to the points of origin of their cutaneous branches.

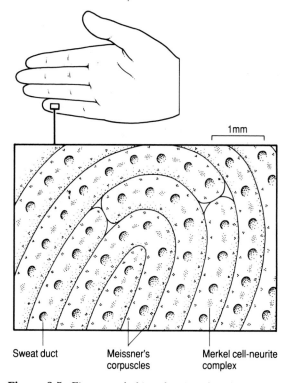

1mm

Sweat duct    Meissner's    Merkel cell-neurite
              corpuscles    complex

**Figure 8.5.** Finger pad skin, showing distribution of Meissner's corpuscles and Merkel cell–neurite complexes.

## REFERENCES

Bannister, L.H. (1976) Sensory terminals of peripheral nerves. In *The Peripheral Nerve* (Landon, D.N., ed.). London: Chapman & Hall.

Breathnach, A.S. (1977) Electronmicroscopy of cutaneous nerves and receptors. *J. Invest. Dermatol.* **69:** 8–26.

Cunningham, F.O. and FitzGerald, M.J.T. (1972) Encapsulated nerve endings in hairy skin. *J. Anat.* **112:** 93–97.

Foreman, J.C. (1987) Peptides and neurogenic inflammation. *Br. Med. Bull.* **43:** 386–400.

Iggo, A. (1985) Sensory receptors in the skin of mammals and their sensory functions. *Rev. Neurol.* **141:** 599–615.

Torebjork, A.B., Vallbo, A.B. and Ochoa, J.L. (1987) Intraneural microstimulation in man: its relation to specificity of tactile sensations. *Brain* **110:** 1509-1529.

# 9

# Autonomic nervous system and visceral afferents

Following an overview of the anatomy of the autonomic nervous system, the chief autonomic transmitters and receptors are described in order to make sense of the physiological effects produced by autonomic activity. An understanding of these effects is a prerequisite for the study of drug actions on this system.

The chapter concludes with some remarks on the visceral afferent system, which uses autonomic pathways to reach the CNS. Visceral afferents participate in important reflexes, and they are a potential source of pain in visceral disorders.

## COMPONENTS OF THE AUTONOMIC NERVOUS SYSTEM

The **autonomic** ('self-regulating') **nervous system** is distributed to the peripheral tissues and organs by way of outlying autonomic ganglia. Controling centers in the hypothalamus and brainstem send *central autonomic fibers* to synapse upon *preganglionic neurons* located in the gray matter of the brainstem and spinal cord. From these neurons *preganglionic fibers* (mostly myelinated) project out of the CNS to synapse upon multipolar neurons in the autonomic ganglia. Unmyelinated *postganglionic fibers* emerge and form terminal networks in the target tissues.

Both anatomically and functionally, the autonomic system is composed of **sympathetic** and **parasympathetic** divisions.

## SYMPATHETIC NERVOUS SYSTEM

The sympathetic system is so called because it acts in sympathy with the emotions. In association with rage or fear, the sympathetic system prepares the body for 'fight or flight': the heart rate is increased, the pupils dilate, the skin sweats. Blood is diverted from the skin and intestinal tract to the skeletal muscles, and the sphincters of the alimentary and urinary tracts are closed.

The sympathetic outflow from the nervous system is *thoracolumbar*, the preganglionic neurons being located in the lateral gray horn of the spinal cord at thoracic and upper two (or three) lumbar segmental levels. From these neurons, preganglionic fibers emerge in the corresponding anterior nerve roots and enter the sympathetic chain. The fibers do one of four things, in accordance with 1–4 in *Figure 9.1:*

1. Some fibers synapse in the nearest ganglion. Postganglionic fibers enter spinal nerves T1–L2 and supply blood vessels and sweat glands in the territory of these nerves.
2. Some fibers *ascend* the sympathetic chain and synapse in the superior or middle cervical ganglion, or in the **stellate ganglion.** (The stellate consists of the fused inferior cervical and first thoracic ganglia; it lies in front of the neck of the first rib.) Postganglionic fibers supply the head, neck, and upper limbs; also

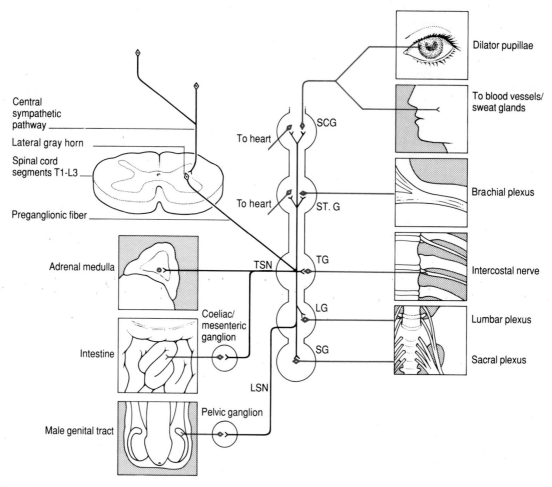

**Figure 9.1.** General plan of the sympathetic system. Ganglionic neurons and postganglionic fibers are shown in red. LG, lumbar ganglia; LSN, lumbar splanchnic nerve; SCG, superior cervical ganglion; SG, sacral ganglia; ST.G, stellate ganglion; TG, thoracic ganglia; TSN, thoracic splanchnic nerve.

the heart. Of particular importance is the supply to the dilator muscle of the pupil (Panel 9.1).

3. Some fibers *descend* to synapse in lumbar or sacral ganglia of the sympathetic chain. Postganglionic fibers enter the lumbosacral plexus for distribution to the blood vessels and skin of the lower limb.

4. Some fibers *traverse* the chain and emerge as the (preganglionic) thoracic and lumbar splanchnic nerves. The **thoracic splanchnic nerves** (usually called, simply, the splanchnic nerves) pass through the lower eight thoracic ganglia, pierce the diaphragm, and synapse in celiac, mesenteric, and renal ganglia within the abdomen. Postganglionic fibers accompany branches of the aorta to reach the gastrointestinal tract, liver, pancreas, and kidneys.

**Lumbar splanchnic nerves** pass through the upper three lumbar ganglia and meet in front of the bifurcation of the abdominal aorta. They enter the pelvis as the **hypogastric nerves** before ending in pelvic ganglia, from which the genitourinary tract is supplied.

The medulla of the adrenal gland is the homolog of a sympathetic ganglion, being derived from the neural crest. It receives a direct input from fibers of the thoracic splanchnic nerve of its own side (see later).

The sympathetic system exerts tonic (continuous) constrictor activity on blood vessels in the limbs. In order to improve the blood flow to the hands or feet, impulse traffic along the sympathetic system can be interrupted surgically (Panel 9.1).

## CLINICAL PANEL 9.1 • SYMPATHETIC INTERRUPTION

### Stellate block

Injection of local anesthetic around the stellate ganglion—*stellate block*—is a procedure used in order to test the effects of sympathetic interruption on blood flow to the hand. Both pre- and postganglionic fibers are inactivated, producing sympathetic paralysis in the head and neck on that side, as well as in the upper limb. A successful stellate block is demonstrated by (a) *a warm, dry* hand, and (b) *Horner's syndrome,* which consists of a constricted pupil due to unopposed action of the pupillary constrictor, and ptosis (drooping) of the upper eyelid due to paralysis of smooth muscle fibers contained in the levator muscle of the upper eyelid (*Figure CP 9.1.1*).

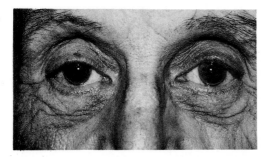

**Figure CP 9.1.1.** Horner's syndrome, patient's right side. Note the *moderate ptosis* of the eyelid, and the *moderate miosis* (pupillary constriction). Horner's syndrome often escapes detection! (Photograph kindly provided by Dr David Russel; permission of Elsevier Science Publishers is acknowledged.)

*Functional sympathectomy* of the upper limb may be carried out by cutting the sympathetic chain below the stellate ganglion. This is not an anatomical sympathectomy because the ganglionic supply to the limb from the middle cervical and stellate ganglia remains intact. It is a functional one because the ganglionic neurons for the limb are deprived of tonic sympathetic drive. Horner's syndrome is avoided by making the cut at the level of the *second* rib: the preganglionic fibers for the head and neck enter the stellate direct from the first thoracic spinal nerve.

Two indications for interruption of the sympathetic supply to one or both upper limbs are painful blanching of the fingers in cold weather *(Raynaud phenomenon)*, and *hyperhidrosis* (excessive sweating) of the hands—usually an embarrassing affliction of teenage girls.

The sympathetic supply to the eye is considered further in Chapter 17.

### Lumbar sympathectomy

In order to improve blood flow in the lower limb, the preganglionic nerve supply may be interrupted by cutting the upper end of the lumbar sympathetic chain. The usual procedure is to remove the 2nd and 3rd lumbar sympathetic ganglia. A bilateral *lumbar sympathectomy* may produce impotence as a side effect owing to interruption of a pathway to erectile tissue (see main text).

## THE PARASYMPATHETIC NERVOUS SYSTEM

The parasympathetic system generally has the effect of counterbalancing the sympathetic system. It adapts the eyes for close-up viewing, slows the heart, promotes secretion of salivary and intestinal juices, and accelerates intestinal peristalsis. A notable instance of *concerted* sympathetic and parasympathetic activity occurs during sexual intercourse.

The parasympathetic outflow from the CNS is *craniosacral* (*Figure 9.2*). Preganglionic fibers emerge from the brainstem in four cranial nerves—the oculomotor, facial, glossopharyngeal, and vagus—and from sacral segments of the spinal cord.

### Cranial parasympathetic system

Preganglionic parasympathetic fibers emerge in four cranial nerves:

1. In the oculomotor nerve, to synapse in the **ciliary ganglion.** Postganglionic fibers inner-

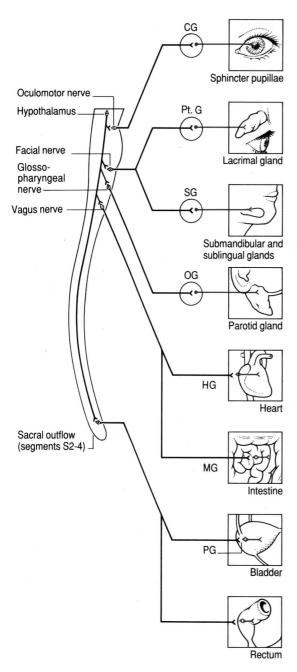

**Figure 9.2.** General plan of the parasympathetic system. Ganglionic neurons and postganglionic fibers are shown in red. CG, ciliary ganglion; HG, heart ganglia; MG, myenteric ganglia; OG, otic ganglion; PG, pelvic ganglion; Pt. G, pterygopalatine ganglion; SG, submandibular ganglion.

vate the sphincter of the pupil and the ciliary muscle. Both muscles act to produce the *accommodation reflex*.

2. In the facial nerve, to synapse in the **pterygopalatine ganglion**, which innervates the lacrimal and nasal glands; and in the **submandibular ganglion,** which innervates the submandibular and sublingual glands.

3. In the glossopharyngeal nerve, to synapse in the **otic ganglion,** which innervates the parotid gland.

4. In the vagus nerve, to synapse in parasympathetic ganglia close to the heart and lungs; and to synapse upon ganglion cells in the wall of the stomach and small intestine, and in the ascending and transverse parts of the colon.

### *Sacral parasympathetic system*

The sacral segments of the spinal cord occupy the conus medullaris (conus terminalis) at the lower extremity of the spinal cord, behind the body of the first lumbar vertebra. From the lateral gray matter of segments S2, S3 and S4, preganglionic fibers descend in the cauda equina within ventral nerve roots. Upon emerging from the pelvic sacral foramina the fibers separate out as the **pelvic splanchnic nerves.** Some fibers of the left and right pelvic splanchnic nerves synapse on ganglion cells in the wall of the distal colon and rectum. The rest synapse in **pelvic ganglia,** which contain sympathetic as well as parasympathetic neurons. Postganglionic parasympathetic fibers supply the detrusor muscle of the bladder; also the tunica media of the internal pudendal artery and of its branches to the cavernous tissue of the penis/clitoris (see later).

### NEUROTRANSMISSION IN THE AUTONOMIC SYSTEM

### *Ganglionic transmission (Figure 9.3)*

The preganglionic neurons of the sympathetic *and* parasympathetic systems are *cholinergic:* the neurons liberate acetylcholine (ACh) onto the ganglion cells at axodendritic synapses. The receptors on the ganglion cells are *nicotinic*—so named because the excitatory effect can be imitated by locally applied nicotine.

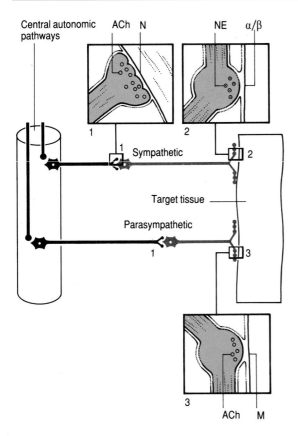

**Figure 9.3.** Autonomic transmitters and receptors. Ganglionic neurons and postganglionic fibers are shown in red. ACh, acetylcholine; M, muscarinic receptors; N, nicotinic receptors; NE, norepinephrine.

## *Junctional transmission (Figure 9.3)*

Postganglionic fibers of the sympathetic and parasympathetic systems form *neuroeffector junctions* with target tissues. Transmitter substances are liberated from innumerable varicosities strung along the course of the nerve fibers.

The chief transmitter at sympathetic neuroeffector junctions is *norepinephrine (noradrenalin)*, which is liberated from dense-cored vesicles. The postganglionic sympathetic system in general is described as *adrenergic*. A notable exception to the adrenergic rule is the *cholinergic* sympathetic supply to the eccrine sweat glands over the body surface.

The chief transmitter at parasympathetic neuroeffector junctions is *acetylcholine*. The post-

ganglionic parasympathetic system in general is *cholinergic*.

## Junctional receptors

Physiological effects of autonomic stimulation depend upon the nature of the *postjunctional receptors* inserted by target cells into their own plasma membranes. In addition, transmitter release is influenced by *prejunctional receptors* in the axolemmal membrane of the nerve terminals.

SYMPATHETIC JUNCTIONAL RECEPTORS (ADRENOCEPTORS) *(FIGURE 9.4)*

Two kinds of *alpha adrenoceptor* and two kinds of *beta adrenoceptor* have been identified for norepinephrine, as follows:

1. Postjunctional, $\alpha_1$ adrenoceptors initiate contraction of smooth muscle in the following locations: peripheral small arteries and large arterioles; the dilator pupillae; the sphincters of the alimentary tract and bladder neck; and the vas deferens.
2. Prejunctional, $\alpha_2$ adrenoceptors are present on parasympathetic as well as on sympathetic terminals. They inhibit transmitter release in both

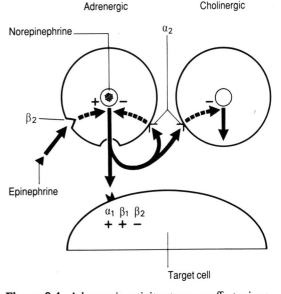

**Figure 9.4.** Adrenergic activity at a neuroeffector junction. Release of norepinephrine is promoted by epinephrine and inhibited by prejunctional $\alpha_2$ receptors, which also inhibit transmitter release from neighboring parasympathetic varicosities.

cases. On sympathetic terminals, they are called *autoreceptors.*

3. Postjunctional, $\beta_1$ adrenoceptors increase pacemaker activity in the heart and increase the force of ventricular contraction. In response to a severe fall of blood pressure, sympathetic activation of $\beta_1$ receptors on the juxtaglomerular cells of the kidney causes secretion of *renin.* Renin initiates production of the powerful vasoconstrictor, angiotensin II.

4. $\beta_2$ receptors respond to circulating *epinephrine (adrenalin)* (*Figure 9.5*) as well as to locally released norepinephrine.

*Postjunctional* $\beta_2$ receptors *relax smooth muscle,* notably in the tracheobronchial tree and in the accommodatory muscles of the eye. Some postjunctional $\beta_2$ receptors are on the surface of hepatocytes in the liver, where they initiate glycogen

breakdown to provide glucose for immediate energy needs.

*Prejunctional* $\beta_2$ receptors on adrenergic terminals promote release of norepinephrine.

Most of the norepinephrine liberated at sympathetic terminals is retrieved by an *amine uptake pump.* Some of it is degraded after uptake by a mitochondrial enzyme, *monoamine oxidase.*

The effects of *drugs* on the sympathetic system are considered in Panel 9.2.

### Parasympathetic junctional receptors *(Figure 9.6)*

Parasympathetic junctional receptors are called *muscarinic* because they can be mimicked by application of the drug muscarine. Parasympathetic stimulation produces the following *muscarinic* effects:

- Slowing of the heart in response to vagal stimulation, and diminished force of ventricular contraction
- Contraction of smooth muscle, with the following effects: intestinal peristalsis, bladder emptying, accommodation of the eye for 'near vision'

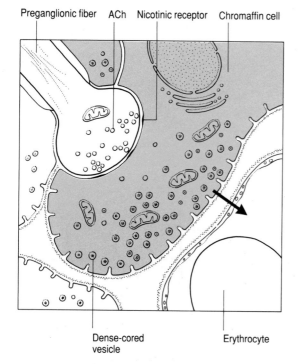

**Figure 9.5.** Chromaffin cell of the adrenal medulla receiving a synaptic contact from a preganglionic fiber of the thoracic splanchnic nerve. Acetylcholine (ACh) activates nicotinic receptors. 80% of the dense-cored vesicles are large and contain epinephrine; 20% are small and contain norepinephrine. Arrow indicates release into capillary bed.

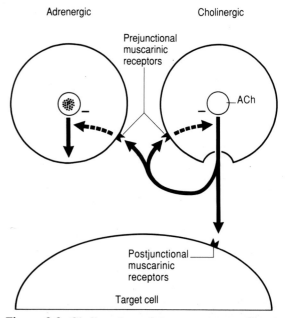

**Figure 9.6.** Cholinergic activity at a neuroeffector junction. Release of excess acetylcholine (ACh) is inhibited by prejunctional muscarinic receptors, which also inhibit transmitter release from neighboring sympathetic varicosities.

## CLINICAL PANEL 9.2 • DRUGS AND THE SYMPATHETIC SYSTEM

Considerable scope is offered for pharmacological interference at sympathetic nerve endings. Drugs which cross the blood–brain barrier (Chapter 26) may exert their effects upon central rather than peripheral adrenoceptors. Potential sites of drug action are numbered in *Figure CP 9.2.1*.

1. Norepinephrine (NE) is loosely bound to a protein in the dense-cored vesicles. It can be unbound by specific drugs, whereupon it diffuses into the axoplasm and is degraded by monoamine oxidase.
2. Exocytosis into the synaptic cleft can be accelerated. Amphetamine, for example, exerts its central stimulant effect by flooding the extracellular space with expelled NE.
3. $\alpha$ or $\beta$ receptors can be selectively either stimulated or blocked. As was mentioned in Chapter 6, a receptor can be likened to a lock, and a drug which operates the lock is an *agonist*. A drug which 'jams' the lock without operating it is a *blocker*. 'Beta agonists' are used to relax the bronchial musculature in asthmatic patients. Cardioselective 'beta blockers' are used to limit access of NE to $\beta_1$ receptors.
4. The amine uptake mechanism can be blocked in the CNS by the tricyclic antidepressant drugs, or by cocaine. As a result, NE accumulates in the brain extracellular fluid.
5. Some antidepressant drugs increase the NE

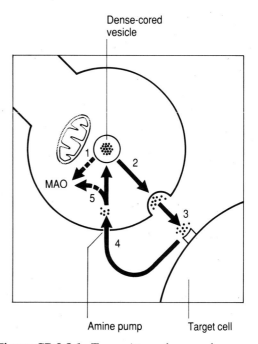

**Figure CP 9.2.1.** Transmitter release and recycling at adrenergic nerve endings. MAO, monoamine oxidase. For numbers, see text.

content of synaptic vesicles by inhibiting monoamine oxidase, which normally degrades some of the transmitter after retrieval.

---

- Glandular secretion
- In addition to the above postjunctional effects, prejunctional muscarinic receptors located on sympathetic varicosities inhibit release of norepinephrine.

The effects of *drugs* on the parasympathetic system are considered in Panel 9.3. Drugs having muscarinic effects are described as cholinergic. Drugs that prevent access of ACh to junctional receptors are anticholinergic.

A major consideration in the use of drugs either to imitate or to suppress sympathetic or parasympathetic activity, is the existence of $\alpha$, $\beta$, and muscarinic receptors in the *central* nervous system. In psychiatric practice, in particular, drugs are

often chosen for their action at central rather than their peripheral receptors.

### 'NANC' neurons in the autonomic nervous system

*Non-adrenergic, non-cholinergic (NANC) neurons* are found in both divisions of the autonomic system. In sympathetic ganglia, small internuncial neurons liberate *dopamine*—a precursor of noradrenaline. Some of the dopamine is secreted into capillaries, the rest binds with dopamine receptors on the main (adrenergic) neurons and exerts a mild inhibitory effect.

NANC neurons are especially numerous among

## CLINICAL PANEL 9.3 • DRUGS AND THE PARASYMPATHETIC SYSTEM

Possible peripheral effects of cholinergic and anticholinergic drugs are listed in *Figure CP 9.3.1.* Some success has been achieved in the search for organ- or tissue-specific drugs. For example, the contribution of the vagus nerve to acid secretion in the stomach involves acti-vation of a muscarinic receptor ($M_1$) which is distinct from the receptor type ($M_2$) found in the heart or on smooth muscle. An $M_1$ receptor blocker is now available for patients suffering from peptic ulcer, for the specific purpose of reducing gastric acidity.

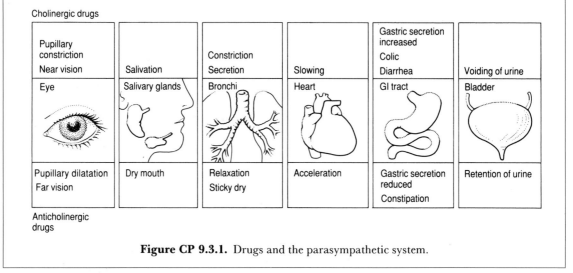

Cholinergic drugs

| Eye | Salivary glands | Bronchi | Heart | GI tract | Bladder |
|---|---|---|---|---|---|
| Pupillary constriction / Near vision | Salivation | Constriction / Secretion | Slowing | Gastric secretion increased / Colic / Diarrhea | Voiding of urine |
| Pupillary dilatation / Far vision | Dry mouth | Relaxation / Sticky dry | Acceleration | Gastric secretion reduced / Constipation | Retention of urine |

Anticholinergic drugs

**Figure CP 9.3.1.** Drugs and the parasympathetic system.

the ganglion cells in the wall of the alimentary tract, and in the pelvic ganglia. More than 50 different *peptide* substances have been identified, either singly or in various combinations, in these neurons. For the most part, they act as *modulators*, acting either pre- or postjunctionally to influence the duration of action of classical transmitters. Some are *cotransmitters* (i.e. released in combination) along with acetylcholine.

*Vasoactive intestinal polypeptide* (VIP) is a cotransmitter in the cholinergic supply to the salivary glands and to sweat glands. VIP is a powerful vasodilator and conveniently opens the local vascular bed (through specific VIP receptors on arterioles) just when the muscarinic ACh receptors are raising glandular metabolism.

### Penile/clitoral erection

VIP is a cotransmitter in the *nervi erigentes* ('erectile nerves'). The nervi erigentes are postganglionic pelvic splanchnic nerve fibers supplying the internal pudendal arteries and their branches to the cavernous tissue of the penis/clitoris. During *erec-tion*, the arteries are forced to relax and the cavernous tissue is flooded with arterial blood.

The sympathetic system, too, is active during sexual arousal. Outflow resistance from the penis/clitoris is increased by sympathetically induced contraction of smooth muscle in the cavernous tissue septa.

Powerful electrical stimulation *either* of the lumbar splanchnic nerves (sympathetic) *or* of the nervi erigentes (parasympathetic) produces erection. However, failure to achieve erections (impotence) may follow a bilateral lumbar sympathectomy, with the nervi erigentes intact. Impotence may also be a feature of long-standing peripheral neuropathies, associated with atrophy of postganglionic fibers in both systems. It should be mentioned that impotence is more often due to psychological problems, such as depression, rather than to interruption of anatomical pathways.

### Notes on seminal emission and ejaculation

The mature sperm are stored in the lower end of the vas deferens and in the tail of the epididymis.

The entire length of the vas is intensely rich in adrenergic nerve endings and $\alpha$ receptors. So too is the smooth muscle of the bladder neck, prostate, and seminal vesicles. The fibers are distributed from sympathetic ganglion cells in the pelvic plexuses.

### EMISSION

At the male climax, peristaltic waves milk the sperm rapidly into the prostatic urethra. The secretions of the prostate and seminal vesicles are squeezed into the urethra as well, to complete the semen, and the bladder neck is sealed off.

### EJACULATION

Contact of the semen with the urethral mucous membrane triggers reflex contractions of the bulbospongiosus muscle, to empty the urethra. The pudendal nerve provides both limbs of this reflex arc.

## Interaction of the autonomic and immune systems

The lymphatic tissues of the thymus, lymph nodes, and respiratory and alimentary mucous membranes are in receipt of adrenergic and cholinergic nerve fibers. They also receive fibers containing various neuronal peptide substances, many of these fibers having their cell bodies in spinal and cranial sensory ganglia. Attempts to incorporate these findings into concepts of normal and disordered immune function are only tentative as yet.

## VISCERAL AFFERENTS

Afferents from thoracic and abdominal viscera utilize autonomic pathways to reach the central nervous system. They participate in important reflexes involved in the control of circulation, respiration, digestion, micturition, and coition. Details on visceral reflexes are to be found in textbooks of physiology.

Visceral activities are not normally perceived, but they do reach conscious levels in a variety of disease states. Visceral pain is of immense importance in the context of clinical diagnosis.

## Visceral pain

There are three fundamental types of visceral pain:

1. Pure visceral pain, felt in the region of the affected organ
2. Visceral referred pain, projected subjectively into the territory of the corresponding nerves
3. Viscerosomatic pain, caused by spread of disease to somatic structures.

### Pure visceral pain

Pure visceral pain is characteristically vague and deep-seated. It is often accompanied by sweating or nausea. It is experienced as the initial pain in association with inflammation and/or ulceration in the alimentary tract; with obstruction of the intestine, bile duct, or ureter; or when the capsule of a solid organ (liver, kidney, pancreas) is stretched by underlying disease. In marked contrast, the viscera are completely *insensitive* to cutting or burning.

### Visceral referred pain

As its severity increases, visceral pain is 'referred' to somatic structures innervated from the same segmental levels of the spinal cord. For example, the pain of myocardial ischemia is referred to the chest wall ('angina pectoris'), pains of biliary or intestinal origin are referred to the anterior abdominal wall, and labor pains are referred to the sacral area of the back.

According to the generally accepted 'convergence–projection' theory of referred pain, the brain falsely interprets the source of noxious stimulation because visceral and somatic nociceptors have some spinothalalamic neurons in common; in previous experience, these neurons habitually signaled somatic pain.

### Viscerosomatic pain

The parietal serous membranes (pleura and peritoneum) receive a rich sensory supply from the overlying intercostal nerves, and they are exquisitely sensitive to acute inflammatory exudates. The extension of an inflammatory process to the surface of stomach, intestine, appendix or gallbladder gives rise to a severe, steady pain in the abdominal wall directly overlying the inflamed organ. With the onset of acute peritonitis, the abdominal wall is 'splinted' by the muscles in a protective reflex.

### Tenderness

*Tenderness is pain elicited by palpation.* In the abdomen, it is sought by pressing the hand and fingers against the abdominal wall. The clinician is, in effect, clothing the finger pads with the patient's parietal peritoneum and using this to seek out an inflamed organ. If the organ is mobile, like the appendix, 'shifting tenderness' may be elicited if the patient is willing to roll from one side to the other.

### Pain and the mind

Although visceral pain has well-established causative mechanisms (inflammation, spasm of smooth muscle, ischemia, distention), thoracic or abdominal pain may be experienced in the complete absence of visceral disease. Pain that recurs or persists over a long period (months) and is not accounted for by standard investigational procedures, is more likely to have a *psychological* rather than a physical explanation. This is not to deny

that the pain is real, but to imply that it originates within the brain itself. An example is the abused child whose abdominal pains represent a cry for help. In adults, recurrent and rather ill-defined pains are a common manifestation of *endogenous depression* (see Chapter 18).

### REFERENCES

Appenzeller, D. (1982) *The Autonomic Nervous System: An Introduction to Basic and Clinical Concepts*, 3rd edn. Amsterdam: Elsevier Biomedical Press.

Burnstock, G. (1986) The changing face of autonomic neurotransmission. *Acta Physiol. Scand.* **126:** 67–91.

Coupland, R.E. (1989) The natural history of the chromaffin cell. *Arch. Histol. Cytol.* **52:** 331–341.

Merskey, H. (1978) Pain and personality. In *The Psychology of Pain* (Sternbach, R.A., ed.). New York: Raven Press.

Paintal, A.S. (1986) The visceral sensations—some basic mechanisms. *Prog. Brain Res.* **67:** 3–18.

Procacci, P., Zoppi, M. and Maresca, M. (1986). Clinical approach to visceral sensation. *Prog. Brain Res.* **67:** 21–28.

Weihe, E., Nohr, D., Michel, S., Muller, S., Zentel, H.-J., Fink, T. and Krekel, J. (1991) Molecular anatomy of the neuro-immune connection. *Int. J. Neurosci.* **59:** 1–23.

CHAPTER SUMMARY

Development of the spinal cord
Adult anatomy
Distribution of spinal nerves
*CLINICAL PANELS*
Spina bifida · Nerve root compression

**10**

# Nerve roots

The development of the spinal cord is first described; the spinal nerves are then considered in the anatomical context of segmental arrangements and in the clinical contexts of nerve root compression syndromes and of anesthetic procedures.

## DEVELOPMENT OF THE SPINAL CORD

### Cellular differentiation

The neural tube of the embryo consists of a pseudostratified epithelium surrounding the neural canal (*Figure 10.1A*). Dorsal to the sulcus limitans the epithelium forms the **alar plate**; ventral to the sulcus it forms the **basal plate.** (The terms 'dorsal' and 'ventral' correspond to 'anterior' and 'posterior' in postnatal anatomy.)

The neuroepithelium contains germinal cells which synthesize DNA before retracting to the innermost, **ventricular zone,** where they divide. The daughter nuclei move outward, synthesize fresh DNA, then retreat and divide again. After several such cycles, postmitotic cells round up in the **intermediate zone.** Some of the postmitotic cells are immature neurons; the rest are **glioblasts** which after further division become astrocytes or oligodendrocytes. Some of the glioblasts form an ependymal lining for the neural canal.

The microglial cells of the CNS are derived from basophil cells of the blood.

Enlargement of the intermediate zone of the alar plate creates the dorsal horn of gray matter. The dorsal horn receives the central processes of dorsal root ganglion cells (*Figure 10.1B*). As explained in Chapter 1, the ganglion cells are derived from the neural crest.

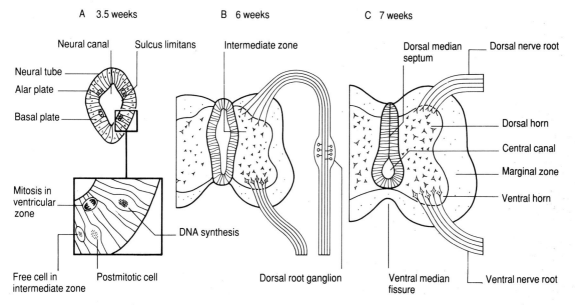

**Figure 10.1.** Cellular differentiation in the embryonic spinal cord.

Partial occlusion of the neural canal by the developing dorsal gray horn gives rise to the dorsal median septum and to the definitive central canal of the cord (*Figure 10.1C*).

Enlargement of the intermediate zone of the basal plate creates the ventral gray horn and the ventral median fissure (*Figure 10.1C*). Axons emerge from the ventral horn and form the ventral nerve roots.

In the outermost, **marginal zone** of the cord, axons run from spinal cord to brain and *vice versa*.

**Caudal cell mass**

The neural tube reaches caudally only to the level of the second lumbar mesodermal somites. Following closure of the posterior neuropore, the ectoderm and mesoderm at the level of the more caudal lumbar and sacral somites blend to form a *caudal cell mass*. This ribbon of cells becomes canalized and links up with the neural tube; it gives rise to the lower end of the spinal cord.

### *Ascent of the cord* (Figure 10.2)

The spinal cord occupies the full length of the vertebral canal until the end of the 12th postconceptual week. The sixth to eighth weeks are marked by *regression of the tail:* the number of coccygeal vertebrae is reduced from six to three, and the enclosed part of the neural tube shrivels to become a neuroglial thread, the **filum terminale.**

After the 12th week the vertebral column grows more rapidly than the spinal cord, and the cord is forced to ascend the vertebral canal. The tip of the cord reaches the 2nd or 3rd lumbar level at the time of birth. The adult level (1st or 2nd lumbar) is reached 3 weeks later.

As a consequence of greater ascent of the lower part of the cord compared to the upper part, the spinal nerve roots show an increasing disparity between their segmental levels of attachment to the cord, and the corresponding vertebral levels (*Figure 10.3*).

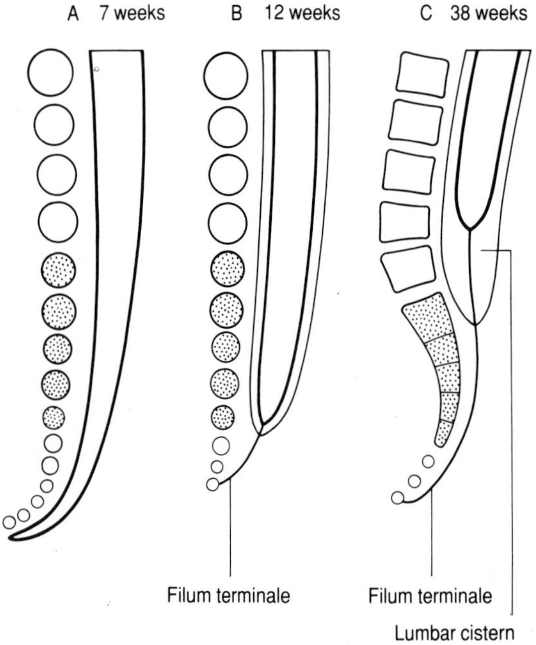

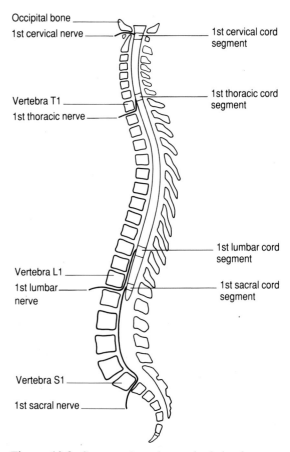

Figure 10.2. (A, B) Regression of coccygeal segments of spinal cord creates the filum terminale; (C) ascent of spinal cord.

**Figure 10.3.** Segmental and vertebral levels compared. Spinal nerves 1–7 emerge above the corresponding vertebrae, the remaining spinal nerves emerge below.

### Neural arches

During the fifth week, the mesenchymal vertebrae surrounding the notochord give rise to *neural arches* for protection of the spinal cord (*Figure 10.4*). The arches are initially bifid (split). Later, they fuse in the midline and form the vertebral spines.

Conditions in which the two halves of the neural arches fail to unite are collectively known as *spina bifida* (Panel 10.1).

## ADULT ANATOMY

The spinal cord and nerve roots are sheathed by pia mater and float in cerebrospinal fluid contained in the subarachnoid space. The **denticulate ligament** pierces the arachnoid so that the cord is anchored to the dura mater on each side. Outside the dura is the **extradural (epidural) venous plexus** (*Figure 10.5*) which harvests the vertebral red marrow and empties into the segmental veins (deep cervical, intercostal, lumbar, sacral). These veins are without valves, and reflux of blood from the territory of segmental veins is a notorious cause of cancer spread from the prostate, lung, breast, and thyroid gland. In fact, nerve root compression from collapse of an invaded vertebra may be the presenting sign of cancer in one of these organs.

The respective anterior and posterior nerve roots join at the intervertebral foramina, where the

---

## CLINICAL PANEL 10.1 • SPINA BIFIDA

Among the more common congenital malformations of the CNS are several conditions included under the general heading, *spina bifida*. The 'bifid' effect is produced by failure of union of the two halves of the neural arches, usually in the lumbosacral region (*Figure CP 10.1.1*)

*Spina bifida occulta* (*A*) is usually symptom-free, being detected incidentally in lumbosacral radiographs.

In *spina bifida cystica* a meningeal cyst protrudes through the vertebral defect. In 10% of these cases the cyst is a *meningocele* containing no nervous elements (*B*). In 90%, unfortunately, the cyst is a *meningomyelocele*, containing either spinal cord or cauda equina (*C*); the lower limbs, bladder and rectum are paralyzed, as in the case illustrated in *Figure CP 10.1.2*, and meningitis is likely to supervene sooner or later. To make matters worse, an Arnold–Chiari syndrome (Chapter 4) is almost always present as well.

The most severe form of spina bifida is *myelocele* (*D*), where the neural folds have remained open and CSF leaks onto the surrounding skin. The clinical outlook is very poor.

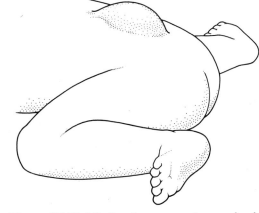

**Figure CP 10.1.2.** Lumbar meningomyelocele (from a photograph). The 'frog leg' posture is characteristic of combined femoral and sciatic nerve paralysis, with preservation of hip flexion by the iliopsoas.

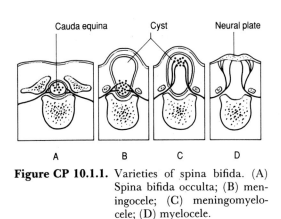

**Figure CP 10.1.1.** Varieties of spina bifida. (A) Spina bifida occulta; (B) meningocele; (C) meningomyelocele; (D) myelocele.

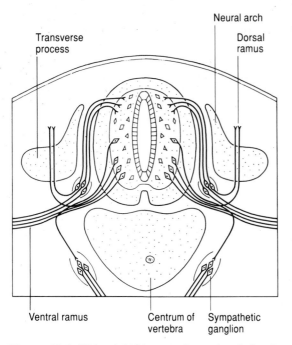

**Figure 10.4.** Normal, bifid stage of neural arch development in an embryo of 8 weeks.

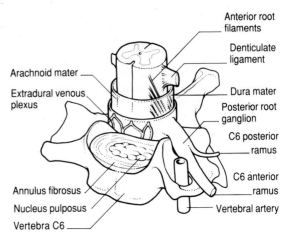

**Figure 10.5.** Relationships of the 6th cervical spinal nerve.

'facet' joints between successive articular processes are each supplied by the nearest three spinal nerves. Pain caused by injury or disease of any of the above structures is referred to the cutaneous territory of the corresponding posterior rami (*Figure 10.7*).

posterior root ganglia are located (*Figure 10.5*). The arachnoid mater blends with the perineurium of the spinal nerve, and the dura mater blends with the epineurium. The nerve roots carry extensions of the subarachnoid space into the intervertebral foramina.

Below the level of the spinal cord, the nerve roots passing to the lower lumbar and sacral intervertebral foramina constitute the **cauda equina** ('horse's tail'). The cauda equina floats in the lumbar subarachnoid cistern (*Figure 10.6*), which reaches to the level of the second sacral vertebra. At its upper end the cauda comprises nerve roots L3–S5 of both sides—a total of 32 roots.

In the center of the cauda equina is the unimportant filum terminale, which pierces the meninges to become attached to the coccyx.

## DISTRIBUTION OF SPINAL NERVES

Each spinal nerve gives off a recurrent branch which provides mechanoreceptors and pain receptors for the dura mater, posterior longitudinal ligament, and intervertebral disc. The synovial

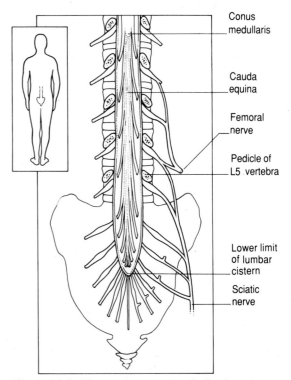

**Figure 10.6.** The cauda equina in the lumbar cistern. Contributions to the femoral and sciatic nerves are shown on the right side.

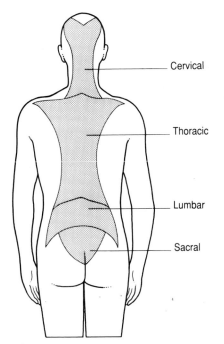

**Figure 10.7.** Cutaneous distribution of posterior rami of spinal nerves.

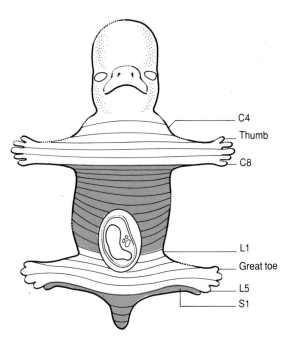

**Figure 10.8.** Embryonic dermatome pattern.

### Segmental sensory distribution: the dermatomes

A *dermatome* is the strip of skin supplied by an individual spinal nerve. The dermatomes are orderly in the embryo (*Figure 10.8*) but they are distorted by the outgrowth of the limbs (*Figure 10.9*). Spinal nerves C5, C6, C7, C8 and T1 are drawn into the upper limb, so that C4 abuts on T2 at the level of the sternal angle. Nerves L2, L3, L4, L5, S1 and S2 are drawn into the lower limb, so that L2 abuts on S3 over the buttock. Maps like those in *Figure 10.10* fail to portray *overlap* in the cutaneous distribution of successive dorsal nerve roots. On the trunk, for example, the skin over an intercostal space is supplied by the nerves immediately above and below as well as by the proper nerve.

### Segmental motor distribution

In the limbs, the individual muscles are supplied by more than one spinal nerve because of interchange in the limb nerve plexuses. The segmental supply of the limbs is expressed in terms of *movements* in *Figure 10.10*.

### Nerve root compression syndromes

Nerve root compression within the vertebral canal is most frequent where the spine is most mobile, namely at lower cervical and lower lumbar levels (Panel 10.2). The effects of root compression may be expressed in five different ways:

1. Pain perceived in the *muscles* supplied by the corresponding spinal nerve(s)
2. *Paresthesia* (numbness or tingling) along the respective dermatome(s)
3. Cutaneous sensory loss—more likely if two successive dermatomes are involved, because of overlap
4. Motor weakness
5. Loss of a tendon reflex if the segmental level is appropriate (*Table 10.1*).

**Table 10.1 Segmental levels of tendon reflexes**

| Segmental level | Reflex |
| --- | --- |
| C5,6 | Biceps |
| C5,6 | Brachioradialis ('supinator reflex') |
| C7 | Triceps |
| L3,4 | Knee jerk |
| S1 | Ankle jerk |

## CLINICAL PANEL 10.2 ● NERVE ROOT COMPRESSION

### Cervical roots

The intervertebral discs and synovial joints of the neck are subject to degenerative disease *(cervical spondylosis)* in 50% of 50-year-old people and in 70% of 70 year olds. Although any or all of the joints may deteriorate, problems are most frequent in relation to vertebra C6, which provides the fulcrum for flexion/extension movements of the neck. Spinal nerve C6 (above) or C7 (below) may be pinched by extruded disc material or by bony excrescences around the synovial joints *(Figure CP 10.2.1)*. Sensory, motor, and reflex disturbances may result in accordance with the data in *Figures* 10.9 and 10.10 and *Table 10.1*.

### Lumbosacral roots

One important cause of low-back pain is a *prolapsed intervertebral disc (herniated nucleus pulposus)*. Fully 95% of all disc prolapses occur immediately above or below the last lumbar vertebra. The typical herniation is *posterolateral*, with compression of the nerve roots passing to the *next* intervertebral foramen *(Figure CP 10.2.2)*. Symptoms include backache caused by rupture of the annulus fibrosus, and pain in the buttock/thigh/leg caused by pressure on posterior root fibers contributing to the sciatic nerve. The pain is increased by stretching the affected root, e.g. by having the straightened leg raised by the examiner.

An L4/5 disc prolapse produces pain/paresthesia over the L5 dermatome. Motor weakness may be detected during dorsiflexion of the great toe (later, of all toes and of the ankle), and during eversion of the foot. Abduction of the hip may also be weak; this movement is tested with the patient lying on one side.

With an L5/S1 prolapse (the commonest of all), symptoms are felt in the back of the leg/sole of foot (S1 dermatome). Plantar flexion may be weak and the ankle jerk reduced or absent.

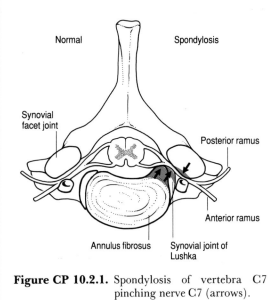

**Figure CP 10.2.1.** Spondylosis of vertebra C7 pinching nerve C7 (arrows).

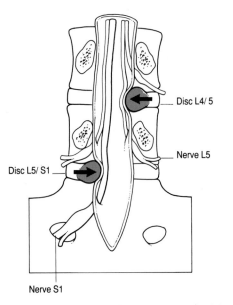
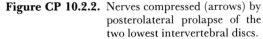

**Figure CP 10.2.2.** Nerves compressed (arrows) by posterolateral prolapse of the two lowest intervertebral discs.

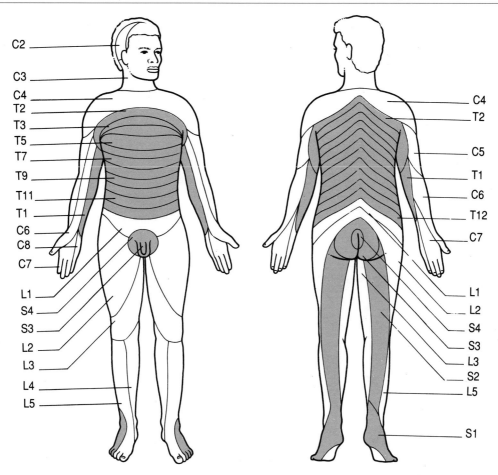

**Figure 10.9.** Adult dermatome pattern.

### Lumbar puncture (spinal tap)

To obtain a sample of cerebrospinal fluid, a needle is passed forward and upward between the spines of vertebrae L3 and L4 or between L4 and L5. The patient lies curled up on one side during the procedure; aseptic precautions are observed and the skin and interspinous ligaments are anesthetized before the needle is inserted. A slight 'give' is felt when the fused dura-arachnoid layer has been penetrated.

A lumbar puncture is *not* performed if there is any reason to suspect the presence of raised intracranial pressure (see Coning, in Chapter 5).

### Anesthetic procedures

A so-called *spinal anesthetic* is often given in preference to a general anesthetic, prior to surgical procedures on the prostate in the elderly. A local anesthetic is injected into the lumbar cistern in order to block impulse conduction in the lumbar and sacral nerve roots. Care is taken that the anesthetic does not reach a high level in the subarachnoid space, for fear of paralyzing the intercostal and phrenic nerve root fibers serving respiration.

### Anesthesia and childbirth

In skilled hands, pain-free labour can be assured by blocking the lumbar and sacral nerve roots extradurally. For *epidural anesthesia*, local anesthetic is carefully introduced into the extradural space by the lumbar route. For *caudal anesthesia* the extradural space is approached in an upward direction, through the sacral hiatus. In both procedures, the anesthetic diffuses through the dural sheath of the nerve roots where they leave the vertebral canal. Labor may be prolonged because of interruption of

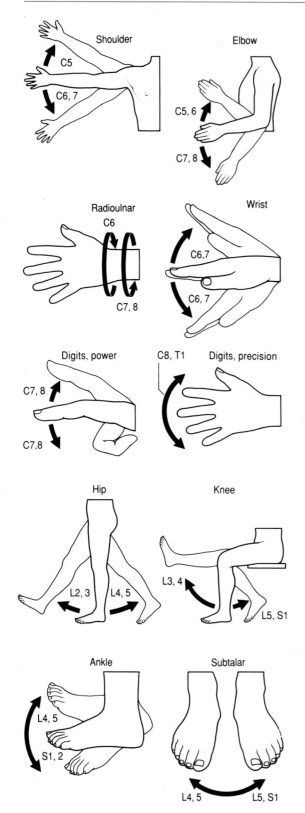

excitatory reflex arcs linking perineum to uterus through the lower end of the spinal cord. However, avoidance of general anesthesia is valuable in allowing immediate bonding to take place between mother and child.

## EXERCISES

1 Bearing in mind the list of five potential effects of combined (anterior and posterior) nerve root compression, use *Figures 10.9* and *10.10*, and *Table 10.1* to list the possible results of:
   (a) Combined prolapse of the intervertebral discs immediately above and below vertebra C6 on the right side;
   (b) Nerve root entrapment on the left side following collapse of vertebra T1;
   (c) Nerve root entrapment on the left side following collapse of vertebra L4;
   (d) Combined prolapse of the intervertebral discs immediately above and below vertebra L5.

2 Automobile accidents are a potential cause of *cauda equina syndromes*, in which the vertebral canal is more or less obliterated by vertebral fragments. Control of the bladder, and of sexual functions, may be severely affected because of interruption of parasympathetic nerve fibers (see Chapter 10).
   How much skin would be rendered completely insensitive by destruction of the sacral nerve roots by a crushed first sacral vertebra? What lower limb movements would be (a) paralyzed, (b) weakened?

## REFERENCES

Adams, C.B.T. and Logue, V. (1971) Studies in cervical spondylitic myelopathy. 1. Movement of the cervical roots, dura, and cord, and their relation to the course of extrathecal roots. *Brain* **94:** 557–568.

**Figure 10.10.** Segmental control of limb movements. (Adapted from Last, R.J. (1973) *Anatomy: Regional and Applied*, 5th edn. Edinburgh: Churchill Livingstone; and Rosse, C. and Clawson, D.K. (1980) *The Musculoskeletal System in Health and Disease*. Hagerstown: Harper & Row.)

Auteroche, P. (1983) Innervation of the zygapophyseal joints of the lumbar spine. *Anat. Clin.* **5:** 17–28.

Barson, A.J. and Logue, V. (1970) The vertebral level of termination of the spinal cord during normal and abnormal development. *J. Anat.* **106:** 489–497.

Groen, D.J., Baljet, R. and Drukker, J. (1990) Nerves and nerve plexuses of the human vertebral column. *Am. J. Anat.* **188:** 282–296.

Russell, E.J. (1990) Cervical disc disease. *Radiology* **177:** 313–325.

Sunderland, S. (1974) Meningeal–dural relationships in the intervertebral foramen. *J. Neurosurg.* **40:** 756–763.

# 11

# Spinal cord: ascending pathways

The spinal cord is the gateway through which sensory information reaches the brain from all parts of the body below the head. It also contains the neural effector apparatus for execution of motor responses, as well as innumerable local circuit neurons serving somatic and visceral reflexes. This chapter concentrates on the ascending pathways that originate in posterior root ganglia and in the posterior horn of gray matter.

## GENERAL FEATURES

The arrangement of gray and white matter at different levels of the spinal cord is shown in *Figure 11.1*. The cervical and lumbosacral enlargements

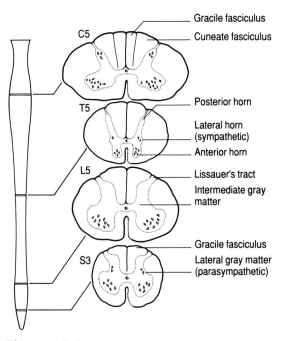

**Figure 11.1.** Representative transverse sections of the spinal cord.

are produced by expansions of the gray matter required to service the limbs. White matter is most abundant in the upper reaches of the cord, which contain the sensory and motor pathways serving all four limbs. In the posterior funiculus, for example, the gracile fasciculus carries information from the lower limb and is present at cervical as well as lumbosacral segmental levels, whereas the cuneate fasciculus carries information from the upper limb and is not seen at lumbar level.

Although it is convenient to refer to different levels of the spinal cord in terms of numbered segments, corresponding to the sites of attachment of the paired nerve roots, the cord shows no evidence of segmentation internally. The nuclear groups seen in transverse sections are in reality cell columns, most of them spanning several segments (*Figure 11.2*).

### Types of spinal neurons

The smallest neurons (soma diameters 5–20 $\mu$m) are *propriospinal*, being entirely contained within the cord. Some are confined within a single segment; others span two or more segments by way of the neighboring **propriospinal tract** (*Figure 11.3*). Many of the smallest neurons participate in spinal reflexes. Others are intermediate cell stations interposed between fiber tracts descending from the brain and motor neurons projecting to the locomotor apparatus. Others again are so

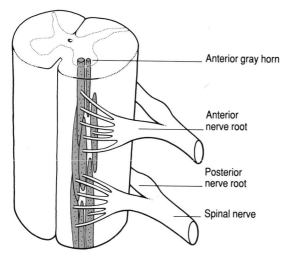

**Figure 11.2.** Two segments of the spinal cord, showing cell columns in the anterior gray horn.

Anterior gray horn

Anterior nerve root

Posterior nerve root

Spinal nerve

placed as to influence sensory transmission from lower to higher levels of the CNS.

Medium-sized neurons (soma diameters 20–50 $\mu$m) are found in all parts of the gray matter except the substantia gelatinosa. Most are *relay (projection) cells* receiving synaptic boutons from posterior root afferents and projecting their axons to the brain. The projections are in the form of *tracts*, a tract being defined as a functionally homogeneous group of fibers. As will be seen, the term 'tract' is

often used loosely because many projections originally thought to be 'pure' contain more than one functional class of fiber.

The largest neurons of all are the alpha motoneurons (somas 50–100 $\mu$m) for the supply of skeletal muscles. Scattered among them are small, gamma motoneurons supplying muscle spindles. In the medial part of the anterior horn are *Renshaw cells*, which exert tonic inhibition upon alpha motoneurons.

Spinal reflex arcs originating in muscle spindles and tendon organs have been described in Chapter 7. Originating in the skin is the *flexor reflex*, whereby the lower limb flexes in response to a noxious stimulus applied to the sole. The reflex is polysynaptic, with propriospinal spread over several segments. The full response involves a *crossed extensor reflex* designed to support the body weight on the opposite leg; the internuncials responsible cross the midline (*Fig. 11.3*).

**Laminae of Rexed**

In thick sections of the spinal cord, the nerve cells exhibit a laminar (layered) arrangement. True lamination is confined to the posterior horn (*Figure 11.4*), but 10 laminae have been defined in the gray matter as a whole in order to correlate findings from animal research in different laboratories.

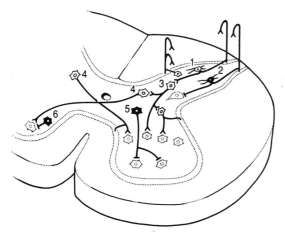

**Figure 11.3.** Propriospinal internuncial neurons. (1) Excitatory substantia gelatinosa neuron; (2) inhibitory substantia gelatinosa neuron; (3) flexor reflex internuncial; (4) neuron serving crossed extensor reflex; (5) Ia inhibitory internuncial; (6) Renshaw cell.

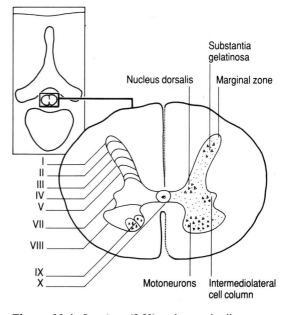

Substantia gelatinosa

Nucleus dorsalis

Marginal zone

Motoneurons

Intermediolateral cell column

**Figure 11.4.** Laminae (I–X) and named cell groups at mid-thoracic level.

### *Spinal ganglia* (Figure 11.5)

The spinal or posterior root ganglia are located in the intervertebral foramina, where the anterior and posterior roots come together to form the spinal nerves. Thoracic ganglia contain about 50 000 unipolar neurons, and those serving the limbs contain about 100 000. The individual ganglion cells are invested with modified Schwann cells called **satellite cells.** The common stem axon of each cell bifurcates, sending a centrifugal process into one or other ramus of the spinal nerve (or into the recurrent branch) and a centripetal ('center-seeking') process into the spinal cord. Following stimulation of the peripheral sensory receptors, trains of nerve impulses traverse the point of bifurcation without interruption, although the cell body is also depolarized. The initial segment of the stem axon does not normally generate impulses but it may do so if the adjacent part of the posterior root is compressed, for example by a prolapsed intervertebral disc.

Traditionally, the centripetal axons of all spinal ganglion cells have been thought to enter posterior nerve roots. It is now known that many visceral afferents (in particular) enter the cord by way of *anterior* roots and work their way to the posterior gray horn. This feature accounts for the frequent failure of *posterior rhizotomy* (surgical section of posterior roots) to relieve pain originating from intra-abdominal cancer.

### Central terminations of posterior root afferents *(Figure 11.6)*

In the *dorsal root entry zone* close to the surface of the cord, the afferent fibers become segregated into medial and lateral streams. The medial stream comprises medium and large fibers which divide within the posterior funiculus into ascending and descending branches. The branches swing into the posterior gray horn and synapse in laminae II, III, and IV. The largest ascending fibers run all the way to the posterior column nuclei (gracilis/cuneatus) in the medulla oblongata. These long fibers form the bulk of the gracile and cuneate fasciculi.

The lateral stream comprises small (Aδ and C) fibers which, upon entry, divide into short ascending and descending branches within the **posterolateral tract** *of Lissauer.* They synapse upon neurons in the **marginal zone** (lamina I) and in the substantia gelatinosa (lamina II); some fibers synapse upon dendrites of cells belonging to laminae III–V.

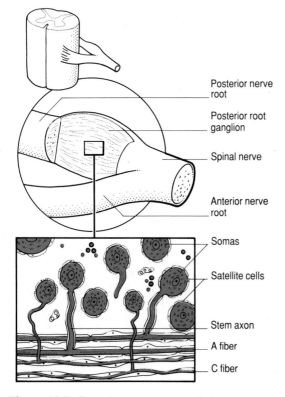

**Figure 11.5.** Posterior root ganglion. In bottom figure note T-shaped bifurcation of stem fibers.

Labels (Figure 11.5): Posterior nerve root; Posterior root ganglion; Spinal nerve; Anterior nerve root; Somas; Satellite cells; Stem axon; A fiber; C fiber

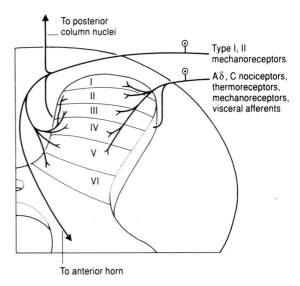

**Figure 11.6.** Terminations of primary afferent neurons in the posterior gray horn.

Labels (Figure 11.6): To posterior column nuclei; Type I, II mechanoreceptors; Aδ, C nociceptors, thermoreceptors, mechanoreceptors, visceral afferents; To anterior horn

## ASCENDING SENSORY PATHWAYS

### *Categories of sensation*

In accordance with the flowchart in *Table 11.1*, neurologists speak of two kinds of sensation, *conscious* and *unconscious*. Conscious sensations are *perceived*, at the level of the cerebral cortex. Unconscious sensations are not perceived; they have reference to the cerebellum (see later).

**Table 11.1** Categories of sensation

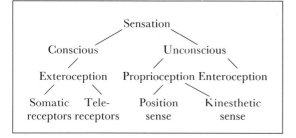

### Conscious sensations

These are of two kinds of conscious sensation, *exteroceptive* and *proprioceptive*. Exteroceptive sensations come from the external world; they impinge either on somatic receptors on the body surface or on *telereceptors* serving vision and hearing. Somatic sensations include touch, pressure, heat, cold and pain.

Conscious proprioceptive sensations arise within the body. The receptors concerned are those of the locomotor system (muscles, joints, bones) and of the vestibular labyrinth. The pathways to the cerebral cortex form the substrate for *position sense* when the body is stationary, and for *kinesthetic sense* during movement.

### Unconscious sensations

These also are of two kinds. *Unconscious proprioception* is the term used to describe afferent information reaching the cerebellum through the spinocerebellar pathways and their brainstem equivalents. This information is essential for smooth motor co-ordination.

Secondly, *enteroception* (Greek, *enteron*, gut) is a little-used term referring to unconscious afferent signals involved in visceral reflexes.

### Sensory testing

Routine assessment of *somatic exteroceptive sensation* includes tests for:

- touch, by grazing the skin with the finger tip or a cotton swab
- pain, by applying the point of a pin
- thermal sense, by applying warm or cold test tubes to the skin.

In alert and co-operative patients, active and passive tests of *conscious proprioception* can be performed. *Active* tests examine the patient's ability to execute set-piece activities *with the eyes closed:*

- in the erect position, to stand still, and to 'toe the line', without swaying
- in the seated position, to bring the index finger to the nose from the extended position of the arm (finger-to-nose test)
- in the recumbent position, to place the heel of the foot on the opposite knee (heel-to-knee test)

*Passive* tests of conscious proprioception include:

- Joint sense. The clinician grasps the thumb or great toe by the sides and moves it while asking the patient to name the direction of movement ('up' or 'down'). Joint sense is mediated in part by articular receptors but mainly by passive stretching of neuromuscular spindles. (If the nerves supplying a joint are anesthetized, or if the joint is completely replaced by a prosthesis, joint sense is only slightly impaired. Alternatively, activation of spindles by means of a vibrator creates the *illusion* of movement when the relevant joint is stationary.)
- Vibration sense. The clinician assesses the patient's ability to detect the vibrations of a tuning fork applied to the radial styloid process or to the shin.

## SOMATIC SENSORY PATHWAYS

Two major pathways are involved in somatic sensory perception. They are the *posterior column–medial lemniscal pathway* and the *spinothalamic pathway*. They have the following features in common (*Figure 11.7*):

- Both comprise first-order, second-order, and third-order sets of sensory neurons.
- The somas of the first-order neurons, or *primary afferents*, occupy posterior root ganglia.

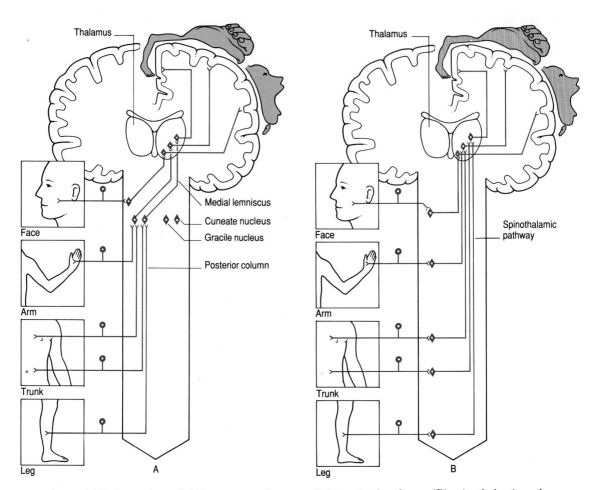

**Figure 11.7.** Basic plans of: (A) posterior column–medial lemniscal pathway; (B) spinothalamic pathway.

- The somas of the second-order neurons occupy CNS gray matter on the same side as the first-order neurons.
- The second-order axons *cross the midline* and then ascend to terminate in the thalamus.
- The third-order neurons project from the thalamus to the somatic sensory cortex.
- Both pathways are *somatotopic:* an orderly map of body parts can be identified experimentally in the gray matter at each of the three loci of fiber termination.
- Synaptic transmission from primary to secondary neurons, and from secondary to tertiary, can be modulated (inhibited or enhanced) by other neurons.

### The posterior column–medial lemniscal pathway (Figure 11.8)

The first order afferents include the largest somas in the posterior root ganglia. Their peripheral processes receive information from the largest sensory receptors: Meissner's and Pacinian corpuscles, Ruffini endings and Merkel cell–neurite complexes, neuromuscular spindles and Golgi tendon organs. The centripetal processes from cells supplying the lower limb and lower trunk send long collaterals in the **gracile fasciculus (fasciculus gracilis)** to reach the gracile nucleus in the medulla oblongata. The corresponding collaterals from the upper limb and upper trunk run in the

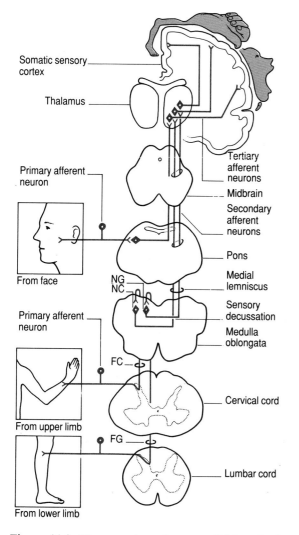

**Figure 11.8.** The posterior column–medial lemniscal pathway. FC, fasciculus cuneatus; FG, fasciculus gracilis; NC, nucleus cuneatus; NG, nucleus gracilis.

cuneate fasciculus (**fasciculus cuneatus**) to reach the cuneate nucleus.

The second-order afferents commence in the posterior column nuclei, namely the **nucleus gracilis** and **nucleus cuneatus.** They pass ventrally in the tegmentum of the medulla oblongata before intersecting their opposite numbers in the great *sensory decussation.* Having crossed the midline, the fibers turn rostrally in the *medial lemniscus.*

The medial lemniscus diverges from the midline as it ascends through the tegmentum of the

pons and midbrain. It terminates in the lateral part of the ventral posterior nucleus of the thalamus (ventral posterolateral nucleus).

Terminating in the medial part of the same nucleus (ventral posteromedial nucleus) is the *trigeminal lemniscus,* which serves the head region.

The third-order afferents project from the thalamus to the somatic sensory cortex.

**Functions**

The chief functions of the posterior column–medial lemniscal pathway are those of *conscious proprioception* and *discriminative touch.* Together, these attributes provide the parietal lobe with an instantaneous *body image* so that we are constantly aware of the position of body parts both at rest and during movement. Without this informational background, the execution of movements is severely impaired. For example, if the posterior columns are sectioned on both sides in a monkey, the animal tends to miss its target when swinging from one bar to another even though its entire motor apparatus remains intact.

In humans, disturbance of posterior column function is most often observed in association with demyelinating diseases such as multiple sclerosis. The classical symptom is known as *sensory ataxia.* This term signifies a movement disorder resulting from sensory impairment, in contrast to *cerebellar ataxia,* in which a movement disorder results from a lesion within the motor system. The patient with a severe sensory ataxia can stand unsupported only with the feet well apart and with the gaze directed downward to include the feet. The gait is broad-based, with a stamping action that maximizes any conscious proprioceptive function that remains (*Figure 11.9*).

Sensory testing in posterior column disease reveals severe swaying when the patient stands with the feet together and the eyes closed. This is *Romberg's sign.* (Inability to 'toe the line' with the eyes closed is *tandem* Romberg's sign.) The finger-to-nose and/or heel-to-knee tests may reveal loss of kinesthetic sense. Joint sense and vibration sense may also be impaired. (*Note:* Romberg's sign may also be elicited in patients suffering from vestibular disorders (Chapter 15); in cerebellar disorders there may be instability of station whether the eyes are open or closed (Chapter 19).)

Tactile, painful and thermal sensations are preserved, but there is impairment of *tactile discrimination.* The patient has difficulty in discriminating

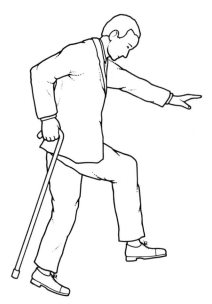

**Figure 11.9.** The 'stamp and stick' gait of sensory ataxia.

between single and paired stimuli applied to the skin; in identifying numbers traced onto the skin by the examiner's finger; and in distinguishing between objects of similar shape but of different textures.

A difficulty in assigning specific functional deficits to posterior column disease is the rarity of pathology affecting the posterior funiculi *alone*. In particular, the posterior part of the lateral funiculus is likely to be involved as well. Postmortem findings, from patients having different degrees of pathology in the posterior and lateral funiculi, suggest that kinesthetic sense from the lower limb may be mediated in part by fibers that leave the gracile fasciculus at thoracic level and relay rostrally in the posterior part of the lateral funiculus.

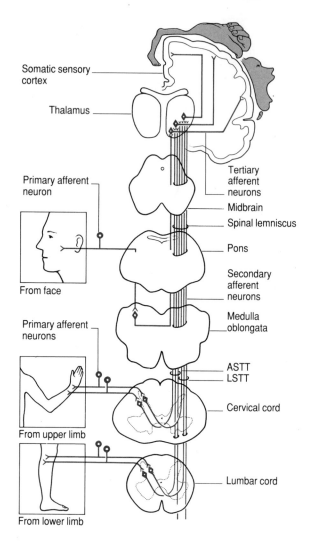

**Figure 11.10.** The spinothalamic pathway. ASTT, anterior spinothalamic tract; LSTT, lateral spinothalamic tract.

### Spinothalamic pathway (Figure 11.10)

The spinothalamic pathway consists of second-order sensory neurons projecting from laminae I, III, IV and V of the posterior gray horn to the contralateral thalamus. The cells of origin receive excitatory and inhibitory synapses from neurons of the substantia gelatinosa (*Figure 11.6*); these have important 'gating' (modulatory) effects on sensory transmission, as explained in Chapter 18.

The axons of the spinothalamic pathway cross the midline in the anterior commissure at all segmental levels. Having crossed, they run up-

ward in the anterolateral part of the cord. This 'anterolateral pathway' (as it is sometimes called) is divisible into an **anterior spinothalamic tract** located in the anterior funiculus and a **lateral spinothalamic tract** located in the lateral funiculus. The two tracts merge in the brainstem as the **spinal lemniscus**. The spinal lemniscus is joined by trigeminal afferents from the head region, and it accompanies the medial lemniscus to the ventral posterior nucleus of the thalamus, terminating immediately behind the medial lemniscus. Third-order sensory neurons project from the thalamus to the somatic sensory cortex.

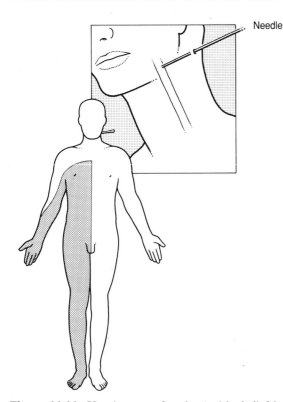

**Figure 11.11.** Usual extent of analgesia (shaded) following cordotomy at C1/2 segmental level.

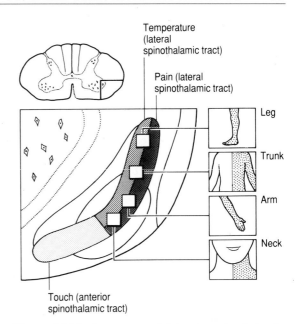

**Figure 11.12.** Sensory modalities in spinothalamic pathway at upper cervical level.

## Functions

The functions of the spinothalamic pathway have been elucidated by the procedure known as *cordotomy*, whereby the spinothalamic pathway is interrupted on one or both sides for the relief of intractable pain. For a *percutaneous cordotomy*, the patient is sedated and a needle is passed between the atlas and the axis, into the subarachnoid space. Under radiological guidance, the needle tip is advanced into the anterolateral region of the cord.

A stimulating electrode is passed through the needle. If the placement is correct a mild current will elicit paresthesia (tingling) on the opposite side of the body. The anterolateral pathway is then destroyed electrolytically. Afterwards, the patient is insensitive to *pinprick, heat, or cold* applied to the opposite side (*Figure 11.11*). Sensitivity to *touch* is reduced. The effect commences several segments below the level of the procedure because of the oblique passage of spinothalamic fibers across the white commissure.

Cordotomy is sometimes performed for patients terminally ill with cancer. It is not used for benign conditions because the analgesic (pain-relieving) effect wears off after about a year. This functional recovery may be due to nociceptive transmission either in uncrossed fibers of the spinoreticular system (see later) or in C fiber collaterals sent to the posterior column nuclei by *some* axons of the lateral root entry stream.

The internal anatomy of the human spinothalamic pathway has been worked out from postoperative sensory testing and is shown in *Figure 11.12*. The picture is one of *modality segregation*. The lateral spinothalamic tract mediates noxious and thermal sensations separately, and the anterior spinothalamic tract mediates touch. The lateral tract is somatotopically arranged, the neck being represented at the front and the leg at the back. The anterior tract is likely (though not proven) to be somatotopic also.

A rare but classical condition illustrating *dissociated sensory loss* is illustrated in Panel 11.1.

## *Spinoreticular tracts* (Figure 11.13)

The **spinoreticular tracts** are the most antique somatosensory pathways. The reticular formation of the brainstem has scant regard for the midline,

## CLINICAL PANEL 11.1 ● SYRINGOMYELIA

Syringomyelia is a disorder of uncertain etiology, characterized by development of a *syrinx* or fusiform cyst, in or beside the central canal, usually in the cervical region (*Figure CP 11.1.1*). Initial symptoms arise from obliteration of spinothalamic fibers decussating in the white commissure.

The early clinical picture is one of *dissociated sensory loss*. Sensitivity is lost to painful and thermal stimuli whereas sensitivity to touch is retained because the posterior column–medial lemniscal pathway is preserved. Typically, the patient develops ulcers on the fingers arising from painless cuts and burns. The joints of the elbow, wrist, and hand may become disorganized over time, or even dislocated, owing to loss of warning sensation from stretched joint capsules.

Progressive expansion of the syrinx may compromise conduction in the long ascending and descending pathways.

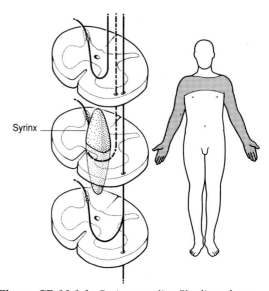

**Figure CP 11.1.1.** Syringomyelia. Shading shows distribution of analgesia.

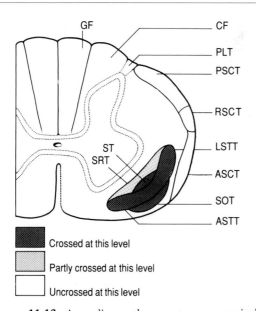

Crossed at this level

Partly crossed at this level

Uncrossed at this level

**Figure 11.13.** Ascending pathways at upper cervical level. ASCT, anterior spinocerebellar tract; ASTT, anterior spinothalamic tract; CF, cuneate fasciculus; GF, gracile fasciculus; LSTT, lateral spinothalamic tract; PLT, posterolateral tract; PSCT, posterior spinocerebellar tract; RSCT, rostral spinocerebellar tract; SOT, spino-olivary tract; SRT, spinoreticular tract; ST, spinotectal tract.

being essentially bilaterally distributed in terms of its ascending and descending connections. Spinoreticular fibers originate in laminae V–VII and accompany the spinothalamic pathway as far as the brainstem. Postmortem studies of nerve fiber degeneration following cordotomy procedures indicate that at least half of the spinoreticular fibers may be *uncrossed*. Accurate estimations based on axonal degeneration are difficult because some spinothalamic fibers give off collaterals to the reticular formation as they pass by.

The spinoreticular tracts terminate at all levels of the brainstem and they are not somatotopically arranged. Impulse traffic is continued rostrally to the thalamus in the *ascending reticular activating system* (Chapter 19). Briefly, the spinoreticular system has two interrelated functions:

1. To *arouse* the cerebral cortex, i.e. to induce or maintain the waking state.
2. To report to the limbic cortex (e.g. the cingulate gyrus) about the *nature* of the stimulus. The emotional response may be pleasurable (e.g. to stroking) or aversive (e.g. to pinprick).

In summary, the phylogenetically old, 'paleospinothalamic' pathways through the reticular formation are concerned with the arousal and affective (emotional) aspects of somatic sensory stimuli. In contrast, the direct, 'neospinothalamic' path-

11/SPINAL CORD: ASCENDING PATHWAYS **95**

way is analytical, encoding information about modality, intensity, and location.

## Spinocerebellar pathways

Four fiber tracts run from the spinal cord to the cerebellum. They are:

- posterior spinocerebellar
- cuneocerebellar
- anterior spinocerebellar
- rostral spinocerebellar.

The first two are principally concerned with unconscious proprioception. The second two report continuously about the state of play among the internuncial neurons of the spinal cord.

## Unconscious proprioception

Unconscious proprioception is served by the **posterior spinocerebellar tract** for the lower limb and lower trunk, and by the **cuneocerebellar tract** for the upper limb and upper trunk. Both are *uncrossed*, in keeping with the known control by each cerebellar hemisphere of its own side of the body.

The *posterior spinocerebellar tract* originates in the **nucleus dorsalis** of Clarke (thoracic nucleus) in lamina VII at the base of the posterior gray horn (*Figure 11.3*). The nucleus dorsalis extends from T1 through L1 segmental levels and the primary afferents from the lower limb enter the gracile fasciculus to reach it (*Figure 11.14*). Nucleus dorsalis receives primary afferents of all kinds from the muscles and joints, including an intense input from muscle spindle primaries. It also receives collaterals from cutaneous sensory neurons. The fibers of the posterior spinocerebellar tract are the largest in the entire CNS, measuring 20 μm in external diameter. Very fast conduction (120 m/s) is required to keep the cerebellum informed about ongoing movements. The tract ascends close to the surface of the cord (*Figure 11.13*) and enters the inferior cerebellar peduncle.

The *cuneocerebellar tract* comes from the **accessory cuneate nucleus,** which lies above and outside the cuneate nucleus. The primary afferent inputs are of the same nature as those for the nucleus dorsalis; they reach it through the cuneate fasciculus. The cuneocerebellar tract enters the inferior cerebellar peduncle.

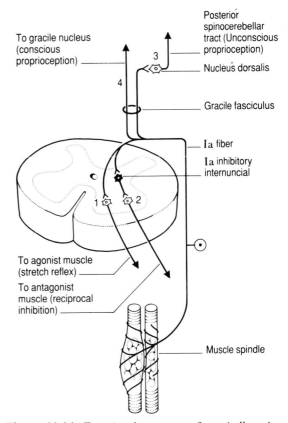

**Figure 11.14.** Functional anatomy of a spindle primary afferent from the lower limb. (1) Stretch reflex; (2) Ia internuncial serving reciprocal inhibition; (3) unconscious proprioception; (4) kinesthesia.

## Information from reflex arcs

Two tracts originate in the intermediate gray matter of the cord. Although they receive some primary afferents of a similar nature to those already mentioned, their main function is to monitor the state of activity of spinal reflex arcs.

From the lower half of the cord, the pathway is the **anterior spinocerebellar tract** (*Figure 11.13*). The component fibers cross initially and run close to the surface as far as the midbrain. They then turn into the *superior* cerebellar peduncle and some of them re-cross within the cerebellar white matter.

From the upper half of the cord, the **rostral spinocerebellar tract** ascends without crossing and enters the superior and inferior cerebellar peduncles.

## OTHER ASCENDING PATHWAYS

The **spinotectal tract** (crossed) runs alongside the spinothalamic pathway (*Figure 11.13*), which it resembles in its origin and functional composition. It ends in the superior colliculus, where it joins crossed visual and auditory inputs involved in turning the eyes/head/trunk toward sources of sensory stimulation.

The **spino-olivary tract** (crossed) sends tactile information to the inferior olivary nucleus in the medulla oblongata. The inferior olivary nucleus has an important function in *motor learning* through its action on the contralateral cerebellar cortex (Chapter 19). The spino-olivary tract may have a role in modifying olivary discharge when a moving part encounters an obstacle (for example, if the toe is stubbed while climbing a stairway).

A *spinocervical tract* is well developed in the cat, where the spinothalamic pathways are small. It seems to be vestigial or absent in humans.

## REFERENCES

Cervero, F. (1986) Dorsal horn neurons and their sensory inputs. In *Spinal Afferent Processing* (Yaksh, T.L., ed.), pp. 197–216. New York: Plenum Press.

Coggeshall, R.E. (1990) Unmyelinated primary afferent fibers in the dorsal column, a possible alternate ascending pathway for noxious information. In *Recent Achievements in Restorative Neurology 3: Altered Sensation and Pain* (Dimitrijivic, S. *et al.*, eds), pp. 128–131. Basel: Karger.

Dykes, R.W. (1983) Parallel processing of somatosensory information: a theory. *Brain Res. Rev.* **6:** 47–115.

Nathan, P.W., Smith, M.C. and Cook, A.W. (1986) Sensory effects in man of lesions of the posterior columns and of some other afferent pathways. *Brain* **109:** 1003–1041.

Smith, M.C. and Deacon, P. (1984) Topographical anatomy of the posterior columns of the spinal cord in man. *Brain* **107:** 671–698.

Willis, W.D. (1985) Ascending somatosensory systems. In *Spinal Afferent Processing* (Yaksh, T.L., ed.), pp. 243–274. New York: Plenum Press.

# 12
# Spinal cord: descending pathways

This chapter describes the general arrangement of neurons in the anterior gray horn of the spinal cord, together with their afferent connections at segmental level. There follows a description of the main supraspinal pathways descending to the spinal gray matter from the brain. Clinical examples illustrate the effects of damage to supraspinal pathways and to anterior horn cells.

## ANATOMY OF THE ANTERIOR GRAY HORN

### Cell columns

Each of the columns of motoneurons in the anterior gray horn supplies a group of muscles having similar functions. The individual muscles are supplied from cell groups (nuclei) within the columns. Axial (trunk) muscles are supplied from medially placed columns, proximal limb segment muscles from the mid-region, and distal limb segment musculature from lateral columns (*Figure 12.1*). Columns supplying extensor muscles lie anterior to columns supplying flexors; hence the presence of ventromedial and dorsomedial columns for the trunk, and ventrolateral and dorsolateral columns for the limbs. A retrodorsolateral nucleus is devoted to the intrinsic muscles of the hand and

foot. An isolated, central nucleus supplies the diaphragm.

The segmental levels of the six somatomotor cell columns are listed in *Table 12.1*. The autonomic nervous system is represented by the intermediolateral cell column.

### Cell types

Large, alpha motoneurons ($\alpha$MNs) supply the extrafusal fibers of the skeletal muscles. Interspersed among them are small, gamma motoneurons ($\gamma$MNs) supplying the intrafusal fibers of neuromuscular spindles.

### Tonic and phasic motoneurons

The $\alpha$MNs have large dendritic trees receiving some 10 000 excitatory boutons from propriospinal neurons and from supraspinal pathways descending from the cerebral cortex and brainstem. The somas of $\alpha$MNs receive some 5000 inhibitory boutons, mostly from propriospinal sources.

Two principal types of $\alpha$MN are recognized, *tonic* and *phasic*. Tonic $\alpha$MNs innervate squads of slow, oxidative–glycolytic (SOG) muscle fibers; they are readily depolarized and have relatively slowly conducting axons with small spike amplitudes. Phasic $\alpha$MNs innervate squads of fast,

**Table 12.1** The somatomotor cell columns

| Cell column | Muscles |
| --- | --- |
| Ventromedial (all segments) | Erector spinae |
| Dorsomedial (T1–L2) | Intercostals, abdominals |
| Ventrolateral (C5–8, L2–S2) | Arm/thigh |
| Dorsolateral (C6–8, L3–S3) | Forearm/leg |
| Retrodorsolateral (C8, T1, S1–2) | Hand/foot |
| Central (C3–5) | Diaphragm |

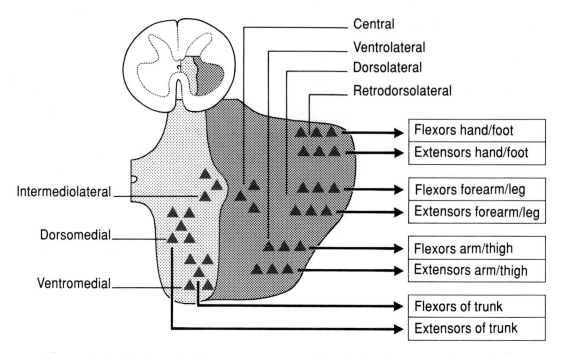

**Figure 12.1.** Cell columns in the anterior gray horn of the spinal cord: somatotopic organization.

oxidative (FO) and fast, oxidative–glycolytic (FOG) muscle fibers. The phasic neurons are larger, have higher thresholds, and have rapidly conducting axons with large spike amplitudes.

Usually tonic neurons are recruited first when voluntary movements are initiated, even if the movement is to be fast.

### Renshaw cells

The axons of the αMNs give off recurrent branches which form excitatory, cholinergic synapses upon inhibitory internuncial neurons called *Renshaw cells* in the medial part of the anterior horn. The Renshaw cells form inhibitory, glycinergic synapses upon the αMNs. This is a classical example of *negative feedback*, or *recurrent inhibition*, through which the discharges of αMNs are self-limiting (see Panel 12.1).

### Segmental-level inputs to alpha motoneurons

At each segmental level, αMNs receive powerful excitatory and inhibitory inputs. Note that any inhibitory effect produced by activity in dorsal

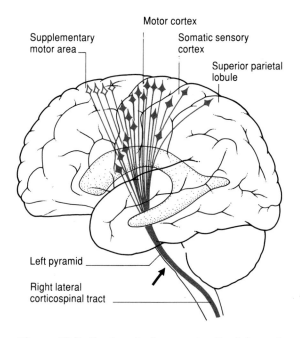

**Figure 12.2.** Corticospinal tract visualized from the left side. The supplementary motor area is on the medial surface of the hemisphere. Arrow indicates level of pyrimidal decussation.

---

**CLINICAL PANEL 12.1 • STRYCHNINE POISONING**

Strychnine is a glycine receptor blocker. The victim of strychnine poisoning suffers agonizing convulsions because of liberation of $\alpha$ motoneurons from the tonic inhibitory control of Renshaw cells. The convulsions resemble those induced by the tetanus toxin, described in Chapter 5. This is no surprise because tetanus toxin prevents the release of glycine from Renshaw cells. Postmortem studies of normal human brain, using radiolabeled strychnine, have shown glycine receptors to be especially abundant in the nucleus of the trigeminal nerve supplying the jaw muscles, and in the nucleus of the facial nerve supplying the muscles of facial expression. These two muscle groups are especially affected in both types of convulsive attack.

---

nerve root fibers requires interpolation of inhibitory internuncials, since all primary afferent neurons are excitatory in nature.

Segmental-level inputs to a *flexor* motoneuron include the following:

- Type Ia and Type II afferents from spindles in the flexor muscles provide the afferent limb of the monosynaptic stretch reflex (for example, the biceps reflex).
- Type Ia afferents from spindles in *extensor* muscles exert reciprocal inhibition upon the flexor motoneurons via Ia inhibitory internuncials.
- Type Ib afferents from Golgi tendon organs in the flexor muscles exert autogenetic inhibition upon the flexor motoneurons.
- Type Ib afferents from Golgi tendon organs in *extensor* muscles exert reciprocal excitation of flexors via excitatory internuncials.
- Afferents from the flexor aspect of relevant synovial joints are stimulated when the capsule becomes taut in extension. They initiate an articular protective reflex, as described in Chapter 8.
- The *flexor reflex* is the withdrawal movement that occurs upon noxious stimulation of skin or muscle. Large numbers of excitatory, 'flexor reflex' internuncials are activated over several spinal segments on the same side as the stimulus, as well as inhibitory internuncials supplying motoneurons to antagonist muscles. In the lower limb, flexion of one leg is accompanied by an *extensor thrust* of the opposite leg, through the activity of excitatory internuncials projecting across the midline.
- Renshaw cells.

A reciprocal list can be drawn up for extensor motoneurons, with substitution of extensor thrust inputs for flexor reflex internuncials.

## DESCENDING MOTOR PATHWAYS

Important pathways descending to the spinal cord are the following:

- corticospinal
- reticulospinal
- vestibulospinal
- tectospinal
- raphespinal
- aminergic
- autonomic.

### *The corticospinal tract*

The **corticospinal tract** is the great voluntary motor pathway. About 80% of its fibers take origin from the motor cortex in the precentral gyrus (area 4). Other sources are the supplementary motor area on the medial side of the hemisphere (area 6), the premotor cortex on the lateral side (area 6), the somatic sensory cortex (areas 3, 1 and 2), and the superior parietal lobule (area 5) (*Figure 12.2*). (The six numbered areas refer to cortical areas defined by Brodmann (see Chapter 23).) The contributions from the two sensory areas mentioned terminate in sensory nuclei of the brainstem and spinal cord, where they modulate sensory transmission.

The corticospinal tract descends through the corona radiata and internal capsule to reach the brainstem. It continues through the crus of the midbrain and the basilar pons to reach the medulla oblongata. Here it forms the pyramid (hence the synonym, **pyramidal tract).**

During its descent through the brainstem, the corticospinal tract gives off fibers which activate motor cranial nerve nuclei, notably those serving the muscles of the face, jaw, and tongue. These fibers are called **corticonuclear**, or *corticobulbar* (*Figure 12.3*).

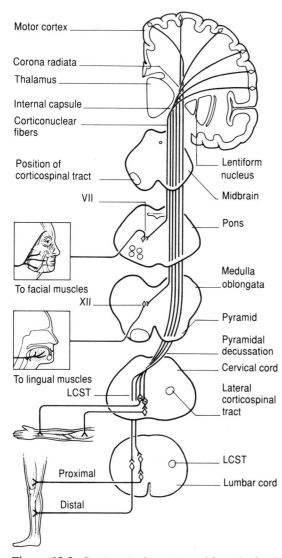

**Figure 12.3.** Corticospinal tract viewed from the front. At spinal cord level only the lateral corticospinal tract is shown. LCST, lateral corticospinal tract; VII, nucleus of facial nerve; XII, hypoglossal nucleus.

Just above the spinomedullary junction (*Figure 12.4*):

- About 80% of the pyramidal fibers cross the midline in the **pyramidal decussation.** These fibers descend on the contralateral side of the spinal cord as the **lateral corticospinal tract** (crossed corticospinal tract).
- About 15% enter the **anterior corticospinal tract**, which occupies the anterior funiculus at cervical and upper thoracic levels. These fibers cross in the white commissure and supply motoneurons serving deep muscles in the neck.
- About 5% of the pyramidal fibers enter the lateral corticospinal tract on the same side. (These are not shown in *Figure 12.3*.)

The corticospinal tract contains about one million nerve fibers. The average conduction velocity is 60 m/s, indicating an average fiber diameter of $10 \, \mu m$ ('rule of six' in Chapter 5). About 3% of the fibers are extra large (up to $20 \, \mu m$); they arise from giant neurons (cells of Betz) in the motor cortex (Chapter 23). All corticospinal fibers are excitatory and appear to use glutamate as their transmitter substance.

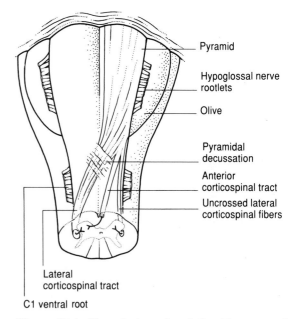

**Figure 12.4.** Ventral view of medulla oblongata and upper spinal cord, showing the three spinal projections of the left pyramid.

## Targets of the lateral corticospinal tract

In the *anterior gray horn*, the axons of the giant cells of Betz synapse upon the dendrites of $\alpha$ and $\gamma$ motoneurons supplying distal limb muscles, i.e. the extrinsic and intrinsic muscles of the hands and feet. A unique property of these *corticomotoneuronal fibers* is that of *fractionation*, whereby small groups of neurons can be selectively activated. This is most obvious in the case of the index finger, which can be flexed or extended quite independently, although three of its long tendons arise from muscle bellies devoted to all four fingers. Fraction-

ation is essential for the execution of skilled movements such as buttoning a coat or tying shoe laces. *Skilled movements are lost, and never recover, following damage to the corticomotoneuronal system anywhere from the motor cortex to the spinal cord.*

As mentioned already in Chapter 7, the $\alpha$ and $\gamma$ motoneurons are coactivated during a given movement, so that spindles in the prime movers are signaling active stretch while those in the antagonists are signaling passive stretch.

Other axons of the corticospinal tract synapse upon Renshaw cells in the anterior horn. The number of possible functions here is large because

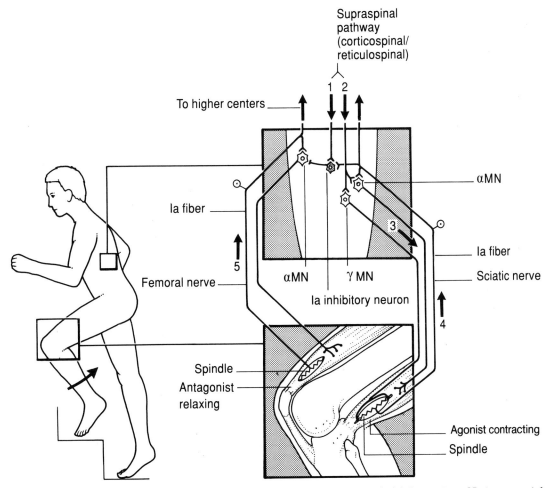

**Figure 12.5.** Sequence of events in a voluntary movement (flexion of the knee). (1) Activation of Ia internuncials to inhibit antagonist $\alpha$ motoneurons ($\alpha$MN); (2) activation of agonist $\alpha$ and $\gamma$ MN; (3) activation of extrafusal and intrafusal muscle fibers; (4) feedback from actively stretched spindles increases excitation of agonist $\alpha$MN and inhibition of antagonist $\alpha$MN; (5) Ia fibers from passively stretched antagonist spindles find the respective $\alpha$MN refractory. *Note:* The sequence $\gamma$MN–Ia fiber–$\alpha$MN is known as the *gamma loop*.

some Renshaw cells synapse mainly upon Ia inhibitory internuncials, and others upon other Renshaw cells. Probably the most important function is to permit *co-contraction* of prime movers and their antagonists, in order to fix one or more joints—for example, when a chopping or shoveling action is required of the hand. Co-contraction is achieved by inactivation of Ia inhibitory internuncials by Renshaw cells.

In the *intermediate gray matter* (and in the base of the anterior horn), motoneurons supplying axial and proximal limb muscles are recruited mainly indirectly, by way of excitatory internuncials. Also located in the intermediate gray matter are the Ia inhibitory internuncials, and these are the *first* neurons to be activated during voluntary movements. Activity of the Ia internuncials causes the antagonist muscles to relax before the prime movers (agonists) contract. In addition, it renders the antagonists' motoneurons refractory to stimulation by spindle afferents passively stretched by the movement. The sequence of events is shown in *Figure 12.5* and its caption, for voluntary flexion of the knee.

In ballistic (fast) movement at any of the major joints, EMG records reveal a 'triphasic response' in the form of a momentary interruption of agonist activity by a twitch of the antagonist muscle group.

In the *posterior gray horn*, there is some suppression of sensory transmission into the spinothalamic pathway during voluntary movement. Modulation is more pronounced at the level of the gracile nucleus, where pyramidal tract fibers (after crossing) are capable of either enhancing sensory transmisssion from the fingers during slow, exploratory movements, or reducing it during rapid movements.

## Upper and lower motor neurons

In the context of disease, clinicians refer to the corticospinal (and corticonuclear) neurons as *upper motor neurons* (Panel 12.2), and those of the brain stem and spinal cord as *lower motor neurons* (Panel 12.3).

---

### CLINICAL PANEL 12.2 • UPPER MOTOR NEURON DISEASE

*Upper motor neuron disease* is a clinical term used to denote interruption of the corticospinal tract somewhere along its course. If the lesion occurs above the level of the pyramidal decussation, the signs will be detected on the opposite side of the body; if it occurs below the decussation, the signs will be detected on the same side.

Sudden interruption of the corticospinal tract is characterized by the following features:

1. The affected limb(s) show an initial flaccid (floppy) paralysis with loss of tendon reflexes. Normal muscle tone—defined as the resistance to passive movement (e.g. flexion/extension of the knee by the examiner)—is lost.
2. After several days or weeks, some return of voluntary motor function can be expected. At the same time, muscle tone increases progressively. The typical long-term effect on muscle tone is one of *spasticity*, with abnormally brisk reflexes (*hyperreflexia*). Classically, spasticity in the leg is 'claspknife' in character: after initial strong resistance to

passive flexion of the knee, the joint gives way.
3. *Clonus* can often be elicited at the ankle/wrist. It consists of rhythmic contraction of the flexor muscles 5–10 times per second in response to sudden passive dorsiflexion.
4. *Babinski sign (extensor plantar response)* consists of dorsiflexion of the great toe and fanning of the other toes in response to a scraping stimulus applied to the sole of the foot. The normal response is flexion of the toes (see *Figure CP 12.2.1*).
5. The *abdominal reflexes* are absent on the affected side. A normal abdominal reflex consists of brief contraction of the abdominal muscles when the overlying skin is scraped.

The above features are most commonly observed after a vascular *stroke* interrupting the corticospinal tract on one side of the cerebrum or brainstem. The usual picture here is one of initial flaccid *hemiplegia* ('half-paralysis'), followed by a permanent spastic *hemiparesis* ('half-weakness'). As illustrated in Chapter 26, Panel

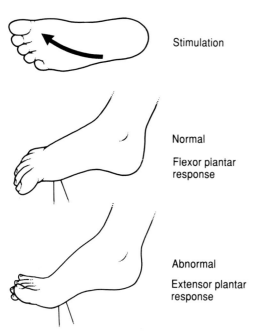

Stimulation

Normal

Flexor plantar
response

Abnormal

Extensor plantar
response

**Figure CP 12.2.1.** The plantar reflex.

26.2, the spasticity following a stroke characteristically affects the antigravity muscles. In the
lower limb these are the extensors of the knee
and the plantar flexors of the foot; in the upper
limb, they are the flexors of the elbow and of the
wrist and fingers. Following complete transection of the spinal cord, on the other hand, there
may be a *paraplegia in flexion* of the lower limbs,
owing to concurrent interruption of the vestibulospinal tract (Panel 12.4).

The 'positive' signs listed under (2), (3), and
(4) cannot be explained on the basis of interruption of the corticospinal tract alone. In the rare
cases in which the human pyramid has been
transected surgically, spasticity and hyperreflexia have not been prominent later on,
although a Babinski sign has been present.

Spasticity and hyperreflexia are largely
explained by the fact that stretch reflexes in
spastic muscle groups are hyperactive. EMG
records of spastic muscles show enhanced
motor unit activity in response to relatively slow
rates of stretch, e.g. slow passive elbow extension. However, this is not the sole basis of
explanation. In patients with spastic hemiparesis, the ankle flexors show increased tone (resistance to passive dorsiflexion) even with *very*
slow rates of stretch—too slow to elicit any
EMG response. The effect is known as *increased
muscle stiffness*, 'muscle stiffness' being the term
used to refer to the intrinsic viscoelastic properties of skeletal muscle. The reason for this
physical change is not yet clear.

### Why are α motoneurons hyperexcitable?

In paraplegic patients, spasticity and hyperreflexia are often accompanied by increased cutaneomuscular reflex excitability, through polysynaptic propriospinal pathways. Pulling on a
pair of trousers may be enough to produce
spasms of the hip and knee flexors, sometimes
accompanied by autonomic effects (sweating,
hypertension, emptying of the bladder). Where
the requisite technical facilities exist, the situation can be dramatically improved by perfusion of the lumbar CSF cistern with minute
amounts of *baclofen,* a GABA mimetic (imita-
tive) drug. The first inference is that the drug
diffuses through the pia-glial membrane of the
spinal cord, activates GABA receptors located
on the surface of primary afferent nerve terminals, and dampens impulse traffic by means
of presynaptic inhibition. The second inference
is that the resident population of GABA neurons in the substantia gelatinosa has fallen silent
in these cases through loss of tonic suraspinal
'drive'. The normal source of supraspinal drive
seems to derive in part from the corticospinal
tract, and in part from corticoreticulospinal
fibers that reach the spinal cord via the tegmentum of the brainstem rather than via the pyramids.

---

## CLINICAL PANEL 12.3 • LOWER MOTOR NEURON DISEASE

Disease of lower motor neurons may be caused by a variety of infectious agents—notably the virus of poliomyelitis. The term *motor neuron disease*, or *MND*, is used to describe a symptom complex characterized by degeneration of upper *and* lower motor neurons in late middle age. The etiology is unknown; the variable manifestations of the disease are suggestive of more than one cause. During the first year or two, lower motor neurons alone may be involved, especially in the upper limbs. This phase is called *progressive muscular atrophy*. It has the following manifestations:

1. Weakness of the muscles affected, together with
2. Wasting. The wasting is not merely a disuse atrophy but results from loss of a trophic (nourishing) factor produced by motoneurons and conveyed to muscle by axonal transport.
3. Loss of tendon reflexes *(areflexia)* in the wasted muscles.
4. *Fasciculations*, which are visible twitchings of small groups of muscle fibers in the early stage of wasting. They arise from spontaneous discharge of motoneurons with activation of motor units. It should be stressed

that fasciculations are sometimes observed in healthy muscle, especially after exercise.
5. *Fibrillations*, which are minute contractions detectable only by needle electromyography (a recording electrode in the form of a needle is inserted into the muscle). Fibrillations are the result of *denervation supersensitivity:* following denervation, additional ACh receptors develop along the surface of muscle fibers, to the extent that the fibers respond to minute amounts of free acetylcholine in the circulating blood.
6. Sooner or later, signs of upper motor neuron disease appear. The lower limbs become weak, with increased muscle tone and brisk reflexes. This condition is called *amyotrophic lateral sclerosis*. Motor cranial nerve nuclei in the pons and medulla oblongata may be involved from the start (*progressive bulbar palsy*, Chapter 14) or only terminally. Death from respiratory complications usually occurs within 5 years of onset.

The absence of significant sensory disturbances is small comfort to these patients. *'Whatever you do, don't get motor neuron disease. It's bloody awful.'*—actor David Niven, who died of it.

---

### The reticulospinal tracts

The reticulospinal tracts originate in the reticular formation of the pons and medulla oblongata. They are partially crossed.

The *pontine reticulospinal tract* descends in the anterior funiculus, and the *medullary reticulospinal tract* descends in the lateral funiculus (*Figure 12.6*). Both tracts are believed to act upon motoneurons supplying axial (trunk) and proximal limb muscles. Access is indirect, by way of internuncial neurons shared with the corticospinal tract.

Information from animal experiments indicates that the pontine reticulospinal tract acts upon extensor motoneurons and the medullary reticulospinal tract upon flexor motoneurons. Both pathways exert reciprocal inhibition.

The reticulospinal system is involved in two different kinds of motor behavior: locomotion, and postural control.

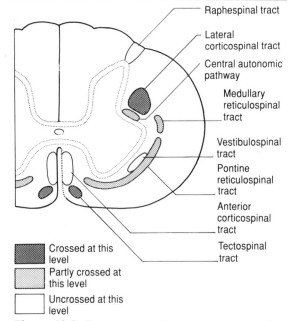

Raphespinal tract

Lateral corticospinal tract

Central autonomic pathway

Medullary reticulospinal tract

Vestibulospinal tract

Pontine reticulospinal tract

Anterior corticospinal tract

Tectospinal tract

Crossed at this level

Partly crossed at this level

Uncrossed at this level

**Figure 12.6.** Descending pathways at upper cervical level.

---

### CLINICAL PANEL 12.4 ● SPINAL CORD INJURY

In the Western world, automobile accidents are the commonest cause of spinal cord injury. More than half of the victims are in the 15–30 year age group, and the cervical cord is most commonly affected.

Injury at thoracic or lumbar segmental level results in *paraplegia* (paralysis of lower limbs). Injury at cervical level causes *tetraplegia (quadriplegia)*, in which the extent of upper limb paralysis depends on the number or level of cervical segments involved.

#### Spinal shock

The following features are found below the segmental level of the injury in the first few days following a complete cord transection:

- Paralysis of movement. The limbs are flaccid and tendon reflexes are absent.
- Anesthesia (loss of all forms of sensation)
- Paralysis of the bladder and rectum.

In addition, the patient develops *postural hypotension* when raised from the recumbent position, because of interruption of the baroreceptor reflex. Wearing an abdominal binder may be sufficient to compensate for the lost reflex.

#### Return of spinal function

Several days or weeks later, reflex functions of the cord become progressively restored, and 'upper motor neuron signs' appear. Muscle tone becomes excessive (spastic). Tendon reflexes become abnormally brisk. A Babinski sign can be elicited on both sides. Ankle clonus

is commonly seen when a patient's leg is lifted into contact with the footplate of a wheelchair.

If extensor spasticity in the lower limbs is dominant, the patient develops *paraplegia in extension*; if flexor spasticity is dominant, *paraplegia in flexion*. An extended posture may permit *spinal standing*; it is promoted by appropriate passive placement of the limbs, and it is the rule following cord injury which is either incomplete or low. A flexed posture is promoted by repetitive *mass flexor reflexes* involving the ankles, knees and hips; mass reflexes can follow any cutaneous stimulation of the legs if the flexor reflex internuncial neurons of the cord are already sensitized by afferent discharges from a bedsore or from an infected bladder.

The condition of the bladder is of great importance because of the twin dangers of infection and formation of bladder stones. For the initial, *atonic* bladder, a sterile catheter is inserted in order to ensure unobstructed drainage. Later, the bladder becomes *automatic*, emptying itself every 4–6 hours through a reflex arc involving the sacral autonomic center in the conus medullaris.

In animals, much of the damage done to the cord by injury has been shown to be secondary to local shifts in electrolyte concentrations, and to vascular changes including arterial spasm and venous thrombosis. Some modest success is being achieved in counteracting these effects. Another line of experimental research is to implant *embryonic* spinal gray matter at the site of injury. These grafts often survive and establish local synaptic connections, but the goal of functional recovery has not been attained.

---

#### Locomotion

Walking and running are rhythmical events involving all four limbs. Movements of the two sides are reciprocal with respect to flexor and extensor contractions and relaxations. In lower animals, locomotion is regulated by a hierarchical system in which the lowest members are internuncial neurons on both sides at cervical and lumbosacral levels, activating the flexors and extensors of the individual limbs. They are called *pattern generators*. Co-ordinating the pattern generators for the individual limbs is a further generator situated in the

intermediate gray matter at the upper end of the spinal cord; it is capable of initiating rhythmical movements after section of the neuraxis at the spinomedullary junction. Locomotion is initiated from a *locomotor center* stretched across the midbrain at the level of the inferior colliculi. In anesthetized animals, electrical stimulation of the mesencephalic locomotor center with pulses of increasing frequency produces walking movements, then trotting, and finally, galloping.

Although the basic locomotor patterns are inbuilt, they are modulated by sensory feedback from the terrain. Overall control of the motor output resides in the premotor cortex, which has direct projections to the pontine and medullary neurons that give rise to the reticulospinal tracts. The tracts are used to steer the animal as it walks or runs, and to override the spinal generators, for example in scaling a wall.

Human locomotion is less 'spinal' than that of quadrupeds. However, the general neuroanatomical framework has been conserved during higher evolution, and the basic physiology seems to be in place as well. In particular, a bilaterally organized motor system controling proximal and axial muscles *must* exist to account for the return of near-perfect locomotor function following removal of an entire cerebral hemisphere during childhood or adolescence. Such people never recover manual skill on the contralateral side, and this reinforces the belief among physical therapists that two distinct pathways are involved in motor control: pyramidal, and 'extrapyramidal.' The latter term denotes the reticulospinal pathway and its controls upstream in the cerebral cortex and basal ganglia.

## Posture

Definitions of *posture* vary with the context in which the term is used. In the general context of standing, sitting, and recumbency, posture may be defined as the position held between movements. In the local context of a single hand or foot, the term denotes *postural fixation*—the immobilization of proximal limb joints by co-contraction of the surrounding muscles, leaving the distal limb parts free to do voluntary business. As will be noted in Chapter 23, there is reason to believe that the human premotor cortex is programmed to select appropriate proximal muscle groups by way of the reticulospinal tracts, to set the stage for any particular movement of the hand or foot.

The interpolation of internuncial neurons between the two main motor pathways acting upon motoneurons serving axial and proximal limb muscles, means that *either* pathway may be in command for a particular movement sequence—the extrapyramidal (reticulospinal) pathway for routine tasks, the pyramidal pathway for tasks requiring close attention—for example, picking one's way along a path strewn with rubble.

## The tectospinal tract

The tectospinal tract is a crossed pathway descending from the tectum of the midbrain to the medial part of the anterior gray horn at cervical

and upper thoracic levels. It is strategically placed for access to axial motoneurons (*Figure 12.6*).

The tectospinal tract is an important motor pathway in the reptilian brain, being responsible for orienting the head/trunk toward sources of visual stimulation (superior colliculus) or auditory stimulation (inferior colliculus). It is likely to have similar automatic functions in humans.

## The vestibulospinal tract

The vestibulospinal tract is an important uncrossed pathway whereby the tone of antigravity muscles is automatically increased when the head is tilted to one side. It descends in the anterior funiculus (*Figure 12.6*) and its function is to keep the center of gravity between the feet. It originates in the vestibular nucleus in the medulla oblongata. (*Note:* As explained in Chapter 15, there are in fact *two* vestibulospinal tracts on each side. The unqualified term refers to the *lateral* vestibulospinal tract.)

## The raphespinal tract

The raphespinal tract originates in and beside the *raphe nucleus* situated in the midline in the medulla oblongata. It descends on both sides within the posterolateral tract of Lissauer. Its function is to modulate sensory transmission between first- and second-order neurons in the posterior gray horn—particularly with respect to pain (see Chapter 18).

## Aminergic pathways

Aminergic pathways descend from specialized cell groups in the pons and medulla oblongata (Chapter 18). The principal neurotransmitters involved are *norepinephrine* and *serotonin*, both of which are classed as *biogenic amines*. The aminergic pathways descend in the outer parts of the anterior and lateral funiculi, and are distributed widely in the spinal gray matter. In general terms, they have inhibitory effects on sensory neurons and facilitatory effects on motor neurons.

## Central autonomic pathways

Central sympathetic and parasympathetic fibers descend beside the intermediate gray matter (*Figure 12.6*). They originate in part from autonomic control centers in the hypothalamus and in part from several nuclear groups in the brainstem. They terminate in the intermediolateral cell columns that give rise to the preganglionic sympathetic and parasympathetic fibers of the peripheral autonomic system.

The central sympathetic pathway is required for normal *baroreceptor reflex* activity. If the spinal cord is crushed in a neck injury, the patient loses consciousness if raised from the recumbent position within the first week or so because a fall of blood pressure in the carotid sinus on sitting up normally causes a compensatory increase in sympathetic activity in order to maintain blood flow to the brain.

The central parasympathetic pathway is required for normal bladder (and rectal) function. The fibers concerned originate in the reticular formation, mainly at the level of the pons (Chapter 18). The pontine center has a tonic inhibitory action on the sacral parasympathetic system. Severe injury to the spinal cord or cauda equina results in reflex voiding when the bladder is only half full (Panel 12.4).

### Note on the rubrospinal tract

The rubrospinal tract is an important motor pathway in cats and dogs, where it arises in the contralateral red nucleus and descends in front of the corticospinal tract. In monkeys this tract is small and in humans it is quite negligible.

## BLOOD SUPPLY OF THE SPINAL CORD

### *Arteries*

Close to the foramen magnum, the two vertebral arteries give off anterior and posterior spinal branches. The anterior branches fuse to form a single **anterior spinal artery** in front of the anterior median fissure (*Figure 12.7*). Branches are given alternately to the left and right sides of the spinal cord. The **posterior spinal arteries** descend along the line of attachment of the dorsal nerve roots on each side.

The three spinal arteries are boosted by several *radiculospinal* branches from the vertebral arteries and from intercostal arteries. They are distinguishable from the small *radicular* arteries which enter every intervertebral foramen to nourish the nerve roots. The largest radiculospinal artery is the *artery of Adamkiewicz,* which arises from a lower intercostal artery or upper lumbar artery on the

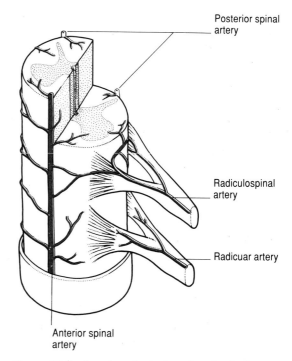

**Figure 12.7.** Arteries of spinal cord and spinal nerve roots.

left side and supplies the lumbar enlargement and conus medullaris.

Vascular disorders of the spinal cord are quite rare. As part of a generalized atherosclerosis, a branch of the anterior spinal artery may become occluded, causing necrosis of the anterior half of the cord on one side. The clinical picture has some resemblance to a one-sided amyotrophic lateral sclerosis owing to destruction of anterior horn motoneurons and diminished function in the lateral corticospinal tract on the same side. However, arterial disease should be suspected here because of the relatively abrupt onset of symptoms and because concurrent damage to the spinothalamic pathway produces loss of pain and of thermal sense on the opposite side, below the level of the lesion.

The artery of Adamkiewicz has to be borne in mind by the vascular surgeon attempting to deal with an abdominal aortic aneurysm. If a clamp is placed across the aorta and the artery happens to arise below that level, the patient is at risk of postoperative paraplegia with incontinence!

### *Veins*

The venous drainage of the cord is by means of anterior and posterior spinal veins, which drain outward along the nerve roots. Any obstruction to the venous outflow is liable to produce edema of the cord, with progressive loss of function.

## EXERCISES

**1** Several conditions, including acute cervical disc prolapse from injury, may damage the anterior and lateral funiculi of the cord on both sides, while leaving the posterior and posterolateral white matter unaffected. Bilateral compression of the corticospinal tracts would produce 'upper motor neuron' signs in the legs. What sensory effects would you anticipate in the legs?

**2** *Hemisection* of the spinal cord produces effects known as the *Brown–Séquard syndrome*. If the left side of the cord was sectioned to the midline by a stab wound at mid-thoracic level, what change(s) of function in each lower limb would you anticipate in terms of (a) motor power, (b) perception of a tuning fork applied to the tibia; (c) perception of pinprick?

## REFERENCES

Abdul-Maguid, T.E. and Bowsher, D. (1979) Alpha- and gamma-motoneurons in the adult human spinal cord and somatic cranial nerve nuclei. *J. Comp. Neurol.* 186: 259–270.

Grillner, S. and Dubuc, R. (1988) Control of locomotion in vertebrates: spinal and supraspinal mechanisms. In *Advances in Neurology, vol. 47: Functional Recovery in Neurological Disease* (Waxman, S.G., ed.), pp. 425–453. New York: Raven Press.

Jeanmonod, D. (1991) Neuroanatomical bases of spasticity. In *Neurosurgery for Spasticity* (Sindou, M., Abbott, R. and Keravel, Y., eds), pp. 3–14. New York: Springer-Verlag.

Massion, J. (1992) Movement, posture and equilibrium: interaction and coordination. *Progr. Neurobiol.* **38:** 35–56.

Meinck, H.M., Benecke, R., Kuster, S. and Konrad, B. (1983) Cutaneomuscular (flexor) reflex organization in normal man and in patients with motor disorders. In *Motor Control Systems in Health and Disease* (Desmedt, J.E., ed.), pp. 787–796. New York: Raven Press.

Nathan, P.W. and Smith, M.C. (1982) The rubrospinal and central tegmental tracts in man. *Brain* **105:** 223–269.

Schoenen, J. and Faull, R.L.M. (1990) Spinal cord: cytoarchitectural, dendroarchitectural, and myeloarchitectural organization. In *The Human Nervous System* (Paxinos, G., ed.), pp. 19–54. San Diego: Academic Press.

Young, W. and Mayer, P. (1988) Neurological and neurophysiological evaluation of spinal cord injury. In *Spinal Cord Dysfunction: Assessment* (Illis, L.S., ed.), pp. 148–165. Oxford: Oxford University Press.

# 13

# Brainstem

**The brainstem of adult anatomy comprises the medulla oblongata, pons, and midbrain. Although each displays special features, all three contain long-fibered pathways linking the spinal cord to the cerebral hemispheres, and vice versa. Nuclear groups include those belonging to 10 of the cranial nerves, as well as major cell groups connected with the cerebellum. Finally, the reticular formation of the brainstem contains regulatory centers controling a variety of visceral functions.**

**The regional anatomy of the brainstem, as seen in transverse sections, is fundamental to an appreciation of the clinical results of branch occlusion within the vertebrobasilar arterial system. The sectional anatomy is also very relevant to the clinical effects produced by patches of demyelination in the course of multiple sclerosis.**

The following description of the internal anatomy of the brainstem is centered on six transverse sections stained by the Weigert method for myelin sheaths. The positions of the more important sensory and motor pathways are indicated, as well as the nuclei of cranial nerves. The *course* of the cranial nerves attached to the brainstem is given in the next four chapters. The reticular formation is described separately in Chapter 18.

## Spinomedullary junction (Figure 13.1)

In the ventral region, the chief feature is the **pyramidal decussation,** which gives rise to the **lateral (crossed) corticospinal tract.** On each side of the decussation at this level is the anterior gray horn of the spinal cord.

In the lateral region, the posterior gray horn of the spinal cord has merged with the **nucleus of the spinal tract of the trigeminal nerve.** *This nucleus is clinically significant in receiving nociceptive information from virtually the entire head and neck.* Nociceptive afferents to the 'spinal nucleus' come from the extracranial and intracranial territories of the trigeminal, glossopharyngeal, vagus, and upper three spinal nerves. The nucleus mediates such diverse pains as headache, toothache, earache, and pain in the neck.

In the dorsal region, the gracile and cuneate fasciculi can be identified. Next to the midline, the

**nucleus gracilis** has made an appearance. In the interval between the two posterior column tracts and the pyramidal decussation is the **central gray matter** surrounding the central canal.

The locations of some smaller ascending and descending pathways are indicated. Most of the small tracts cannot be identified individually on the basis of the Weigert stain alone.

## Middle of medulla oblongata (Figure 13.2)

In the ventral region, the two **pyramids** are separated by the **anterior median sulcus.** Immediately behind each pyramid is the lower end of the inferior olivary nucleus (see next section).

In the lateral region the spinal tract and nucleus of the trigeminal nerve can be identified. On their lateral side is the posterior spinocerebellar tract.

In the dorsal region are the **gracile** and **cuneate nuclei.** These nuclei receive the first-order afferents serving conscious proprioception and discriminative touch. They give rise to second-order afferents which cross the midline and ascend to the contralateral thalamus. Initially, the second-order afferents comprise **internal arcuate fibers** sweeping ventrally and medially between the spinal trigeminal nucleus and the central gray matter. They intersect with their opposite numbers in the great **sensory decussation.** Having

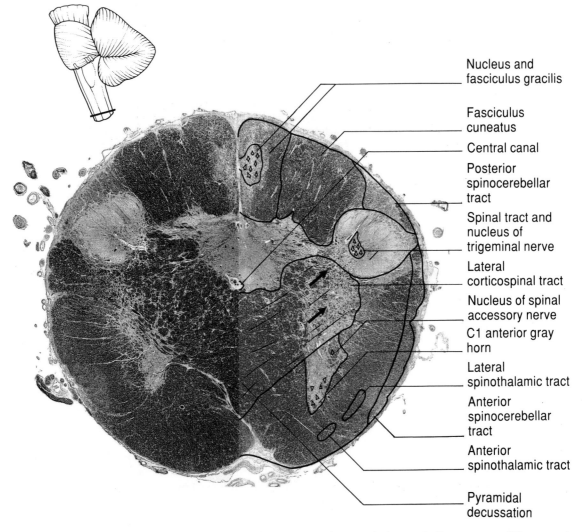

Nucleus and
fasciculus gracilis

Fasciculus
cuneatus

Central canal

Posterior
spinocerebellar
tract

Spinal tract and
nucleus of
trigeminal nerve

Lateral
corticospinal tract

Nucleus of spinal
accessory nerve

C1 anterior gray
horn

Lateral
spinothalamic tract

Anterior
spinocerebellar
tract

Anterior
spinothalamic tract

Pyramidal
decussation

**Figure 13.1.** Cross section at level of spinomedullary junction (see inset). Arrows indicate course of fibers crossing from the pyramid to form the lateral corticospinal tract. (*Note:* The photographs in this chapter are reproduced from *The Human Brain*, by N. Gluhbegovic and T.H. Williams, by kind permission of the authors and of J.B. Lippincott, Inc.)

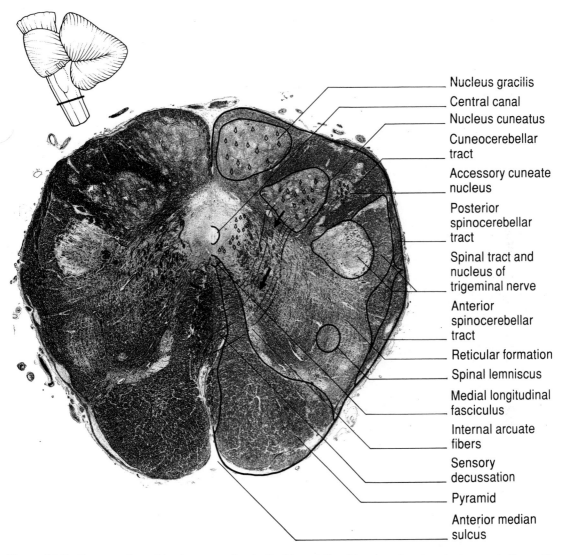

Nucleus gracilis
Central canal
Nucleus cuneatus
Cuneocerebellar tract
Accessory cuneate nucleus
Posterior spinocerebellar tract
Spinal tract and nucleus of trigeminal nerve
Anterior spinocerebellar tract
Reticular formation
Spinal lemniscus
Medial longitudinal fasciculus
Internal arcuate fibers
Sensory decussation
Pyramid
Anterior median sulcus

**Figure 13.2.** Cross section of brainstem at level of mid-medulla oblongata (see inset). Arrows indicate fibers entering the sensory decussation from the cuneate nucleus.

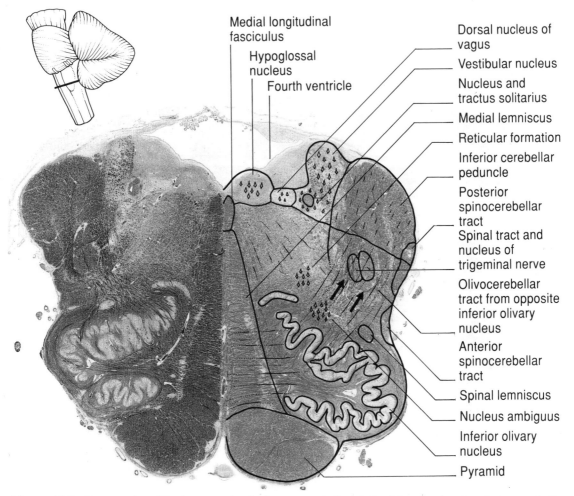

**Figure 13.3.** Cross section of brainstem at level of upper part of medulla oblongata (see inset). Arrows indicate course of olivocerebellar fibers derived from the opposite inferior olivary nucleus.

crossed, they turn rostrally as the **medial lemniscus** (see next section).

Density of staining in Weigert sections reflects thickness of myelin sheaths. As mentioned in Chapter 7, myelin thickness is in proportion to the length of the internodal segments of nerve fibers, and therefore to velocity of conduction. The fastest (darkest) fibers are those of the posterior spinocerebellar tract and fasciculus gracilis. The spinal tract of the trigeminal nerve is light because of the preponderance there of unmyelinated (Group C) fibers.

### Upper part of medulla oblongata (Figure 13.3)

The most striking feature is the wrinkled **inferior olivary nucleus** (ION), which creates the *olive* of gross anatomy. The principal cells of the ION give rise to the **olivocerebellar tract,** which intersects with other pathways before entering the opposite inferior cerebellar peduncle. The ION receives afferents from the motor cortex and red nucleus of its own side, and it has a powerful excitatory effect on the principal (Purkinje) cells of the cerebellar cortex. There is reason to believe that the ION is involved in some way when novel motor skills are being acquired (see Chapter 19).

Medial to the main inferior olivary nucleus are two **accessory olivary nuclei,** which are older phylogenetically.

Dorsal to the pyramid is the **medial lemniscus,** which is disposed dorsoventrally. Dorsal to the lemniscus in turn is the **medial longitudinal fasciculus** (MLF). The MLF runs the entire length of the brainstem and links the vestibular nucleus to the ocular motor nuclei (cranial nerves III, IV and VI). Its chief component in the medulla is the **medial vestibulospinal tract**, which regulates the posture of the head in relation to the trunk (Chapter 15).

The central canal has opened into the caudal part of the **fourth ventricle.** In the central gray matter lining the floor of the ventricle are three cranial nerve nuclei:

1. Near the midline is the **hypoglossal nucleus,** which gives rise to the **hypoglossal nerve** for the supply of the lingual muscles.
2. Lateral to the hypoglossal nucleus is the **dorsal nucleus of the vagus.** This is a parasympathetic motor nucleus supplying preganglionic

fibers to autonomic ganglia in the wall of the gastrointestinal tract.
3. The most lateral nucleus at this level is the **vestibular nucleus,** which receives special sense afferents from the vestibular labyrinth. As well as the medial vestibulospinal tract, this nucleus gives rise to the larger, **lateral vestibulospinal tract,** which helps to sustain the upright posture by acting upon motoneurons supplying extensor (antigravity) muscles.

Ventral to the vestibular nucleus is the **nucleus solitarius,** which surrounds the **tractus solitarius.** The solitary tract contains several kinds of primary afferent fibers terminating at different levels of the nucleus. The largest number are *visceral afferents* from the territory of the glossopharyngeal and vagus nerves.

The final nucleus to be mentioned here is the **nucleus ambiguus,** located in the tegmentum dorsal to the inferior olivary nucleus. The nucleus ambiguus gives rise to the cranial accessory nerve, which is distributed by the vagus. It also contains the *cardioinhibitory center* (Chapter 14).

*Figure 13.4* shows the position of the various nuclei in a dorsal view of the brainstem.

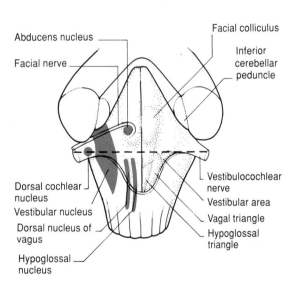

**Figure 13.4.** Cranial nerve nuclei beneath the floor of the fourth ventricle. Dashed line indicates pontomedullary junction. *Left:* position of the nuclei and of the facial nerve. *Right:* surface appearances, with descriptive anatomical terms.

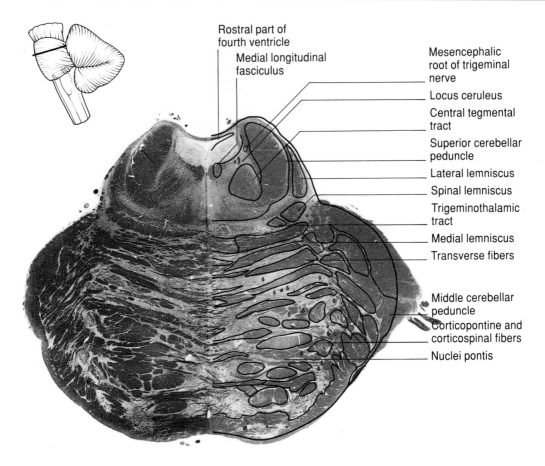

Rostral part of
fourth ventricle

Medial longitudinal
fasciculus

Mesencephalic
root of trigeminal
nerve

Locus ceruleus

Central tegmental
tract

Superior cerebellar
peduncle

Lateral lemniscus

Spinal lemniscus

Trigeminothalamic
tract

Medial lemniscus

Transverse fibers

Middle cerebellar
peduncle

Corticopontine and
corticospinal fibers

Nuclei pontis

**Figure 13.5.** Cross section through the upper part of the pons (see inset).

### Pons *(Figure 13.5)*

The section is taken through the upper part of the pons, where the **superior cerebellar peduncles** are converging as they run upward on either side of the fourth ventricle.

The ventral two-thirds of the section are taken up by the massive *basilar pons,* in which two sets of myelinated fibers are obvious. One set consists of the **transverse fibers of the pons,** which originate in **nuclei pontis** on one side and cross over to enter the opposite **middle cerebellar peduncle.** The other set is seen in cross section and comprises corticopontine and corticospinal fibers.

The **corticopontine fibers** descend from association areas of the cerebral cortex and synapse in the nuclei pontis. Together with the transverse set, they make up the *corticopontocerebellar pathway,* through which the cerebral cortex informs

the contralateral cerebellar hemisphere about intended movements (*Figure 13.6*).

The *corticospinal fibers* constitute the **corticospinal (pyramidal) tract.** The tract is separated into individual fascicles by the transverse fibers. At this level, the corticospinal and corticopontine fascicles look alike.

Dorsal to the basilar region, the profile of the medial lemniscus is horizontal. At its outer border is the **spinal lemniscus** (conjoint anterior and lateral spinothalamic tracts). Alongside these is the **trigeminothalamic tract,** containing second-order sensory neurons from the head and neck. Outside the superior cerebellar peduncle is the **lateral lemniscus,** consisting of *auditory* fibers ascending to the inferior colliculus of the midbrain.

Medial to the peduncle is the **central tegmental tract,** containing fibers descending from the red nucleus to the inferior olivary nucleus.

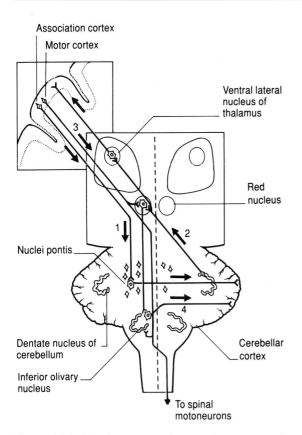

**Figure 13.6.** The four principal motor decussations of the brainstem. Contributory pathways are numbered in accordance with their usual sequence of activation in voluntary movements. (1) Corticopontocerebellar; (2) dentato-thalamo-cortical; (3) corticospinal; (4) olivocerebellar. Also shown is the rubro-olivary connection.

## Isthmus (Figure 13.7)

The **isthmus rhombencephali** is the relatively narrow junctional region of the pons with the midbrain. The ventral region shows the same features as the previous section (transverse fibers, corticopontine and corticospinal fibers). The intermediate, tegmental region is massively invaded by the **decussation of the superior cerebellar peduncles.** These consist of heavily myelinated axons that arise in the central cerebellar nuclei of one side and project to the opposite thalamus and red nucleus.

Dorsal to the decussation, the tegmentum contains the medial longitudinal fasciculus and the central tegmental tract. The medial and spinal lemnisci have been displaced to the side, and the lateral lemniscus is approaching the **inferior colliculus** of the midbrain.

The central canal has narrowed to form the caudal end of the **aqueduct.** The **periaqueductal gray matter** is bounded on each side by the **locus ceruleus** and the **mesencephalic trigeminal nucleus.** The locus ceruleus contains much the largest collection of *noradrenergic neurons* in the CNS. (These and other *aminergic neurons* are described in Chapter 18.)

## Midbrain (Figure 13.8)

The section is taken from the upper part of the midbrain, where the tegmentum is blending with the thalamus.

Most ventral is the **crus cerebri,** which contains all of the 20 million corticopontine fibers descending to the nuclei pontis, and the one million fibers of the corticospinal tract (including corticonuclear fibers distributed to motor cranial nerve nuclei). The medial part of the crus contains corticopontine fibers from the frontal lobe; the lateral part contains corticopontine fibers from the parietal, occipital, and temporal lobes. The middle of the crus contains the corticospinal tract, mingled to some extent with neighboring corticopontine fibers.

The most ventral part of the tegmentum contains the **substantia nigra** ('black substance'). The pigment is *neuromelanin,* produced during synthesis of *dopamine* transmitter. The *nigrostriatal pathway* runs from here to the corpus striatum in the base of the cerebral hemisphere. Clinically, the nigrostriatal pathway is highly significant in relation to Parkinson's disease (Chapter 24). A second set of dopaminergic neurons projects from the *ventral tegmental area* (dorsal to the substantia nigra) to the limbic lobe of the brain. This is the *mesolimbic* dopaminergic pathway, which seems to be significant in relation to psychiatric disorders including schizophrenia (Chapter 18).

The medial part of the tegmentum contains the **red nucleus,** whose content of iron gives it a pink hue in the fresh state. The red nucleus receives ascending afferents from the contralateral central cerebellar nuclei. It receives descending fibers from the motor cortex, many of these being collaterals of corticospinal and corticobulbar fibers.

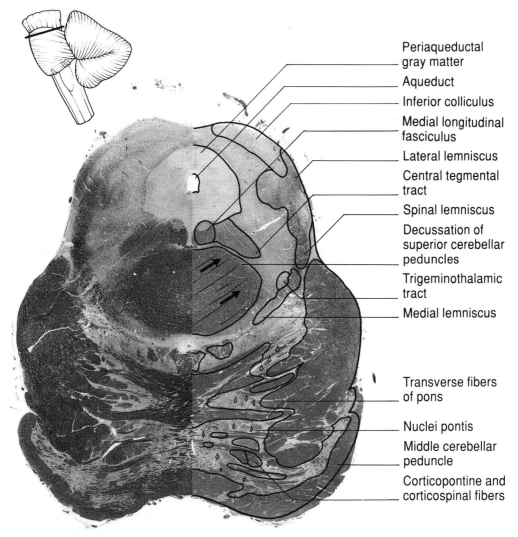

Periaqueductal
gray matter

Aqueduct

Inferior colliculus

Medial longitudinal
fasciculus

Lateral lemniscus

Central tegmental
tract

Spinal lemniscus

Decussation of
superior cerebellar
peduncles

Trigeminothalamic
tract

Medial lemniscus

Transverse fibers
of pons

Nuclei pontis

Middle cerebellar
peduncle

Corticopontine and
corticospinal fibers

**Figure 13.7.**  Cross section of the brainstem at the level of the isthmus (see inset). Arrows indicate the course of fibers emerging from the decussation of the superior cerebellar peduncles.

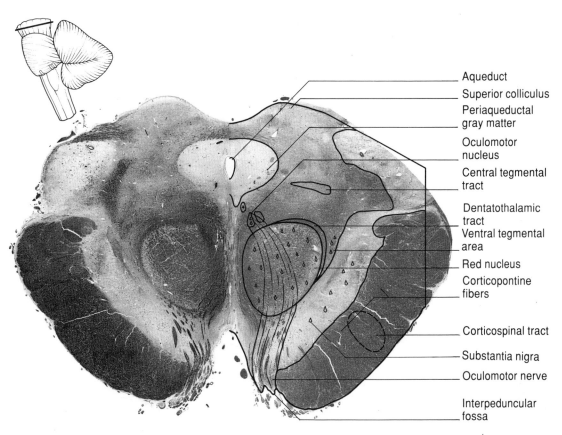

**Figure 13.8.** Cross section of the brainstem at the level of the upper part of the midbrain (see inset).

The human red nucleus is almost entirely *parvocellular* (small-celled), and projects to the ipsilateral inferior olivary nucleus, to the cerebellum and reticular formation, and to the thalamus. The minute *magnocellular* part projects to the caudal part of the reticular formation. In laboratory mammals such as the cat, the magnocellular part of the nucleus is substantial and projects as the *rubrospinal tract* to motoneurons at all levels of the spinal cord. In humans this tract is, at most, negligible.

The lateral part of the tegmentum contains cerebellothalamic fibers; also the medial and spinal lemnisci and the trigeminothalamic tract. The dorsal part contains the central tegmental tract and the medial longitudinal fasciculus.

Ventral to the periaqueductal gray matter is the **oculomotor nucleus**, which gives rise to the **oculomotor nerve**. The nerve passes through the medial part of the tegmentum and emerges from the brain into the interpeduncular fossa.

Dorsal to the periaqueductal gray matter is the **superior colliculus**, the principal subcortical center for visual reflexes. The central tegmental tract no longer contains rubro-olivary fibers but it becomes continuous at higher levels with the medial forebrain bundle (see Chapter 20).

### Orientation of brainstem 'slices' in MR images

*Figure 13.9* shows the orientation of brainstem 'slices' in MR images (see also *Figure 4.6*). The orientation is the opposite of that in the sections. This is because, in illustrations, ventral structures are represented *below*. In the case of the brainstem and spinal cord, the ventral aspect is *anterior* during life. In radiographs, anterior structures are represented *above* (cf. CT scans of the abdomen).

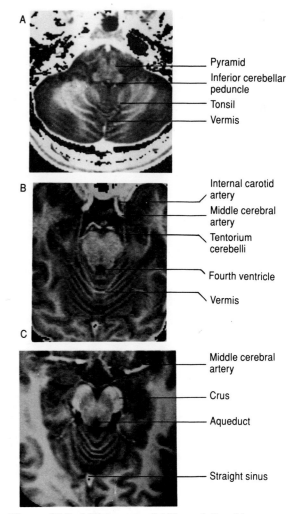

Figure labels: Pyramid, Inferior cerebellar peduncle, Tonsil, Vermis, Internal carotid artery, Middle cerebral artery, Tentorium cerebelli, Fourth ventricle, Vermis, Middle cerebral artery, Crus, Aqueduct, Straight sinus

**Figure 13.9.** MR images of (A) medulla oblongata, (B) pons, (C) midbrain in the standard radiological orientation. (From a series kindly provided by Dr Paul Finn, Department of Radiology, New Deaconess Hospital, Boston.)

### BLOOD SUPPLY OF THE BRAINSTEM *(Figure 13.9)*

The brainstem and cerebellum are supplied by the vertebral and basilar arteries and their branches.

The two vertebral arteries arise from the subclavian arteries and ascend the neck in the foramina transversaria of the upper six cervical vertebrae. They enter the skull through the foramen magnum and unite at the lower border of the pons to form the basilar artery. The basilar artery ascends to the upper border of the pons and divides into two posterior cerebral arteries (*Figure 13.10*).

All of the primary branches of the vertebral and basilar arteries give branches to the brainstem.

### Vertebral branches

● The *posterior inferior cerebellar* artery supplies the side of the medulla before giving branches to the cerebellum.

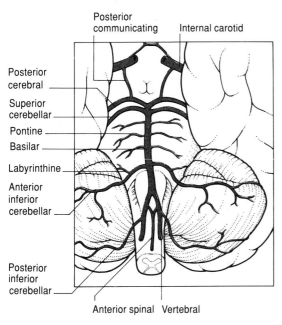

**Figure 13.10.** Arterial supply of brainstem.

- *Anterior* and *posterior spinal* arteries supply the ventral and dorsal medulla, respectively, before descending through the foramen magnum.

### Basilar branches

- The *anterior inferior cerebellar* and *superior cerebellar* arteries supply the side of the pons before giving branches to the cerebellum. The anterior inferior cerebellar usually gives off the labyrinthine artery to the inner ear.
- About a dozen *pontine arteries* supply the full thickness of the medial part of the pons.
- The midbrain is supplied by the *posterior cerebral artery,* and by the *posterior communicating artery* linking the posterior cerebral to the internal carotid.

Some vascular disorders of the brainstem are described in Chapters 14–17.

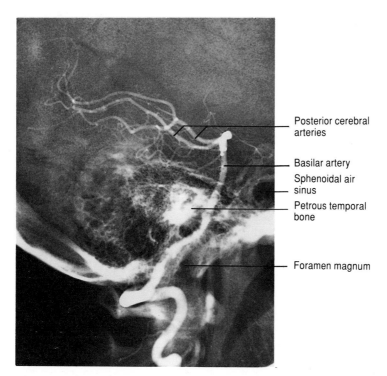

**Figure 13.11.** Vertebral angiogram. Dye injected into the right vertebral artery has entered both posterior cerebral arteries via the basilar. (Photograph kindly provided by Dr. Larry Ginsberg, Department of Radiology, Bowman Gray School of Medicine, Winston-Salem, North Carolina.)

## REFERENCES

Gluhbegovic, N. and Williams, T.H. (1980). *The Human Brain: a Photographic Guide.* New York: Harper & Row.

Nieuwenhuys, R., Voogd, J. and van Huijzen, C. (1988) *The Human Nervous System: a Synopsis and Atlas*, 3rd edn. Berlin: Springer Verlag.

Nathan, P.W. and Smith, M.C. (1982) The rubrospinal and central tegmental tracts in man. *Brain* **105:** 223–269.

Toole, J.F. (1990) *Cerebrovascular Disorders*, 4th. edn. New York: Raven Press.

# 14

# The last four cranial nerves

The overall patterns of development and distribution of cranial nerves III to XII are reviewed first. These patterns account for similarities and differences in the anatomy of the individual nerves. Here and in Chapters 15–17, the nerves mentioned above are described in ascending order, in conformity with the account of the brainstem given in Chapter 13.

## GENERAL ARRANGEMENT OF THE CRANIAL NERVES

In the thoracic region of the developing spinal cord, four distinct cell columns can be identified in the gray matter on each side (*Figure 14.1A,B*). In the basal plate, the *general somatic efferent* column supplies the striated muscles of the trunk and limbs. The *general visceral efferent* column contains preganglionic neurons of the autonomic system. In the alar plate, the *general visceral afferent* column receives afferents from thoracic and abdominal organs. A *general somatic afferent* column receives afferents from the body wall.

In the brainstem, these four cell columns can be identified. However, they are fragmented, and not all of them contribute to each cranial nerve. Their connections are as follows:

- *General somatic efferent*: supplies the striated musculature of the orbit and of the tongue.
- *General visceral efferent:* gives rise to the cranial parasympathetic system described in Chapter 9. The target ganglia are the ciliary, pterygopalatine, otic, and submandibular ganglia in the head, and the vagal ganglia in the thorax and abdomen.
- *General visceral afferent:* receives afferents from the visceral territory of the vagus.
- *General somatic afferent:* receives afferents from skin and mucous membranes, mainly in the territory of the trigeminal nerve.

Additional cell columns are present for branchial arch tissues and for the inner ear (*Figure 14.1C,D*):

- *Special visceral efferent:* supplies the branchial arch musculature of the face, jaws, larynx and pharynx. These striated muscles have visceral functions in relation to food and air intake (hence the name).
- *Special visceral afferent:* receives afferents from taste buds located in the endoderm lining the branchial arches.
- *Special sense afferent:* receives afferents from the inner ear.

### Cell columns in the medulla oblongata (Figure 14.1D)

The somatic efferent cell column is represented by the **hypoglossal nucleus.**

The special visceral efferent cell column is represented by the **nucleus ambiguus,** which migrates to a position dorsal to the inferior olivary nucleus.

The general visceral efferent cell column is represented by the **dorsal nucleus of the vagus,** and by the most rostral part of the nucleus ambiguus.

The general visceral afferent cell column is represented by the lower end of the **nucleus solitarius.**

The special visceral afferent cell column is rep-

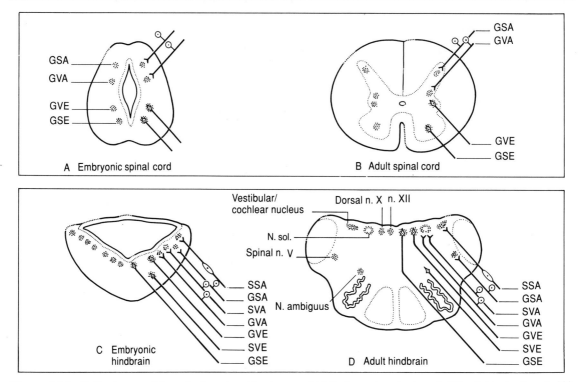

**Figure 14.1.** Cell columns of the spinal cord and brainstem. (A) Embryonic spinal cord; (B) adult spinal cord; (C) embryonic hindbrain; (D) adult hindbrain. *Afferent cell columns*: GSA, general somatic afferent; GVA, general visceral afferent; SSA, special somatic afferent; SVA, special visceral afferent. *Efferent cell columns*: GSE, general somatic efferent; GVE, general visceral efferent; SVE, special visceral efferent. N. sol., nucleus solitarius.

resented by the upper end of the **nucleus solitarius.**

The general somatic afferent cell column is represented by the **spinal trigeminal nucleus,** which migrates to a lateral position.

The special somatic afferent cell column is represented by the **vestibular** and **cochlear nuclei,** located at the pontomedullary junction.

The hypoglossal (XII), accessory (XI), vagus (X), and glossopharyngeal (IX) nerves will now be described. The emphasis will be on functional aspects of the component fibers, at the expense of topographic detail.

## HYPOGLOSSAL NERVE

The hypoglossal nerve (cranial nerve XII) contains somatic efferent fibers for the supply of the extrinsic and intrinsic muscles of the tongue. Its nucleus lies close to the midline and extends the full length of the medulla (*Figure 14.2*). The nerve

emerges as a series of rootlets in the interval between the pyramid and the olive. It crosses the subarachnoid space and leaves the skull through the hypoglossal canal. Just below the skull it lies

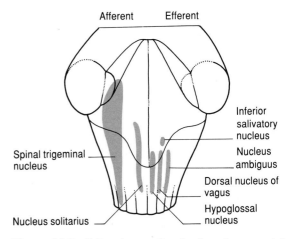

**Figure 14.2.** Cell columns for the last four cranial nerves.

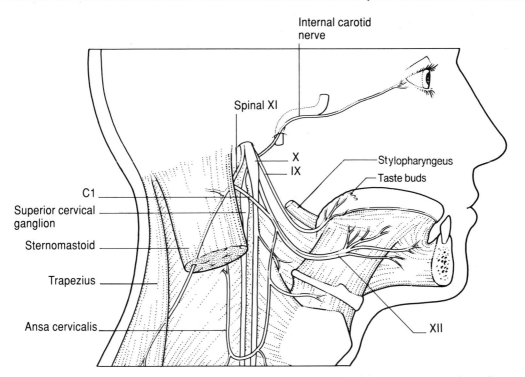

**Figure 14.3.** The last four cranial nerves and the internal carotid branch of the superior cervical ganglion.

close to the vagus and spinal accessory nerves (*Figure 14.3*). It descends on the carotid sheath to the level of the angle of the mandible, then passes forward on the surface of the hyoglossus muscle where it gives off its terminal branches.

In the neck, proprioceptive fibers enter the nerve from the cervical plexus, for distribution to about 100 muscle spindles in the same half of the tongue.

### Phylogenetic note

In reptiles, the lingual muscles, the geniohyoid muscle and the infrahyoid muscles develop together from the uppermost mesodermal somites. The somatic efferent neurons supplying this *hypobranchial muscle sheet* form a continuous ribbon of cells extending from lower medulla to spinal segment C3. In mammals, the hypoglossal nucleus is located more rostrally and its rootlets emerge separately from the cervical rootlets. However, the caudal limit of the hypoglossal nucleus remains linked to the cervical motor cell column by the *supraspinal nucleus*, from which the thyrohyoid muscle is supplied via the first cervical ventral root. In rodents, some of the intrinsic muscle fibers of the tongue receive their motor supply indirectly, from axons which leave the most caudal cells of the hypoglossal nucleus and emerge in the first cervical nerve to join the hypoglossal nerve trunk in the neck. Whether this arrangement holds for primates is not yet known.

### Motor supply to the hypoglossal nucleus

The hypoglossal nucleus receives inputs from the reticular formation, whereby it is recruited for stereotyped motor routines in eating and swallowing. The delicate movements of the tongue during speech require a corticobulbar supply to the nucleus from the large area of the motor cortex involved in this function (*Figure 14.4*). Most of the corticobulbar fibers for the tongue cross over in the upper part of the pyramidal decussation; some remain uncrossed and supply the ipsilateral nucleus.

Supranuclear, nuclear, and infranuclear lesions of the hypoglossal nerve are described together with lesions of the accessory nerve (see Panels 14.1–14.3).

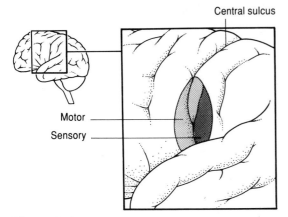

**Figure 14.4.** Areas of the precentral gyrus and post-central gyrus containing cortical representations of the tongue. The cells concerned are interspersed among others devoted to the face. (Adapted from Picard, C. and Olivier, A. (1983), *J. Neurosurg.* **59:** 781–789.)

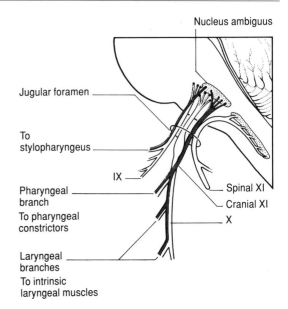

**Figure 14.5.** Course and distribution (in red) of special visceral efferent fibers derived from the nucleus ambiguus.

### Notes on the terms 'corticobulbar' and 'supranuclear'

The *'bulb'* is an archaic term for the medulla oblongata. In clinical usage, it includes the pons as well. *Corticobulbar* or *supranuclear fibers* are fibers of the pyramidal tract which act upon the motor cranial nerve nuclei of the pons (trigeminal and facial) and medulla (hypoglossal and nucleus ambiguus). The spinal accessory nucleus is also included, although it occupies the spinal cord.

Neither term is used with respect to the ocular motor nuclei (oculomotor, trochlear, abducens) because their cortical supply is separate from the pyramidal tract (see Chapter 17).

## SPINAL ACCESSORY NERVE

The spinal accessory (cranial nerve XI) is a purely motor nerve attached to the uppermost five segments of the spinal cord. The nucleus of origin is a column of $\alpha$ and $\gamma$ motoneurons in the base of the anterior gray horn.

The nerve runs upward in the subarachnoid space, behind the denticulate ligament. It enters the cranial cavity through the foramen magnum and leaves it again through the jugular foramen. While in the jugular foramen, it shares a dural sheath with the cranial accessory nerve, but there is no exchange of fibers (*Figure 14.5*). Upon leaving the cranium it crosses the transverse process of the atlas and enters the sternomastoid in company with twigs from roots C2 and C3 of the cervical plexus. It emerges from the posterior border of the sternomastoid and crosses the posterior triangle of the neck to reach the trapezius. It pierces the trapezius in company with twigs from roots C3 and C4 of the cervical plexus. In the posterior triangle the nerve is vulnerable, being embedded in prevertebral fascia and covered only by investing cervical fascia and skin.

The spinal accessory nerve provides the extrafusal and intrafusal motor supply to the sternomastoid and trapezius. The branches from the cervical plexus are proprioceptive in function to the sternomastoid and to the craniocervical part of the trapezius. The thoracic part of the trapezius, which arises from the spines of all the thoracic vertebrae, receives its proprioceptive innervation from the posterior rami of the thoracic spinal nerves. Some of the afferents supplying muscle spindles in the thoracic trapezius do not meet up with the fusimotor supply before reaching the spindles. This is the only instance, in *any* muscle, where the fusimotor and afferent fibers to some spindles travel by completely independent routes.

## GLOSSOPHARYNGEAL, VAGUS, AND CRANIAL ACCESSORY NERVES

Especially relevant to nerves IX, X, and cranial XI are the nucleus solitarius and the nucleus ambiguus. These two nuclei will be described before the three individual nerves are considered.

### Nucleus solitarius

In the center of this nucleus is the **tractus solitarius**, so named because it is made 'solitary' by the sleeve of neurons surrounding it. The original and meaningful name of the neuronal sleeve was *nucleus of the tractus solitarius*.

The nucleus solitarius extends from the lower border of the pons to the level of the nucleus gracilis. Its lower end reaches the midline and forms the *commissural nucleus*. Neuronal packing density in the nucleus solitarius is high and there is neurochemical diversity.

Anatomically, the nucleus is divisible into eight parts. Functionally, four *regions* have been clarified, in accordance with *Figure 14.6:*

1. The uppermost region is the *gustatory nucleus*, which receives primary afferents supplying taste buds in the tongue and palate.
2. The lateral mid-region is the *dorsal respiratory nucleus* (see Chapter 18).
3. The medial midregion is the *baroreceptor nucleus*, which receives the primary afferents supplying the blood pressure detectors in the carotid sinus and aortic arch (see later).
4. The most caudal region, including the commissural nucleus, is the major *visceral afferent nucleus* of the brainstem. It receives primary afferents supplying the alimentary tract and respiratory tract.

### Nucleus ambiguus

Originally of uncertain function (hence the name), the nucleus ambiguus lies immediately behind the inferior olive. Functionally, two regions have been clarified (*Figure 14.6*):

1. The most rostral cells are *parasympathetic*. They give rise to the preganglionic nerve supply to the heart.
2. The remaining cells of the nucleus are *special visceral efferent*. They supply the branchial

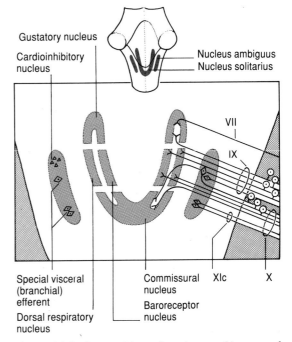

**Figure 14.6.** Composition of nucleus ambiguus and nucleus solitarius.

muscles of the pharynx (stylopharyngeus and the three pharyngeal constrictors) and of the larynx (the intrinsic muscles); also the levator palati.

### Glossopharyngeal nerve

The glossopharyngeal nerve is almost exclusively sensory. It carries no less than five different kinds of afferent fibers traveling to five separate afferent nuclei in the brainstem. The largest of its peripheral territories is the oropharynx, which is bounded in front by the back of the tongue; hence the name for the nerve.

The glossopharyngeal rootlets are attached behind the upper part of the olive. The nerve accompanies the vagus through the anterior compartment of the jugular foramen (the posterior compartment contains the bulb of the internal jugular vein). Within the foramen, the nerve shows small superior and inferior ganglia; these contain unipolar sensory neurons.

Immediately below the skull, the glossopharyngeal nerve finds itself in the company of three other nerves (*Figure 14.3*): the vagus, the spinal accessory, and the internal carotid (sympathetic)

## CLINICAL PANEL 14.1 • SUPRANUCLEAR LESIONS OF THE TENTH, ELEVENTH AND TWELFTH CRANIAL NERVES

The corticonuclear supply to the tenth, eleventh, and twelfth cranial nerves is shown in the accompanying diagram. Supranuclear lesions of all three are commonly seen following vascular strokes damaging the pyramidal tract in the cerebrum or brainstem.

### Effects of unilateral supranuclear lesions

*Figure CP 14.1.1* shows the supranuclear supply to the last four cranial nerve nuclei.

1. The supranuclear supply to the hypoglossal nucleus is *mainly crossed*. The usual picture following a hemiplegic stroke is as follows: during the first few hours or days the tongue, when protruded, deviates toward the paralyzed side because of the stronger pull of the healthy genioglossus. Later, the tongue does not deviate on protrusion.
2. The supranuclear supply to the nucleus ambiguus is *bilateral*. Phonation and swallowing will therefore not be affected.
3. The supranuclear supply to the spinal XI nucleus is *uncrossed for sternomastoid* motoneurons and *crossed for trapezius* motoneurons. The explanation for this arrangement is as follows. When an object in the (say) left hand is held up for inspection, the left trapezius is used to support the weight of the object and the right sternomastoid is used to turn the head. Both actions are effected by the right pyramidal tract.

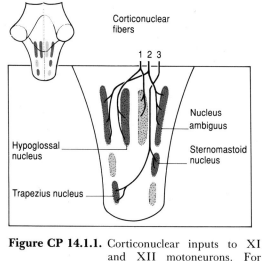

**Figure CP 14.1.1.** Corticonuclear inputs to XI and XII motoneurons. For numbers see text.

### Effects of bilateral supranuclear lesions

The supranuclear supply to the hypoglossal nucleus and nucleus ambiguus may be compromised *bilaterally* by thrombotic episodes in the brainstem in patients suffering from arteriosclerosis of the vertebrobasilar arterial system. The motor nuclei of the trigeminal nerve (to the masticatory muscles) and of the facial nerve (to the facial muscles) may be affected as well. The characteristic picture, known as *pseudobulbar palsy*, is that of an elderly patient who has spastic (tightened) oral and pharyngeal musculature, with consequent difficulty with speech articulation, chewing, and swallowing. The gait is slow and shuffling because of involvement of corticospinal fibers descending to the spinal cord.

---

branch of the superior cervical ganglion. Together with the stylopharyngeus, it slips between the superior and middle constrictor muscles to reach the mucous membrane of the oropharynx.

### Functional divisions and branches

1. Before emerging from the jugular foramen the IX nerve gives off a **tympanic branch** which ramifies on the tympanic membrane and is a potential source of referred pain (see later). The central processes of the tympanic branch synapse in the spinal nucleus of the trigeminal nerve, which receives nociceptive and thermal information from almost the entire head and neck (Chapter 16).
2. Some fibers of the tympanic branch are parasympathetic. They pierce the roof (tegmen tym-

---

**CLINICAL PANEL 14.2 • NUCLEAR LESIONS OF THE TENTH, ELEVENTH, AND TWELFTH CRANIAL NERVES**

Lesions of the hypoglossal nucleus and nucleus ambiguus occur together in *progressive bulbar palsy,* a variant of progressive muscular atrophy (Chapter 12) in which the cranial motor nuclei of the pons and medulla are attacked at the outset. The patient quickly becomes distressed by a multitude of problems: difficulty in chewing and articulation (mandibular and facial nuclei, Chapter 16) and difficulty in swallowing and phonation (hypoglossal and cranial accessory nuclei).

*Unilateral* lesions at nuclear level may be caused by thrombosis of the vertebral artery or of one of its branches (see Lateral Medullary Syndrome in Chapter 15). The distribution of motor weakness is the same as for infranuclear lesions (see Panel 14.3).

---

pani) of the middle ear as the **lesser petrosal nerve**, leave the skull through the foramen ovale, and synapse in the **otic ganglion**. Post-ganglionic fibers supply secretomotor fibers to the parotid gland. The preganglionic fibers originate in the **inferior salivatory nucleus,** which is adjacent to the nucleus ambiguus.

3. The branch to the stylopharyngeus comes from the nucleus ambiguus.
4. Branches serving 'common sensation' (touch) supply the mucous membranes bounding the oropharynx (throat), including the posterior one-third of the tongue. The neurons synapse centrally in the commissural nucleus. The glossopharyngeal branches provide the afferent limb of the *gag reflex*—contraction of the pharyngeal constrictors in response to stroking the wall of the oropharynx. (The gag reflex is unpleasant because of accompanying nausea. To test the integrity of the IX nerve, it is usually sufficient to test sensation on the pharyngeal wall.) Generalized stimulation of the oropharynx elicits a complete *swallowing reflex,* through a linkage between the commissural nucleus and a specific swallowing center nearby (Chapter 18).
5. Gustatory neurons supply the taste buds contained in the circumvallate papillae; they terminate centrally in the gustatory nucleus.
6. An important *carotid* branch descends to the bifurcation of the common carotid artery. This branch contains two different sets of afferent fibers. One set ramifies in the wall of the carotid sinus (at the commencement of the internal carotid artery), terminating in stretch receptors responsive to systolic blood pressure; these *baroreceptor* neurons terminate centrally in the medial part of the nucleus solitarius.

7. The second set of afferents in the carotid branch supplies glomus cells in the carotid body. These nerve endings are *chemoreceptors* monitoring the carbon dioxide and oxygen levels in the blood. The central terminals enter the dorsal respiratory nucleus.

### Vagus and cranial accessory nerves

The vagus is *the* parasympathetic nerve. Its preganglionic component has a huge territory which includes the heart, the lungs, and the alimentary tract from esophagus through transverse colon (Chapter 9). At the same time the vagus is the largest visceral afferent nerve; afferents outnumber parasympathetic fibers by four to one. Overall, the vagus contains the same seven fiber classes as the glossopharyngeal, and they will be listed in the same order.

The rootlets of the vagus and cranial accessory nerves are in series with the glossopharyngeal, and the three nerves travel together into the jugular foramen. At this point the cranial accessory shares a dural sheath with the spinal accessory, but there is no exchange of fibers (*Figure 14.5*). Just below the foramen, the cranial accessory is incorporated into the vagus. The vagus itself shows a small, jugular, and a large, nodose ganglion; both are sensory.

### Functional divisions and branches

1. An **auricular branch** supplies skin lining the outer ear canal, and a **meningeal branch** ramifies in the posterior cranial fossa. Both branches have their cell bodies in the jugular ganglion; the central processes enter the spinal trigeminal nucleus.

## CLINICAL PANEL 14.3 • INFRANUCLEAR LESIONS OF THE LAST FOUR CRANIAL NERVES

### Jugular foramen syndrome

The last four cranial nerves, and the internal carotid (sympathetic) nerve nearby, are at risk of entrapment by a tumor spreading along the base of the skull. The tumor may be a primary one in the nasopharynx, or a metastatic one within lymph nodes of the upper cervical chain. In the second case the primary tumor may be in an air sinus or in the tongue, larynx, or pharynx. In either case a mass can usually be felt behind the ramus of the mandible. The symptomatology varies with the number of nerves caught up in the tumor, and the degree to which the nerves are compromised.

### Symptoms

- Pain in or behind the ear, attributable to irritation of the auricular branches of the ninth and tenth nerves. *Whenever an adult complains of constant pain in one ear, without evidence of middle ear disease, a cancer of the pharynx must be suspected.*
- Headache, from irritation of the meningeal branch of the vagus.
- Hoarseness, due to paralysis of laryngomotor fibers.
- Dysphagia (difficulty in swallowing) due to paralysis of pharyngomotor fibers.

**Signs** (see *Figure CP 14.3.1*)

- Horner's syndrome (ptosis of the upper eyelid, with some pupillary constriction) from interruption of the internal carotid nerve.
- Infranuclear paralysis of the hypoglossal nerve, with wasting of the affected side of the tongue and deviation of the tongue to the affected side on protrusion.
- When the patient is asked to say 'Aahh' the uvula is pulled *away* from the affected side by the unopposed healthy levator palati.
- Sensory loss in the nasopharynx on the affected side.
- On laryngoscopic examination, inability to adduct the vocal cord to the midline.

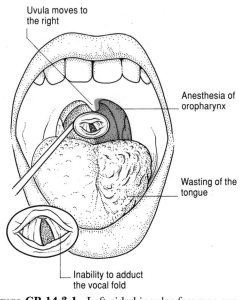

Uvula moves to the right

Anesthesia of oropharynx

Wasting of the tongue

Inability to adduct the vocal fold

**Figure CP 14.3.1.** Left-sided jugular foramen syndrome. A laryngeal mirror is being used to inspect the vocal folds during an attempt to cough.

- Interruption of the spinal accessory nerve produces weakness and wasting of the sternomastoid and trapezius.

A jugular foramen syndrome may also be caused by invasion of the jugular foramen *from above*, for instance by a tumor extending from the cerebellopontine angle (Chapter 16). In this case the sympathetic and spinal accessory nerves will be out of reach, and unaffected.

### Isolated lesion of the spinal accessory nerve

The surface marking for the spinal accessory nerve in the posterior triangle of the neck is a line drawn from the posterior border of the sternomastoid one-third of the way down to the anterior border of the trapezius two-thirds of the way down. It may be injured in this part of its course by a stab wound, or during a surgical procedure for removal of cancerous lymph

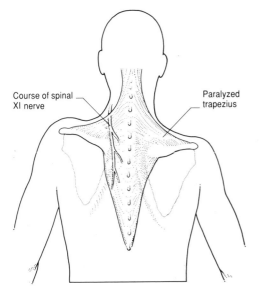

Course of spinal XI nerve

Paralyzed trapezius

nodes. The trapezius is selectively paralyzed, whereupon the scapula and clavicle sag noticeably because trapezius normally helps to carry the upper limb. Shrugging of the shoulder is weakened because the levator scapulae must work alone. Progressive atrophy of the muscle leads to characteristic scalloping of the contour of the neck (see *Figure CP 14.3.2*).

**Figure CP 14.3.2.** Visible effects of right-sided spinal XI paralysis: scalloping of the neck and drooping of the shoulder.

2. *Cardioinhibitory* neurons of the nucleus ambiguus synapse in cardiac ganglia close to the great veins and coronary sinus. The parasympathetic neurons for the respiratory and alimentary tracts originate from the dorsal nucleus of the vagus.
3. Special visceral efferent neurons of the nucleus ambiguus make up the *entire* cranial accessory nerve. The fibers constitute the motor elements in the pharyngeal and laryngeal branches of the vagus. They supply the following striated muscles of branchial origin: levator palati; pharyngeal constrictors; intrinsic muscles of the larynx; upper third of esophagus.
4. General visceral afferent fibers from the heart, and from the respiratory and alimentary tracts have their cell bodies in the nodose ganglion and synapse centrally in the commissural nucleus. They serve important reflexes including the *Bainbridge reflex* (cardiac acceleration brought about by distension of the right atrium); the *cough reflex* (stimulation of a coughing center (Chapter 18) by irritation of the tracheobronchial tree); and the *Hering–Breuer reflex* (inhibition of the dorsal respiratory center by pulmonary stretch receptors). In addition, afferent information from the stomach (in par-

ticular) is forwarded to the hypothalamus and influences feeding behavior (Chapter 20).
5. A few taste buds on the epiglottis report to the gustatory center.
6. Some *baroreceptors* in the aortic arch, and
7. *Chemoreceptors* in the tiny aortic bodies, supplement the corresponding receptors at the carotid bifurcation.

Supranuclear, nuclear, and infranuclear lesions of the ninth, tenth, and eleventh nerves are described in the Clinical Panels.

## REFERENCES

FitzGerald, M.J.T. and Sachithanandan, S.R. (1979) The structure and source of lingual proprioceptors in the monkey. *J. Anat.* **128:** 523–552.

FitzGerald, M.J.T., Comerford, P.T. and Tuffery, A.R. (1982) Sources of innervation of the neuromuscular spindles in sternomastoid and trapezius. *J. Anat.* **134:** 174–190.

Patten, J.P. (1980) *Neurological Differential Diagnosis.* London: Harold Stark.

Sawchenko, P.E. (1983) Central connections of the sensory and motor nuclei of the vagus nerve. *J. Auton. Nerv. Syst.* **9:** 13–26.

# 15

# Vestibulocochlear nerve

**The vestibulocochlear (eighth cranial) nerve consists of two essentially independent nerves. The vestibular nerve supplies sensory end organs signaling head position and head movement. The cochlear nerve is the nerve of hearing. Because of the close anatomical proximity of the two nerves, and of their end organs within the petrous temporal bone, disease processes often produce concurrent clinical effects.**

The vestibulocochlear nerve is primarily composed of the centrally directed axons of bipolar neurons situated in the internal acoustic meatus of the petrous temporal bone (*Figure 15.1*). The peripheral processes are applied to neuroepithelial cells in the cochlea and vestibular labyrinth. The nerve enters the brainstem at the junctional region of the pons and medulla oblongata. The functional anatomy of the two component nerves and end organs will be considered separately.

## VESTIBULAR SYSTEM

The **bony labyrinth** of the inner ear is a very dense shell containing *perilymph*, which resembles extracellular fluid in general. The perilymph provides a water jacket for the **membranous labyrinth,** which encloses the sense organs of balance and of hearing. The sense organs are bathed in *endolymph*. The endolymph resembles intracellular fluid, being potassium-rich and sodium-poor.

The vestibular labyrinth comprises the **utricle**, the **saccule,** and three **semicircular ducts** (*Figure 15.2*). The utricle and saccule each contain a $3 \times 2$ mm$^2$ **macula.** Each semicircular duct contains an **ampulla** at one end, and the ampulla houses a **crista**.

The two maculae are the sensory end organs of the *static* labyrinth, which signals *head position*. The three cristae are the end organs of the *kinetic* or *dynamic* labyrinth, which signals *head movement*.

The bipolar cells of the **vestibular ganglion** occupy the internal acoustic meatus. Their peripheral processes are applied to the five sensory end

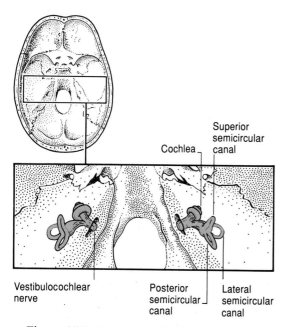

**Figure 15.1.** Bony labyrinth, viewed from above.

Superior
semicircular
canal

Cochlea

Vestibulocochlear
nerve

Posterior
semicircular
canal

Lateral
semicircular
canal

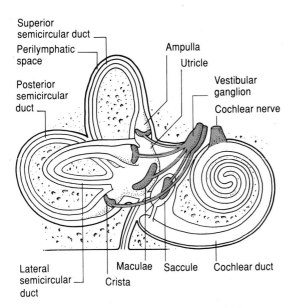

**Figure 15.2.** Locations of the five vestibular sense organs.

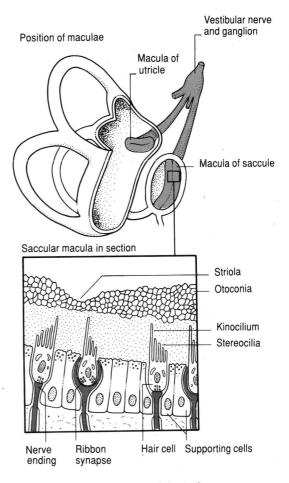

**Figure 15.3.** Static labyrinth.

organs. Their central processes, which constitute the **vestibular nerve,** cross the subarachnoid space and synapse in the vestibular nucleus.

The **vestibular nucleus** is made up of four individual nuclei, **lateral, medial, inferior,** and **superior.**

### Static labyrinth: anatomy and actions

The position and structure of the **maculae** are shown in *Figure 15.3*. The **utricular macula** is relatively horizontal, the **saccular macula** is relatively vertical. The cuboidal cells lining the membranous labyrinth become columnar **supporting cells** in the maculae. Among the supporting cells are so-called **hair cells,** to which vestibular nerve endings are applied. Some hair cells are almost completely enclosed by large nerve endings whereas others (phylogenetically older) receive only small contacts. At the cell bases are *ribbon synapses*, the synaptic vesicles being lined up along *synaptic bars*. Projecting from the free surface of each hair cell are about 100 stereocilia and, close to the cell margin, a single, long *kinocilium.* The hair cells discharge continuously, the resting rate being about 100 Hz.

The cilia are embedded in a gelatinous matrix containing protein-bound calcium carbonate crystals called **otoconia** ('ear sand'). (The term 'oto-

lith', when used, refers to the larger, 'ear stones' of reptiles.) The otoconia exert gravitational drag on the hair cells. Whenever kinocilia are dragged *away* from stereocilia, depolarization is facilitated. As indicated in *Figure 15.3*, the macula has a central groove (*striola*) and the hair cell orientations have a mirror arrangement in relation to the groove. Electrical activity of hair cells is facilitated on one side of the groove by a given gravitational vector, and disfacilitated on the other side.

The maculae also respond to linear acceleration of the head in the horizontal plane (e.g. during walking) or in the vertical (gravitational) plane. Also, when the *tilted* head is stationary in a flexed or extended position the facilitated half of the utricular macula discharges intensely in both ears; the saccular ones are more responsive when the head is held to the side. Both receptors are linked by the vestibular nerve to the lateral, medial and inferior vestibular nuclei.

The primary function of the static labyrinth is to signal the position of the head relative to the trunk. In response to this signal, the vestibular nucleus initiates compensatory movements, with the effect of maintaining the center of gravity between the feet (in standing) or just in front of the feet (during locomotion), and of keeping the head horizontal. These effects are mediated by the vestibulospinal tracts.

The lateral **vestibulospinal tract** *(Deiterospinal tract)* arises from large neurons in the lateral vestibular nucleus of Deiters. The fibers descend in the anterior funiculus on the same side and synapse upon extensor (antigravity) motoneurons in the spinal cord. Both $\alpha$ and $\gamma$ motoneurons are excited, and a significant part of the increased muscle tone is exerted by way of the gamma loop (Chapter 12). During standing, the tract is tonically active on both sides of the spinal cord. During walking, activity is selective for the quadriceps motoneurons of the leading leg; this commences at the moment of heel strike and continues during the stance phase (when the other leg is off the ground). Deiters' nucleus is somatotopically organized, and the functionally appropriate neurons are selected by the flocculonodular lobe of the cerebellum. The flocculonodular lobe (Chapter 19) has two-way connections with all four vestibular nuclei.

Antigravity action is triggered mainly from the horizontal macula of the utricle. The vertical macula of the saccule, on the other hand, is maximally activated by a *free fall*. The shearing effect produces powerful extensor thrust in anticipation of a hard landing.

A small, **medial vestibulospinal tract** arises in the medial and inferior vestibular nuclei. It descends in the medial longitudinal fasciculus and terminates ipsilaterally upon *inhibitory* internuncials in the cervical part of the cord. It operates *head-righting reflexes*, which serve to keep the head — and the gaze — horizontal when the body is craned forward or to one side. Good examples of head-righting reflexes are to be seen around pool tables and in bowling alleys. An added twist can be provided, if required, by torsion of the eyeballs (up to 10°) within the orbital sockets. This *eye-righting reflex* is mediated by axons *ascending* the medial longitudinal fasciculus from the *lateral* vestibular nucleus to reach nuclei controling the extraocular muscles. Evidence derived from unilateral vestibular destruction (Panel 15.1) indicates that the horizontal position of the eyes when the head is upright is the result of a canceling effect of bilateral tonic activity in these *Deitero-ocular* pathways.

The medial vestibulospinal tract is also activated by the kinetic labyrinth.

*The static labyrinth contributes to the sense of position.* The sense of position of the body in space is normally provided by three sensory systems: the visual system, the conscious proprioceptive system, and the vestibular system. Deprived of one of the three, the individual can stand and walk by using information provided by the other two. Following loss of *vision*, for example, the subject can get about, although the constraints imposed by blindness are known to all. Following loss of *conscious proprioception* instead, the subject uses vision as a substitute for proprioceptive sense, and is disabled by closure of the eyes (*sensory ataxia*, Chapter 11). If the *static labyrinths* alone are inactive, closure of the eyes may lead to a heavy fall.

### Kinetic labyrinth: anatomy and action

Basic features of macular epithelium are repeated in the three cristae. Again there are supporting cells, and hair cells to which vestibular nerve endings are applied. The kinocilia of the hair cells are long, penetrating deeply into a gelatinous projection called the *cupula* (*Figure 15.4*). The cupula is bonded to the opposite wall of the ampulla.

The cristae are sensitive to angular acceleration of the labyrinths. Angular acceleration occurs during rotary 'yes' and 'no' movements of the head. The endolymph tends to lag behind because of its inertia, and the cupula balloons like a sail when thrust against it. The disposition of the kinocilia is uniform across each crista, and is such that the *lateral* ampullary crista is facilitated by cupular displacement *toward* the utricle; the *superior* and *posterior* cristae are facilitated by cupular displacement *away from* the utricle. In practical terms, the left lateral ampulla is activated by turning the head to the left; both superior ampullae are activated by flexion of the head; and both posterior ampullae by extension of the head.

Afferents from the cristae terminate in the medial and superior vestibular nuclei. As with the macular afferents, there are two-way connections with the flocculonodular lobe of the cerebellum.

The function of the kinetic labyrinth is to provide information for compensatory movements of the eyes in response to movement of the head.

## CLINICAL PANEL 15.1 • VESTIBULAR DISORDERS

### Unilateral vestibular disease

Acute failure of one vestibular labyrinth may follow spread of disease from the middle ear or thrombosis of the labyrinthine artery. A common cause of unilateral vestibular symptoms in the elderly is a *transient ischemic attack* involving the vertebrobasilar arterial system. Transient ischemic attacks last 15 minutes or less and leave no residual neurological deficit. However, they are commonly followed by a vascular thrombosis somewhere in the brain within 6 months.

The effects of unilateral vestibular disease are well demonstrated when the vestibular system is inactivated surgically, either during removal of an acoustic neuroma (Chapter 16) or as a last resort in treating paroxysmal attacks of vertigo. During the immediate postoperative period, the patient shows triple effects of loss of tonic input from the static labyrinth:

- Loss of function in the Deitero-ocular pathway on one side leads to about 10° of torsion of *both* eyeballs toward that side. The patient's perception of the horizontal shows a corresponding tilt, so that reaching movements become inaccurate.
- The head tilts to the same side, being no longer controled on that side by the head-righting reflex.
- The patient tends to fall to the same side, because the Deiterospinal tract no longer compensates for tilting of the head.

Because function continues in the *normal* lateral semicircular canal, there is a nystagmus to the normal side.

Within a week or two, static labyrinthine function returns and the patient is able to get about. This is due to resumption of activity in the deafferented vestibular nucleus, possibly because of intrinsic membrane properties of the chief neurons. However, *kinetic* labyrinthine function remains disordered (see below).

### Bilateral vestibular disease

Following total loss of *static* labyrinthine function, visual guidance becomes important, and the patient dare not walk out-of-doors after twilight. By day, any distraction causing the patient to look overhead may result in a heavy fall. Loss of *kinetic* labyrinthine function makes it impossible to fix the gaze on an object while the head is moving. During walking, the scene bobs up and down as if it were being viewed through a hand-held camera.

---

*Vestibulo-ocular reflexes* operate to maintain the gaze on a selcted target. A simple example is our ability to gaze at the period (full stop) at the end of a sentence, while moving the head about. The two eyes move *conjugately*, i.e. in parallel.

*Figure 15.4* shows the effect on the semicircular canals of a head turn to the right while looking at a fixed point. The corresponding vestibulo-ocular reflex is shown in *Figure 15.5*. Under cerebellar guidance, the medial vestibular nucleus projects to the contralateral abducens nucleus where it selects two kinds of neurons: (a) motoneurons to abduct the left eye, and (b) *internuclear* neurons which send large axons along the medial longitudinal bundle to the right oculomotor nucleus, where they seek out motoneurons which adduct the right eye.

The superior vestibular nucleus simultaneously *inhibits* the motoneurons serving the antagonist muscles (left medial and right lateral rectus).

Appropriate point-to-point connections also exist between the vestibular nuclei and motoneurons of the oculomotor and trochlear nerves for similar reflexes in the vertical plane.

In order to control the vestibulo-ocular reflexes, the cerebellum needs to be informed about the initial position of the head in relation to the trunk. This information is provided by a great wealth of muscle spindles in the deep muscles surrounding the cervical vertebral column. The spindle afferents enter the rostral spinocerebellar tract and relay in the accessory cuneate nucleus.

### Nystagmus

A horizontal vestibulo-ocular reflex can be elicited by warming or cooling the endolymph in the semicircular canals. In routine tests of vestibular function, advantage is taken of the proximity of the lateral semicircular canal to the middle ear. The

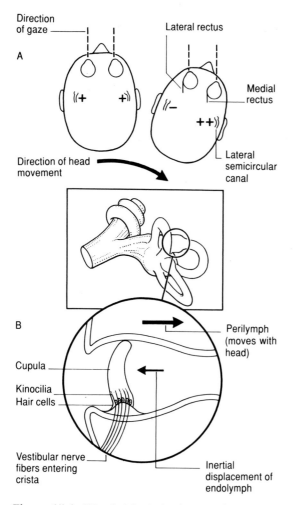

**Figure 15.4.** Kinetic labyrinth, showing the response of the lateral semicircular duct and crista to a rightward turn of the head.

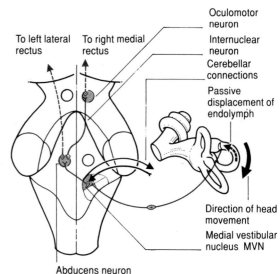

**Figure 15.5.** Minimal pathway for a horizontal vestibulo-ocular reflex originating in the right semicircular canal.

fast phases are repeated several times per second. This is *vestibular nystagmus*. The direction of the nystagmus is named in accordance with the fast phase because of the obvious 'beat'. A warm caloric test applied to the right ear should produce a right-beating nystagmus ('nystagmus to the right').

Subjectively, nystagmus is accompanied by *vertigo*—a sense of rotation of self in relation to the external world, or *vice versa*.

Unilateral and bilateral vestibular syndromes are considered in Panel 15.1. A vascular syndrome involving the vestibular system in the medulla oblongata is described in Panel 15.2.

## Vestibulocortical connections

Second-order sensory neurons project from the vestibular nucleus to the contralateral thalamus. The fibers terminate in company with trigeminothalamic fibers in the ventral posterior nucleus. The main cortical area in receipt of third-order vestibular fibers seems to be a patch immediately behind the face representation on the somatic sensory cortex. In conscious patients with the cortex exposed at operation, a mild electrical stimulus to this patch may elicit a sensation of vertigo.

canal is angled at 30° to the horizontal plane. Tilting the head back by 60° brings the canal into the vertical plane, with the ampulla uppermost. In the *warm caloric test,* water at 44°C is then instilled into the ear. The air in the middle ear is heated, and heat transfer to the lateral canal produces convection currents within the endolymph. Whether through displacement of the cupula or by some other mechanism, the crista of the warmer lateral ampulla becomes more active than its opposite number. The result is a slow drift of the eyes away from the stimulated side. It is *as if* the head had been turned to the side being tested. The drift is followed by a recovery phase in which the eyes snap back to the resting position. Slow and

## CLINICAL PANEL 15.2 • LATERAL MEDULLARY SYNDROME

Thrombosis of the vertebral or posterior inferior cerebellar artery may produce an infarct (area of necrosis) in the lateral part of the medulla. The clinical picture depends on the extent to which the various nuclei and pathways are damaged. Brainstem pathology must always be suspected when a cranial nerve lesion on one side is accompanied by 'upper motor neuron signs' on the other side—so-called *alternating* or *crossed hemiplegia.*

**Lateral medullary syndrome** (see *Figure CP 15.2.1*)

1. Damage to the vestibular nucleus leads to vertigo (often with initial vomiting), together with the symptoms of unilateral disconnection of the labyrinth described in Panel 15.1.
2. Interruption of posterior and rostral spinocerebellar fibers may produce signs of cerebellar ataxia in the ipsilateral limbs. Cerebellar ataxia is a prominent feature if blood flow is interrupted in the posterior inferior cerebellar artery.
3. Damage to the spinal tract of the trigeminal nerve interrupts fine primary afferent fibers descending the brainstem from the trigeminal ganglion (Chapter 16). These fibers are functionally equivalent to those of Lissauer's tract in the spinal cord (Chapter 11). The result of interruption is loss of pain and thermal senses from the face on the same side.

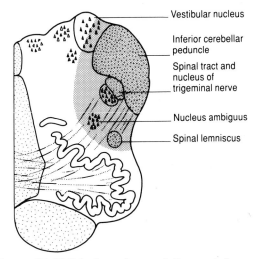

**Figure CP 15.2.1.** Lateral medullary infarct (shaded).

4. Interruption of the central sympathetic pathway to the spinal cord produces a complete Horner's syndrome (ptosis, miosis, anhidrosis).
5. Damage to the nucleus ambiguus causes hoarseness, and sometimes difficulty in swallowing.
6. The only *contralateral* sign is loss of pain and temperature sense in the trunk and limbs, resulting from damage to the lateral spinothalamic tract. There is *no* motor weakness because the corticospinal tract is spared.

## AUDITORY SYSTEM

The auditory system comprises the cochlea, the cochlear nerve, and the central auditory pathway from the cochlear nucleus in the brainstem to the cortex of the temporal lobe. The central auditory pathway is more elaborate than the somatosensory or visual pathway. This is because the same sounds are detected by both ears. In order to signal the location of a sound, a very complex neuronal network is in place, with numerous connections (mainly inhibitory) between the two central pathways in order to magnify minute differences in intensity and timing of sounds that exist during normal, *binaural* hearing.

### The cochlea

The main features of cochlear structure are seen in *Figures 15.6* and *15.7*. The cochlea is pictured as though it were upright, but in life it lies on its side, as shown in *Figure 15.1*. The central bony pillar of the cochlea (the **modiolus**) is in the axis of the internal acoustic meatus. Projecting from the modiolus, like the flange of a screw, is the **osseous**

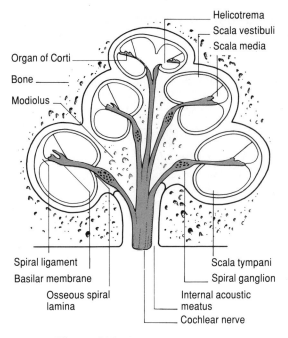

Helicotrema
Scala vestibuli
Scala media
Organ of Corti
Bone
Modiolus

Spiral ligament
Basilar membrane
Osseous spiral lamina
Scala tympani
Spiral ganglion
Internal acoustic meatus
Cochlear nerve

**Figure 15.6.** The cochlea in section.

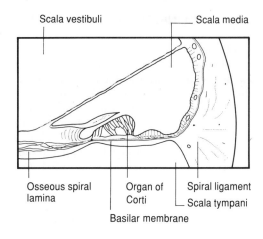

Scala vestibuli
Scala media
Osseous spiral lamina
Organ of Corti
Spiral ligament
Scala tympani
Basilar membrane

spiral lamina. The **basilar membrane** is attached to the tip of this lamina; it reaches across the cavity of the bony cochlea to become attached to the **spiral ligament** on the outer wall. The osseous spiral lamina and spiral ligament become progressively smaller as one ascends the two and one half turns of the cochlea, and the fibers of the basilar membrane become progressively longer.

The basal lamina and its attachments divide the cochlear chamber into upper and lower compartments. These are the **scala vestibuli** and the **scala tympani,** respectively, and they are filled with perilymph. They communicate at the apex of the cochlea, through the **helicotrema.** A third compartment, the **scala media** (cochlear duct), lies above the basilar membrane and is filled with endolymph. It is separated from the scala vestibuli by the delicate **vestibular membrane.**

Sitting on the basilar membrane is the **spiral organ** (*organ of Corti*). The principal sensory receptor epithelium consists of a single row of **inner hair cells,** each one having up to 20 large afferent nerve endings applied to it. The hair cells rest upon supporting cells, and there are ancillary cells as well. The organ of Corti contains a central tunnel, filled with perilymph diffusing through the basilar membrane. On the outer side of the tunnel are several rows of **outer hair cells,** attended by supporting and ancillary cells.

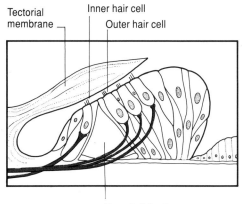

Tectorial membrane
Inner hair cell
Outer hair cell

Tunnel of Corti

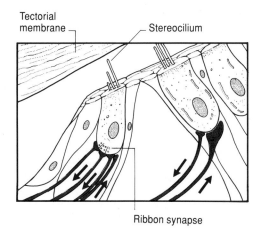

Tectorial membrane
Stereocilium

Ribbon synapse

**Figure 15.7.** Organ of Corti at three levels of magnification. Arrows indicate directions of impulse traffic.

All of the hair cells are surmounted by stereocilia. Unlike the vestibular hair cells, they have no kinocilium in the adult state. The stereocilia of the outer hair cells are embedded in the overlying tectorial membrane. Those of the inner hair cells lie immediately below the membrane.

The outer hair cells are contractile (at least in tissue culture), and they have substantial efferent nerve endings (*Figure 15.7*). In theory at least, oscillatory movents of outer hair cells could influence the sensitivity of the inner hair cells through effects on the tectorial or basilar membrane.

### Sound transduction

The vibrations of the tympanic membrane in response to sound waves are transmitted along the ossicular chain. The foot plate of the stapes fits snugly into the oval window, and vibrations of the stapes are converted to pressure waves in the scala vestibuli. The pressure waves are transmitted through the vestibular membrane to reach the basilar membrane. High frequency pressure waves, created by high-pitched sounds, cause the short fibers of the basilar membrane in the basal turn of the cochlea to resonate and absorb their energy. Low frequency waves produce resonance in the apical turn where the fibers are longest. The basilar membrane is therefore *tonotopic* in its fiber sequence. Not surprisingly, the inner hair cells have a similar tonotopic sequence. In response to local resonance, the cells become depolarized and liberate excitatory transmitter substance from synaptic ribbons (*Figure 15.7*).

The nerve fibers supplying the hair cells are the peripheral processes of the bipolar **spiral ganglion** cells lodged in the base of the osseous spiral lamina.

### Cochlear nerve

The bulk of the cochlear nerve consists of the myelinated central processes of some 30 000 large bipolar neurons of the spiral ganglion. Unmyelinated fibers come from small ganglion cells supplying dendrites to the outer hair cells. (Motor fibers do not travel in the cochlear nerve trunk.) The nerve traverses the subarachnoid space in company with the vestibular and facial nerves, and it enters the brainstem at the pontomedullary junction.

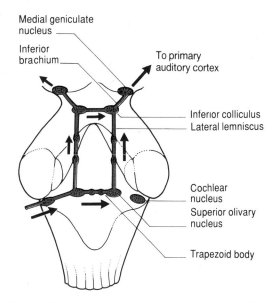

**Figure 15.8.** Dorsal view of brainstem showing basic plan of central auditory pathways.

### Central auditory pathways

The general plan of the central auditory pathway from the left cochlear nerve to the cerebral cortex is shown in *Figure 15.8*. The first cell station is the **cochlear nucleus,** where all cochlear nerve fibers terminate upon entry to the brainstem. From here, some second-order fibers project all the way to the opposite **inferior colliculus** by way of the **trapezoid body** and **lateral lemniscus**. The **inferior brachium** links the inferior colliculus to the **medial geniculate body**, which projects to the **primary auditory cortex** in the temporal lobe.

A small but important *purely ipsilateral* relay passes from the superior olivary nucleus to the higher auditory centers.

### Functional anatomy *(Figure 15.9)*

COCHLEAR NUCLEUS
The cochlear nucleus comprises dorsal and ventral nuclei, on the corresponding surfaces of the inferior cerebellar peduncle. Many incoming fibers of the cochlear nerve bifurcate and enter both nuclei. The cells in both are tonotopically arranged.

Responses of many cells in the ventral nucleus are called primary-like, because their frequency (firing rate) resembles that of primary afferents. Most of the output neurons project to the nearby superior olivary nucleus.

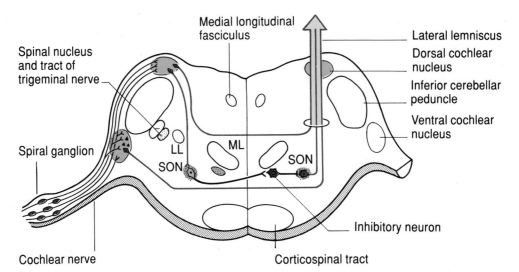

**Figure 15.9.** Transverse section of lower end of pons showing central connections of cochlear nerve. LL, lateral lemniscus; ML, medial lemniscus; SON, superior olivary nucleus.

The cells of the dorsal nucleus are heterogeneous. At least six different cell types have been characterized by their morphology and electrical behavior. Most of the output neurons project to the contralateral inferior colliculus. Individually, they exhibit an extremely narrow range of tonal responses, being 'focused' by collateral inhibiton.

SUPERIOR OLIVARY NUCLEUS
The superior olivary complex of nuclei is relatively small in the human brain. It contains *binaural* neurons affected by inputs from both ears. Ipsilateral inputs are excitatory to the binaural neurons whereas contralateral inputs are inhibitory. The inhibitory effect is mediated by internuncial neurons in the *nucleus of the trapezoid body.*

The superior olivary nucleus is responsive to differences in intensity and timing between sounds entering both ears simultaneously. On the side ipsilateral to a sound, stimulation of the cochlea, and of the nucleus, is earlier and more intense than on the contralateral side. By exaggerating these differences through crossed inhibition, the superior olivary nucleus helps to indicate the spatial direction of incoming sounds. At the same time, the excited nucleus projects to the inferior colliculus of *both* sides, giving rise to binaural responses in the neurons of the inferior colliculus and beyond.

LATERAL LEMNISCUS
Fibers of the lateral lemniscus arise from the dorsal and ventral cochlear nuclei and from the superior olivary nuclei—in both cases, mainly contralater-

ally. The tract terminates in the central nucleus of the superior colliculus. Nuclei within the lateral lemniscus participate in reflex arcs (see later).

INFERIOR COLLICULUS
Spatial information from the superior olivary nucleus, intensity information from the ventral cochlear nucleus, and pitch information from the dorsal cochlear nucleus are integrated in the inferior colliculus. The main (central) part of the nucleus is laminated in a tonotopic manner. Within each tonal lamina, cells differ in their responses: some have a characteristic 'tuning curve' (they respond only to a particular tone); some fire spontaneously but are inhibited by sound; and some respond only to a moving source of sound.

As well as projecting to the medial geniculate nucleus, the inferior colliculus exerts inhibitory effects on its opposite number through the *inferior collicular commissure (Figure 15.8).* It also contributes to the tectospinal tract.

MEDIAL GENICULATE NUCLEUS
The medial geniculate nucleus is the specific thalamic nucleus for hearing. The main (ventral) nucleus is laminated and tonotopic, and the principal neurons project as the **auditory radiation** to the primary auditory cortex.

PRIMARY AUDITORY CORTEX
The upper surface of the temporal lobe shows one or two **transverse temporal gyri.** The anterior one (the gyrus of Heschl) contains the **primary**

**auditory cortex** (see Chapter 23). Tonotopic arrangement is preserved in Heschl's gyrus, its posterior part being responsive to high tones and its anterior part to low tones. The cortex responds to auditory stimuli within the *contralateral sound field*. In cats, destruction of a patch of primary cortex on one side produces a *sigoma* or 'deaf spot' in the contralateral sound field. In humans, ablation of the superior temporal gyrus (in the course of tumor removal) does *not* cause deafness, but it significantly reduces ability to judge the direction and distance of a source of sound.

## Brainstem acoustic reflexes

Fibers emerge from the lateral lemniscus and form the internuncial linkage for certain reflex arcs:

- Fibers entering the motor nuclei of the trigeminal and facial nerves link up with motoneurons supplying the tensor tympani and stapedius, respectively. These muscles exert a damping action on the ossicles of the middle ear. The tensor tympani is activated by the subject's own voice, the stapedius by external sounds.

- Fibers entering the reticular formation have an important *arousal* effect on the state of consciousness, as exemplified by the alarm clock. Sudden loud sounds cause the subject to flinch; this is the 'startle response', mediated by outputs from the reticular formation to the spinal cord and to the motor nucleus of the facial nerve.

### Descending auditory pathways

A cascade of descending fibers runs from the primary auditory cortex to the medial geniculate nucleus and inferior colliculus, and from the inferior colliculus to the superior olivary nucleus. The *olivocochlear bundle* emerges in the vestibular nerve and carries efferent, cholinergic fibers to the cochlea, with some for the vestibular labyrinth. The cochlear fibers apply large synaptic boutons to outer hair cells, and small boutons to the afferent nerve endings on inner hair cells.

The olivocochlear bundle may be involved in the mechanism whereby certain sounds may be

---

## CLINICAL PANEL 15.3 • TWO KINDS OF DEAFNESS

All forms of deafness can be grouped into two categories. *Conductive deafness* is caused by disease in the outer ear canal or in the middle ear. *Sensorineural deafness* is caused by disease in the cochlea or in the neural pathway from cochlea to brain.

Common causes of conductive deafness include accumulation of cerumen (wax) in the outer ear, and *otitis media* (inflammation in the middle ear). *Otosclerosis* is a disorder of the oval window in which the capsule of the synovial joint between the footplate of the stapes and the vestibule of the bony labyrinth is progressively replaced by bone. The stapes becomes immobilized, with severe impairment of hearing throughout the full tonal range. Replacement of the stapes by a prosthesis (artificial substitute) often restores normal hearing.

Sensorineural deafness usually originates within the cochlea. The commonest form is the high-frequency hearing loss of the elderly, resulting from deterioration of the organ of Corti in the basal turn. As a result, the elderly have difficulty in distinguishing among high-frequency consonants (d, s, t); vowels, which are low frequency, are quite audible. The elderly should be addressed *distinctly* rather than loudly.

*Occupational deafness* arises from a noisy environment at work. A persistent noise, especially indoors, may eventually lead to degeneration of the organ of Corti in the region corresponding to the particular frequency.

*Ototoxic deafness* may follow administration of drugs, including streptomycin, neomycin, and quinine.

*Infectious deafness* may follow more or less complete destruction of the cochlea by the virus of mumps or congenital rubella (German measles).

An important cause of sensineural deafness in adults is an *acoustic neuroma*. Because the trigeminal and facial nerves may be affected as well as the cochlear and vestibular, this tumor is described in Chapter 16.

deliberately selected for attention — for example, a particular voice in a jumble of conversation (the 'cocktail party effect'). Experimental evidence indicates an involvement in enhancing detection of faint sounds.

## Deafness

Deafness is a widespread problem in the community. About 10% of adults suffer from it in some degree. The cause may lie in the outer, middle, or inner ear, or in the cochlear neural pathway. The two fundamental types of deafness are described in Panel 15.3.

## REFERENCES

### Vestibular system

Anniko, M. (1988) Functional morphology of the vestibular system. In *Physiology of the Ear* (Jahn, A.F. and Santos-Sacchi, J., eds), pp. 457–475. New York: Raven Press.

Markham, C.H. (1987) Vestibular control of muscular tone and posture. *Can. J. Neurol. Sci.* **14:** 493–496.

Smith, P.F. and Darlington, C.L. (1991) Neurochemical mechanisms of recovery from peripheral vestibular lesions. *Brain Res. Rev.* **16:** 117–133.

Spoendlin, H. (1988) Neural anatomy of the inner ear. In *Physiology of the Ear* (Jahn, A.F. and Santos-Sacchi, J., eds), pp. 201–219. New York: Raven Press.

### Auditory system

Adams, J.C. (1986) Neuronal morphology in the human cochlear nucleus. *Arch. Otolaryngol. Head Neck Surg.* **112:** 1253–1261.

Aitkin, L.M. (1989) The auditory system. In *Handbook of Chemical Neuroanatomy, Vol. 7: Integrated Systems of the CNS, Part II* (Bjorklund, A., Hokfeld, T. and Swanson, L.W., eds), pp. 165–218. New York: Elsevier.

Corwin J.T. and Warchol, M.E. (1991) Auditory hair cells: structure, function, development, and regeneration. *Ann. Rev. Neurosci.* **14:** 301–333.

Phillips, D.P. (1988) Introduction to anatomy and physiology of the central auditory nervous system. In *Physiology of the Ear* (Jahn, A.F. and Santos-Sacchi, J., eds), pp. 407–427. New York: Raven Press.

# 16

# Trigeminal and facial nerves

Although the principal territory of the trigeminal and facial nerves is the splanchnocranium, i.e. the 'visceral' tissues related to the facial skeleton, the two nerves have little in common. The trigeminal supplies the muscles used in eating whereas the facial supplies the mimetic muscles, so named because they mirror the emotional state. Also, the trigeminal supplies the skin of the face whereas the cutaneous element of the facial nerve is minute, being confined to the outer ear canal.

## TRIGEMINAL NERVE

The trigeminal nerve has a very large sensory territory which includes the skin of the face, the oronasal mucous membranes and the teeth, the dura mater and major intracranial blood vessels. The nerve is also both motor and sensory to the muscles of mastication. The **motor root** lies medial to the large **sensory root** at the site of attachment to the pons. The **trigeminal** (Gasserian) **ganglion,** near the apex of the petrous temporal bone, gives rise to the sensory root and consists of unipolar neurons.

Details of the distribution of the ophthalmic, maxillary, and mandibular divisions are available in gross anatomy textbooks. Accurate appreciation of their respective territories on the face is essential if *trigeminal neuralgia* is to be distinguished from other forms of facial pain (Panel 16.1).

## Motor nucleus of the V nerve *(Figure 16.1)*

The motor nucleus is the special visceral nucleus supplying the muscles derived from the embryonic mandibular arch. These comprise the masticatory muscles attached to each half of the mandible (*Figure 16.2*), along with the tensor tympani and tensor palati. The nucleus occupies the lateral pontine tegmentum. Embedded in its upper pole is a node of the reticular formation, the *supratrigeminal nucleus*, which acts as a pattern generator for masticatory rhythm.

Voluntary control is provided for by corticonuclear projections from each motor cortex to both motor nuclei.

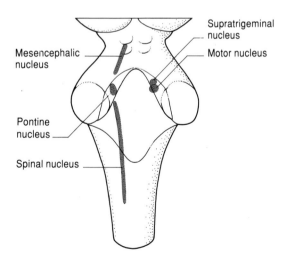

**Figure 16.1.** Trigeminal nuclei. *Left:* sensory nuclei; *right:* motor nucleus, supratrigeminal nucleus.

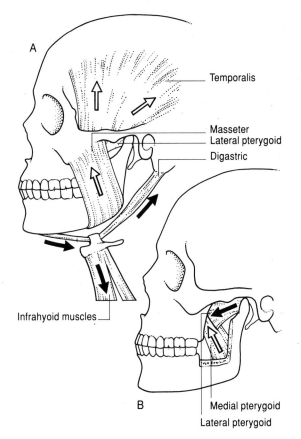

**Figure 16.2.** (A) Masticatory and infrahyoid muscles viewed from the left side; (B) medial view of the pterygoid muscles of the right side. Clear arrows indicate directions of pull of jaw-closing muscles. Black arrows indicate directions of pull of jaw openers.

### *Sensory nuclei of the V nerve*

Three sensory nuclei are associated with the trigeminal nerve: **mesencephalic, pontine,** and **spinal.**

### Mesencephalic nucleus

The mesencephalic nucleus is unique in being the only nucleus in the CNS that is composed of unipolar neurons. In humans their peripheral processes enter the sensory root via the *mesencephalic tract* of the trigeminal. Some travel in the mandibular division to supply stretch receptors (neuromuscular spindles) in the masticatory muscles. Others travel in the maxillary and mandibular divisions to supply stretch receptors (Ruffini endings) in the periodontal ligaments of the teeth.

The central processes of the mesencephalic afferent neurons descend through the pontine tegmentum in the small *tract of Probst.* Most fibers of this tract terminate in the supratrigeminal nucleus; others end in the motor nucleus or in the pontine sensory nucleus; a few travel as far as the dorsal nucleus of the vagus.

### Pontine nucleus

The pontine nucleus is homologous with the posterior column nuclei (gracilis and cuneatus). It processes discriminative tactile information from the skin of the face.

### Spinal nucleus

The spinal nucleus is so called because its caudal end is continuous with the posterior gray horn of the spinal cord. It extends from the lower part of the pons to the third cervical segment of the spinal cord.

Two minor nuclei in its upper part (called pars oralis and pars interpolaris) receive afferents from the mouth. The main spinal nucleus (called pars caudalis) receives tactile, nociceptive, and thermal information from the entire trigeminal area, and even beyond.

In section, the main spinal nucleus is seen to be an expanded continuation of the outer laminae (I–III) of the posterior horn of the cord (*Figure 16.3*). The inner three laminae (IV–VI) are relatively compressed. Laminae III and IV are referred to as the magnocellular part of the nucleus.

In animals, nociceptive-specific neurons are found in lamina I. 'Polymodal' neurons are found in the magnocellular nucleus and probably correspond to lamina V neurons of the spinal cord; they respond to tactile stimuli applied to the trigeminal skin as well as to noxious mechanical stimuli (pinching the skin with a forceps). The two sets of neurons mentioned give rise to the caudal part of the trigeminothalamic tract. Whereas the nociceptive-specific neurons have small receptive fields confined to one territory (a patch of skin or mucous membrane), many of the polymodal neurons show the phenomenon of *convergence* to a marked degree. In anesthetized animals, a single neuron may be responsive to noxious stimuli applied to a tooth, to facial skin, and to the temporomandibular joint. This finding provides a plau-

## CLINICAL PANEL 16.1 ● TRIGEMINAL NEURALGIA

*Trigeminal neuralgia* is an important condition, characterized by attacks of excruciating pain in the territory of one or more divisions of the trigeminal nerve. The patient (who is usually more than 60 years old) is able to map out the affected division(s) accurately. Because the condition has to be distinguished from many other causes of facial pain, the clinician should be able to mark out a trigeminal sensory map (see *Figure CP 16.1.1*). Sometimes there is an underlying osteitis of the petrous temporal bone, or compression of the sensory root by an arterial loop, but usually no explanation is found.

Most patients respond well to drug therapy. For those who do not, the usual practice is to carry out electrocoagulation of the affected division, through a needle electrode inserted through the foramen ovale from below. The intention is to heat the nerve sufficiently to destroy only the finest fibers, in which case analgesia is produced but touch (including the corneal reflex) is preserved. An alternative procedure is *medullary tractotomy:* the spinal root is

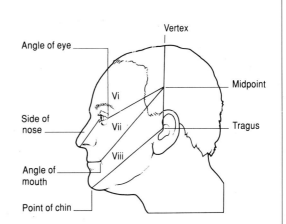

**Figure CP 16.1.1.** Five lines used to delineate the divisions of the trigeminal nerve on the face.

sectioned through the dorsolateral surface of the medulla. In successful cases, pain and temperature sensitivity is lost from the face but touch (mediated by the pontine nucleus) is preserved.

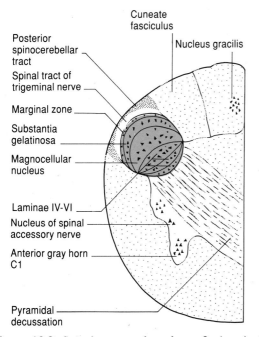

**Figure 16.3.** Spinal tract and nucleus of trigeminal nerve, at level of spinomedullary junction.

sible basis of explanation for erroneous localization of pain by patients. Examples are given in Panel 16.2.

Arrangements for pain modulation appear to be the same as for the spinal cord (see Chapter 18). They include the presence of enkephalinergic and GABAergic internuncials in the substantia gelatinosa, and aminergic projections from the nucleus raphe magnus (partly serotonergic) and the locus ceruleus (noradrenergic).

Afferents to the spinal nucleus come from three sources (*Figure 16.4*):

1. Trigeminal afferents are the central processes of Gasserian ganglion cells. The peripheral processes terminate in tactile and nociceptive endings in the territory of the three divisions of the nerve. Most often involved clinically are the nociceptive terminals in (a) the teeth, (b) the cornea, (c) the temporomandibular joint, and (d) the dura mater of the anterior and middle cranial fossae. Topographic representation of the trigeminal territory is onion-like (*Figure 16.5*); the mandibular fibers terminate in the

---

### CLINICAL PANEL 16.2 ● REFERRED PAIN IN DISEASES OF THE HEAD AND NECK

#### Cervical headache

Experiments in healthy volunteers have demonstrated that noxious stimulation of tissues supplied by the upper three cervical nerves may induce pain referred to the head. Tissues tested include the ligaments of the upper cervical joints, the suboccipital muscles, and the sternomastoid and trapezius. The pain is primarily occipital, as would be expected from the cutaneous distribution of nerves C2 and C3, but it may radiate to the forehead. A common source of cervical headache in the elderly is *spondylosis*, a degenerative arthritis in which bony excrescences compress the emerging spinal nerves (Chapter 10). Another source appears to be myofascial disease of the sternomastoid–trapezius continuum close to the base of the skull. *Trigger points*—tender nodules within the muscles which give rise to occipital pain when compressed—are often detected by physical therapists during palpation of these muscles.

#### Earache

Earache is most often due to an acute infection of the outer ear canal or middle ear. However, pain may be *referred* to a perfectly healthy ear from a variety of sources. The outer ear skin receives small sensory branches from the mandibular, facial, vagus, and upper cervical nerves; the middle ear epithelium is supplied by the glossopharyngeal and vagus. Earache may be a leading symptom of disease in the territory of one of these nerves. Important examples include:

- Cancer of the pharynx—perhaps concealed in the piriform fossa beside the larynx, or near the tonsil.
- An impacted wisdom tooth in the mandible.
- Temporomandibular joint disease.
- Spondylosis of the upper cervical spine.

#### Pain in the face

Important causes of pain referred to the face below the eye include:

- Dental caries or an impacted wisdom tooth in the upper jaw.
- Cancer in a mucous membrane supplied by the maxillary nerve: maxillary air sinus, nasal cavity, nasopharynx.
- Acute maxillary sinusitis.
- Trigeminal neuralgia affecting the maxillary nerve.

---

rostral part of the nucleus, the maxillary fibers in the midregion, and the ophthalmic fibers caudally.

2. Cervical afferents come from the territory of the first three cervical posterior nerve roots. (The first posterior nerve root is either small or absent.) Most often involved clinically are nociceptive fibers supplying (a) the intervertebral joints and spinal dura mater, and (b) the dura mater of the posterior cranial fossa, reached by cervical fibers ascending through the hypoglossal canal.

3. Nociceptive afferents from the mucous membranes of the pharyngotympanic tube, middle ear, pharynx and larynx. These afferents are often involved in acute inflammatory processes during wintertime. Their cell bodies occupy the sensory ganglia of the glossopharyngeal and vagus nerves.

#### Innervation of the teeth

From the superior and inferior alveolar nerves, A$\delta$ and C fibers enter the root canals of the teeth and form a dense plexus within the pulp. Individual fibers terminate in the pulp, in the predentin, and in dentinal tubules. Most dentinal tubules underlying the occlusal surfaces of the teeth contain single nerve fibers; however, the fibers are restricted to the inner ends of the tubules whereas pain can be elicited from the outer surface of dentin after removal of the enamel. Hydrodynamic and chemical factors have been invoked to fill the gap, as well as possible participation of odontoblasts as intermediaries.

The periodontal ligaments are richly innervated by the nerves supplying the oral epithelium including the gums. Some of the nerve endings are a potential source of pain during dental extraction

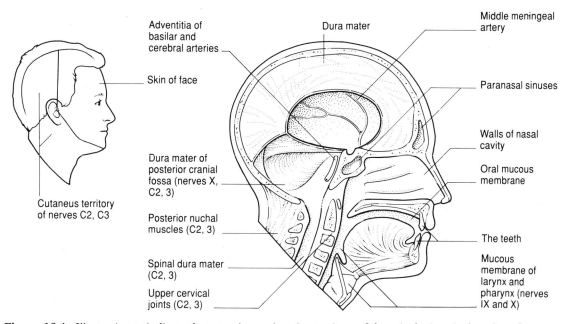

**Figure 16.4.** Illustration to indicate the extensive nociceptive territory of the spinal trigeminal nucleus. Structures labeled without qualification are supplied directly by the trigeminal nerve. The remainder are supplied by other nerves having central nociceptive projections to the spinal trigeminal nucleus.

or periodontal disease. Others function as tension receptors comparable to Ruffini endings found in joint capsules; tension receptors would be anticipated because the ligaments are arranged like hammocks around the roots of the teeth.

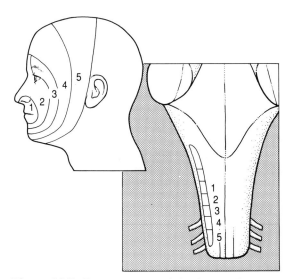

**Figure 16.5.** Representation of the face in the spinal trigeminal nucleus. (Adapted from Sears and Franklin (1980).)

### Innervation of cerebral arteries

The ophthalmic divison of the trigeminal comes close to the internal carotid artery in the cavernous sinus. Here it gives off afferent fibers which accompany the artery to its point of bifurcation into anterior and middle cerebral branches. The nerve fibers accompany these, and also reach the posterior cerebral artery. Several peptide substances have been detected in these axons; they include substance P, the peptide particularly associated with nociceptive transmission.

The function of the *trigeminovascular neurons* (as they are called) is the subject of speculation. Their presence accounts well for the *frontal headache* associated with distortion of the cerebral arteries by space-occupying lesions.

### Trigeminothalamic tract (Figure 16.6)

The *trigeminothalamic tract* originates in the supratrigeminal, pontine, and spinal trigeminal nuclei. Nearly all of its fibers cross the midline before ascending to the ventral posterior nucleus of the thalamus. The tract has features in common with the medial lemniscus (it mediates conscious proprioception and discriminative touch) and the

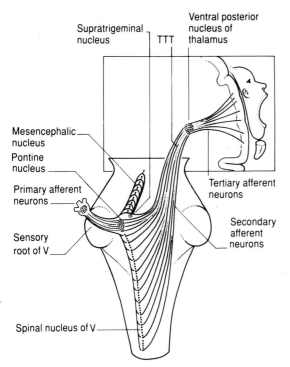

**Figure 16.6.** Primary, secondary, and tertiary trigeminal afferents. TTT, trigeminal tract.

spinal lemniscus (it mediates tactile, nociceptive, and thermal sense). At the level of the midbrain, it is also called the **trigeminal lemniscus.**

From the thalamus, third-order afferents project to the large area of facial representation in the lower half of the somatic sensory cortex.

*Trigeminoreticular* fibers synapse in the parvocellular reticular formation on both sides of the brainstem. They are counterparts of the spinoreticular tract, and they mediate the *arousal* effect of stroking or slapping the face, and of the old-fashioned 'smelling salts' (the ammonia irritates trigeminal afferents in the nose).

### *Mastication*

Mastication is a complex activity requiring orchestration of the nuclear groups supplying the muscles that move the mandible, tongue, cheeks and hyoid bone. The chief controling center seems to be an area of the premotor cortex directly in front of the face representation on the motor cortex. Stimulation of this area produces masticatory cycles.

Brainstem control of mandibular activity resides in the *supratrigeminal nucleus*, which functions as a pattern generator. The supratrigeminal nucleus receives proprioceptive information from the spindle-rich jaw closing muscles (masseter, temporalis, medial pterygoid) and from the periodontal ligaments. The supratrigeminal nucleus also receives tactile information (food in the mouth) from the pontine nucleus, and nociceptive information from the spinal nucleus. It gives rise to an ipsilateral trigeminocerebellar projection and a contralateral trigeminothalamic projection, both of which contain proprioceptive information. It controls mastication directly by means of excitatory and inhibitory inputs to the trigeminal motor nucleus.

The *jaw-closing reflex* is initiated by contact of food with the oral mucous membrane. The response of the pattern generator is to activate the jaw-closing motoneurons so that the teeth are brought into occlusion.

The *jaw-opening reflex* is initiated by periodontal stretch afferents activated by dental occlusion. The pattern generator responds by inhibiting the closure motoneurons and activating the jaw openers. Muscle spindles are especially numerous in the anterior part of the masseter, and when stretch reaches a critical level the pattern generator is switched to a jaw-closing mode.

### The jaw jerk

The *jaw jerk* is a tendon reflex elicited by tapping the chin with a downward stroke. The normal response is a twitch of the jaw-closing muscles, because muscle spindle afferents make some direct synaptic contacts upon trigeminal motoneurons. Supranuclear lesions of the motor nucleus (e.g. pseudobulbar palsy, Chapter 14) may be accompanied by an 'exaggerated' (abnormally brisk) jaw jerk.

The supratrigeminal nucleus is seldom dormant. In the erect posture, it activates the jaw closers to keep the mandible elevated. During sleep, it activates the lateral pterygoid so that the pharynx is not occluded by the tongue. (The root of the tongue is anchored to the mandible.) However, the nucleus is *inactivated by general anesthetics,* in which circumstance the ramus of the mandible must be held forward constantly in order to prevent choking.

## FACIAL NERVE

The facial (7th cranial) is the nerve of supply to the second branchial arch. *The facial nerve proper* supplies the muscles of facial expression, as well as the stapedius, stylohyoid, and posterior digastric. Accompanying the facial nerve proper for part of its course is the *nervus intermedius* which supplies secretomotor fibers to glands in the eye, nose and mouth, and taste fibers to the tongue and palate.

The facial nerve is of clinical importance in being the most frequently paralyzed of all the peripheral nerves.

### *Facial nerve proper*

The *facial nerve proper* arises from the branchial (special visceral) efferent cell column caudal to the motor nucleus of the trigeminal. The *facial motor nucleus* occupies the lateral region of the tegmentum in the caudal part of the pons (*Figure 16.7*). Before emerging from the brainstem, the nerve loops around the abducens nucleus, creating the **facial colliculus** in the floor of the fourth ventricle (Chapter 13).

The facial nerve emerges at the lower border of the pons together with the nervus intermedius. The two nerves cross the subarachnoid space in company with the vestibulocochlear nerve to reach the internal acoustic meatus. The facial nerve enters a narrow bony canal above the vestibule of the labyrinth, bends backward at the **genu**, and descends to the stylomastoid foramen in the interval between the middle ear and the mastoid process. In this interval, it supplies the stapedius muscle.

Upon leaving the skull, the facial nerve supplies the posterior belly of the occipitofrontalis, the stylohyoid, and the posterior belly of the digastric. It then turns forward within the substance of the parotid gland and breaks up into the five named branches which supply the muscles of facial expression (*Figure 16.8*).

### Supranuclear connections

All of the cells of the main motor nucleus receive a corticonuclear supply from the 'face' area of the contralateral motor cortex. In addition, the cells supplying the muscles of the upper face (occipitofrontalis and orbicularis oculi) receive an equal supply from the *ipsilateral* motor cortex. The bilateral supply for the upper facial muscles is reflected in their normally paired activities in wrinkling the

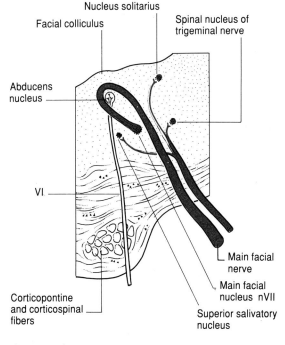

**Figure 16.7.** Transverse section of the pons showing components of the facial nerve and of the nervus intermedius.

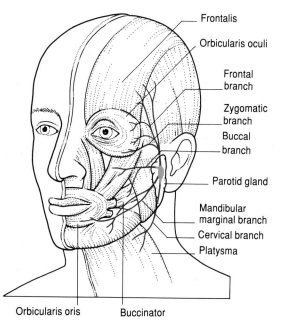

**Figure 16.8.** Principal extracranial branches of the facial nerve.

## CLINICAL PANEL 16.3 • LESIONS OF THE FACIAL NERVE

### Supranuclear lesions

Much the commonest cause of a supranuclear lesion of the seventh nerve is a vascular *stroke*, in which corticonuclear and corticospinal fibers are interrupted at the level of the internal capsule or cerebral cortex. The usual effect of a stroke is to produce a contralateral motor weakness of the *lower* part of the face and of the limbs. The upper face escapes because of the bilateral supranuclear supply to the upper part of the facial nucleus.

### Nuclear lesions

The main motor nucleus may be involved in thrombosis of one of the pontine branches of the basilar artery. As might be anticipated from the relationships depicted in *Figure 16.7*, the usual result of such a lesion is an *alternating hemiplegia:* complete paralysis of the facial and/or abducens nerve on one side combined with motor weakness of the limbs on the opposite side.

### Infranuclear lesions

*Bell's palsy* is a common disorder caused by a neuritis (possibly viral in origin) of the facial nerve. The inflammation causes the nerve to swell, and conduction is compromised by the tight fit of the nerve in the bony canal between the geniculate ganglion and the stylomastoid foramen. There may be some initial pain in the ear, but the condition is otherwise painless.

Facial paralysis is usually complete. On the affected side the patient is unable to raise the eyebrow, close the eye, or retract the lip. Tears may spill from the lax lower eyelid, and saliva may drool from the corner of the mouth. The patient may experience *hyperacusis:* ordinary sounds may be unpleasantly loud due to loss of the damping action of the stapedius muscle.

The segment of nerve between geniculate ganglion and stylomastoid foramen is usually compromised. Tests may reveal blockage of nervus intermedius fibers on the affected side, in the form of reduced lacrimal salivary secretions and loss of taste from the anterior part of the tongue.

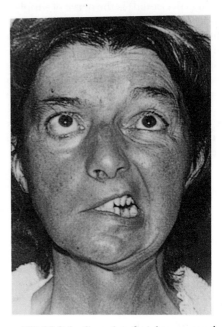

**Figure CP 16.3.1.** Complete facial nerve paralysis, patient's right side. The patient has been asked to show her teeth and to look upward. To compare the two sides, cover the left and right halves of the photograph alternately with a card. On the paralyzed side, note (paralyzed muscles in parentheses): inability to raise the eyebrow (frontalis muscle); drooping of the lower eyelid (orbicularis oculi); inability to retract the mouth (buccinator); no webbing of the neck (platysma). The patient was also unable to abduct the right eye (abducens nerve paralysis, Chapter 17). Together with a history of other disturbances, the clinical picture was suggestive of multiple sclerosis with a current patch of demyelination deep to the facial colliculus, affecting the emerging fibers of the facial and abducens nerves (cf. *Figure 16.7*). (Photograph reproduced from Parsons, M. (1987) *Diagnostic Picture Test in Clinical Neurology.* London: Wolfe Medical Publications, with the kind permission of the author and publisher.)

Four out of five cases recover completely within a few weeks because the nerve has only suffered a conduction block or *neuropraxia*. In the remainder, the nerve undergoes Wallerian degeneration (Chapter 6); recovery takes about 3 months and is often incomplete. During regeneration, some preganglionic fibers of the nervus intermedius may enter the greater petrosal nerve instead of the chorda tympani, with the result that the lacrimal gland becomes active at mealtimes (so-called 'crocodile tears').

Other causes of infranuclear palsy include a patch of demyelination in the course of multiple sclerosis (*Figure CP 16.3.1*), tumors in the cerebellopontine angle (Panel 16.4), middle ear disease, and tumors of the parotid gland. *Herpes zoster oticus* is a rare but well recognized viral infection of the geniculate ganglion. Severe pain in one ear precedes the appearance of a vesicular rash in and around the external acoustic meatus. Swelling of the geniculate ganglion may be sufficient to cause a complete facial palsy (Ramsay Hunt syndrome).

forehead, or blinking, or squeezing the eyes shut. The muscles around the mouth, in contrast, can be activated discretely. The partial bilateral supply helps to distinguish a supranuclear from a nuclear or infranuclear lesion of the facial nerve (Panel 16.3).

More than any other muscle group, the muscles of facial expression are responsive to emotional states. A *limbic* contribution to the supranuclear supply is to be expected, and its most likely source is the **nucleus accumbens** at the base of the forebrain. The nucleus accumbens is linked to ventral parts of the basal ganglia, which in turn influence the motor cortex (Chapter 24). That circuit is compromised in Parkinson's disease, which is characterized by a mask-like, emotionless demeanor.

## Nuclear connections

Five *reflex arcs* involving the facial nucleus are listed in Table 16.1. Most important clinically is the corneal reflex.

### CORNEAL REFLEX

The usual test is to touch the cornea with a cotton wisp. This should elicit a bilateral blink response. The afferent limb of the reflex is the ophthalmic division of the trigeminal nerve (nasociliary branch). The efferent limb is the facial nerve (branch to palpebral element of orbicularis oculi). Since the reflex can still be elicited following section of the spinal tract of the trigeminal nerve (tractotomy operation), internuncials projecting from the pontine nucleus to both facial nuclei must be sufficient to complete the reflex arc.

The corneal reflex may be lost following a lesion of either the ophthalmic or facial nerves. A gradual compression of ophthalmic fibers in the sensory root of the trigeminal nerve may damage corneal neurons selectively. For this reason, the corneal reflex must be tested in patients under suspicion of an acoustic neuroma (Panel 16.4).

**Table 16.1** Brainstem reflexes involving the facial nerve

|  | Corneal reflex | Sucking reflex | Blinking to light | Blinking to noise | Sound attenuation |
|---|---|---|---|---|---|
| Receptor | Cornea | Lips | Retina | Cochlea | Cochlea |
| Afferent | Ophthalmic nerve | Mandibular nerve | Optic nerve | Cochlear nucleus | Cochlear nucleus |
| First synapse | Spinal nucleus of trigeminal | Pontine nucleus of trigeminal | Superior colliculus | Inferior colliculus | Superior olivary nucleus |
| Second synapse | Facial nucleus | Facial nucleus | Facial nucleus | Facial nucleus | Facial nucleus |
| Orbicularis oculi | Orbicularis oculi | Orbicularis oculi | Orbicularis oculi | Orbicularis oculi | Stapedius |

## CLINICAL PANEL 16.4 • SYNDROMES OF THE CEREBELLOPONTINE ANGLE

The *cerebellopontine angle* is the recess between the hemisphere of the cerebellum and the lower border of the pons. The petrous temporal bone, laterally, completes a *triangle* having the fifth nerve at its upper corner and the ninth and tenth at its lower corner; the triangle is bisected by the seventh and eighth nerves (*Figure CP 16.4.1*).

Several kinds of space-occupying lesions may compromise one or more nerves in the angle. The most frequent is an *acoustic neuroma,* which is a slow-growing benign tumor of Schwann cells (a neurolemmoma). The tumor originates in the vestibular nerve within the internal acoustic meatus, but the initial symptoms are more often cochlear than vestibular. *An acoustic neuroma must be suspected in every middle-aged or elderly patient presenting with auditory or vestibular symptoms.* Early diagnosis is important because of the difficulty of removing a large neuroma extending into the posterior cranial fossa; also because the cumulative motor and sensory disturbances may not show significant improvement after surgery.

The following is a fairly typical sequence of symptoms and signs in a case escaping early detection:

- *Tinnitus* is experienced on the affected side, in the form of a high-pitched ringing or fizzing sound.
- *Deafness* on the affected side is slowly progressive over a period of months or years.
- *Vertigo* occurs episodically. Severe vertigo with nystagmus signifies compression of the brainstem.
- *Loss of the corneal reflex* is an early sign of distortion of the fifth nerve by a tumor emerging from the internal acoustic meatus into the posterior cranial fossa.
- *Weakness of the masticatory muscles* is a later sign of trigeminal nerve involvement. The jaw deviates toward the affected side when the mouth is opened, because the normal lateral pterygoid is unopposed. Wasting of the masseter may be obvious on palpation of the cheek.
- *Weakness of the facial musculature* develops as the seventh nerve becomes stretched.
- *Anesthesia of the oropharynx* signifies involvement of the ninth nerve.
- *Ipsilateral 'cerebellar signs'* in the arm and leg appear when the cerebellum is compressed.
- *'Upper motor neuron signs'* in the limbs signify compression of the brainstem.
- *Signs of raised intracranial pressure* (headache, drowsiness, papilledema) signify obstruction of cerebrospinal fluid circulation either inside or around the brainstem.

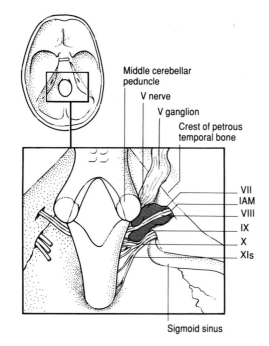

Middle cerebellar peduncle
V nerve
V ganglion
Crest of petrous temporal bone

VII
IAM
VIII
IX
X
XIs

Sigmoid sinus

**Figure CP 16.4.1.** An acoustic neuroma invading the right posterior cranial fossa. XIs, spinal XI nerve.

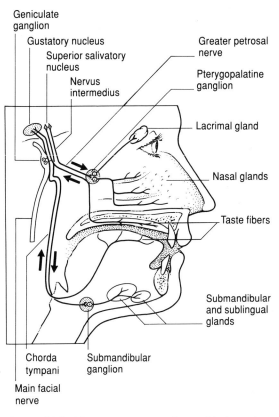

Geniculate ganglion
Gustatory nucleus
Superior salivatory nucleus
Nervus intermedius
Greater petrosal nerve
Pterygopalatine ganglion
Lacrimal gland
Nasal glands
Taste fibers
Submandibular and sublingual glands
Chorda tympani
Submandibular ganglion
Main facial nerve

**Figure 16.9.** The nervus intermedius and its branches. Arrows indicate direction of impulse traffic.

### Nervus intermedius

The *nervus intermedius* enters the facial nerve proximal to the genu. It contains two sets of parasympathetic fibers and two sets of special sense fibers (*Figure 16.9*).

The *parasympathetic root* of the nerve arises from the **superior salivatory nucleus** in the pons. It forms the motor component of the greater petrosal and chorda tympani nerves. The greater petrosal fibers synapse in the pterygopalatine ganglion whose postganglionic fibers supply the lacrimal and nasal glands. The chorda tympani fibers synapse in the **submandibular ganglion** whose postganglionic fibers supply the submandibular and sublingual glands.

The *special sense root* of the nerve has unipolar cell bodies in the **geniculate ganglion** of the facial nerve. The peripheral processes of the ganglion cells supply taste buds in the palate via the great petrosal nerve, and taste buds in the anterior two-thirds of the tongue via the chorda tympani. The central processes enter the gustatory nucleus, which also receives fibers from the glossopharyngeal nerve (Chapter 14). From here, second-order neurons accompany the contralateral medial lemniscus. One cortical locus for taste is adjacent to the tongue area in the postcentral gyrus; another is in the insula.

A few cells of the geniculate ganglion supply skin in and around the external acoustic meatus.

### REFERENCES

### Trigeminal nerve

Bogduk, N., Corrigan, B., Kelly, P., Schneider, G. and Farr, R. (1985) Cervical headache. *Aust. J. Med.* **143:** 202–207.

Dubner, R., Sharav, Y., Gracely, R.H. and Price, D.D. (1987) Idiopathic trigeminal neuralgia: sensory features and pain mechanisms. *Pain* **31:** 23–33.

Sears, E.S. and Franklin, G.M. (1980) Diseases of the cranial nerves. In *Neurology* (Rosenberg, R.N., ed.), pp. 471–494. New York: Grune & Stratton.

Sessle, B.J. (1990) Anatomy, physiology and pathophysiology of orofacial pain. In *Headache and Facial Pain* (Jacobson, A.L. and Donlon, W.C., eds), pp. 1–24. New York: Raven Press.

Yokota, T. (1988) Anatomy and physiology of intra- and extracranial nociceptive afferents and their central projections. In *Basic Mechanisms of Headache* (Olesen, J. and Edvinsson, L., eds), pp. 117–128. Amsterdam: Elsevier.

### Facial nerve

Lang, J. (1984) Clinical anatomy of the cerebellopontine angle and internal acoustic meatus. *Adv. Oto-Rhino-Laryng.* **34:** 8–24.

Manni, J.J. and Stennert, E. (1984) Diagnostic methods in facial nerve pathology. *Adv. Oto-Rhino-Laryng.* **34:** 202–213.

Parnes, S. M. (1988) The facial nerve. In *Physiology of the Ear* (Jahn, A.F. and Santos-Sacchi, J., eds), pp. 125–142. New York: Raven Press.

# 17

# Ocular motor nerves

The eyes have a large repertoire of movements, all of them concerned with 'fixation'. When an object is fixated, the light reflected from its center impinges on the fovea centralis of the retina, the point of most acute vision.

Since the two eyes always move together, appropriate sets of ocular motoneurons on both sides must be picked out simultaneously by the premotor controling centers. Different premotor centers are dominant for different kinds of ocular movement. For example, the automatic scanning of a piece of text has a control quite different to that used to track a fly moving across the page.

As well as the extraocular muscles, the eye possesses intrinsic, smooth muscles that regulate the size of the pupil and the thickness of the lens. The smooth muscles are controlled by the sympathetic and parasympathetic systems, as outlined in Chapter 9.

Because of the immense diagnostic and therapeutic importance of ocular innervation, and because of the complexity of the subject when considered in detail, neurophthalmology has become a branch of medicine in its own right.

## INTRODUCTION

The ocular motor nerves comprise the oculomotor (3rd cranial), trochlear (4th cranial) and abducens (6th cranial) nerves. They provide the motor nerve supply to the four recti and two oblique muscles controling movements of the eyeball on each side (*Figure 17.1*). The oculomotor nerve contains two additional sets of neurons: one to supply the levator of the upper eyelid, the other to control the sphincter of the pupil and the ciliary muscle.

The nuclei serving the extraocular muscles (extrinsic muscles of the eye) belong to the somatic efferent cell column of the brainstem, in line with the nucleus of the hypoglossal nerve. The oculomotor nucleus has an additional, parasympathetic nucleus which belongs to the general visceral efferent cell column.

### Oculomotor nerve

The nucleus of the third nerve is at the level of the superior colliculi. It is partly embedded in the periaqueductal gray matter (*Figure 17.2A*). It is composed of five individual nuclei for the supply of striated muscles, and one parasympathetic nucleus.

The nerve passes through the tegmentum of the midbrain and emerges into the interpeduncular

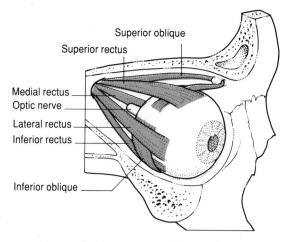

**Figure 17.1.** Extrinsic ocular muscles.

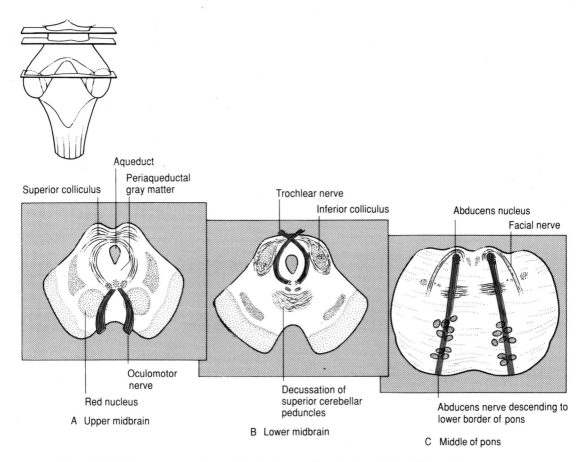

Aqueduct

Periaqueductal
gray matter

Superior colliculus

Trochlear nerve

Inferior colliculus

Abducens nucleus

Facial nerve

Oculomotor
nerve

Red nucleus

A  Upper midbrain

Decussation of
superior cerebellar
peduncles

B  Lower midbrain

Abducens nerve descending to
lower border of pons

C  Middle of pons

**Figure 17.2.** Transverse sections of the brainstem showing the origins of the ocular motor nerves.

arachnoid cistern. It crosses the apex of the petrous temporal bone, pierces the dural roof of the cavernous sinus, runs in the lateral wall of the sinus and breaks into upper and lower divisions within the superior orbital fissure. The upper division supplies the superior rectus and the levator palpebrae superioris; the lower division supplies the inferior and medial recti and the inferior oblique.

The parasympathetic fibers originate in the *Edinger–Westphal* nucleus. They accompany the main nerve as far as the orbit, then leave the branch to the inferior oblique and synapse in the **ciliary ganglion.** Postganglionic fibers emerge from the ganglion in the **short ciliary nerves,** which pierce the lamina cribrosa ('sieve-like layer') of the sclera and supply the *ciliaris* and *sphincter pupillae.*

### Trochlear nerve

The nucleus of the fourth nerve is at the level of the inferior colliculus. The nerve itself is unique in two respects (*Figure 17.2B*): it is the only nerve to emerge from the back of the brainstem; and it crosses the midline.

The trochlear nerve winds around the crus of the midbrain and travels through the cavernous sinus in company with the third nerve (*Figure 17.3*). It passes through the superior orbital fissure and supplies the superior oblique muscle.

### Abducens nerve

The nucleus of the sixth nerve is at the level of the facial colliculus, in the middle of the pons (*Figure*

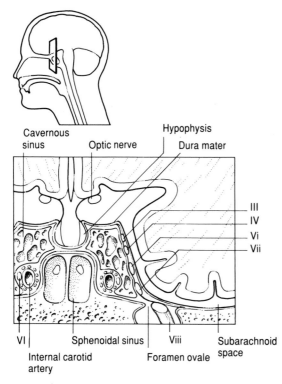

Cavernous sinus

Optic nerve

Hypophysis

Dura mater

III
IV
Vi
Vii

VI

Sphenoidal sinus

Viii

Foramen ovale

Subarachnoid space

Internal carotid artery

**Figure 17.3.** Coronal section of the cavernous sinus and related structures. III, oculomotor nerve; IV, trochlear nerve; VI, abducent nerve; Vi, Vii, Viii, ophthalmic, maxillary, mandibular divisions of trigeminal nerve.

*17.2C).* The nerve emerges at the lower border of the pons and runs up the pontine subarachnoid cistern, beside the basilar artery. It angles over the apex of the petrous temporal bone and passes through the cavernous sinus beside the internal carotid artery (*Figure 17.3*). It enters the orbit through the superior orbital fissure and supplies the lateral rectus, which abducts the eye.

### Nerve endings

#### Motor endings

All of the ocular motor units are small, containing 5–10 muscles fibers apiece (compared with 1000 or more in the tibialis anterior). Three categories have been described for human extraocular muscles:

- Type A: large-diameter muscle fibers having single motor end plates

- Type B: intermediate-diameter muscle fibers having several plates each
- Type C: small-diameter muscle fibers having numerous plates strung along them like beads.

Type A fibers produce the fast twitches required for saccadic movements. Type B are slow-twitch and may be used for smooth pursuit. Type C show only local contractions beneath the individual plates. Type C fibers may be involved in keeping the visual axes of the two eyes parallel with one another. Since the visual axes diverge following administration of muscle relaxants, keeping them parallel must require continuous muscle action, even during sleep.

### Sensory endings

In addition to neuromuscular spindles of standard type, numerous *palisade endings* exist in the form of nerve spirals around individual muscle fibers.

The extraocular muscle proprioceptors are the peripheral terminals of neurons in the mesencephalic nucleus of the trigeminal nerve. In monkeys, some of the central processes of these neurons reach as far caudally as the accessory cuneate nucleus in the medulla oblongata. This nucleus also receives proprioceptive terminals from the neck muscles, and it projects both to the ipsilateral cerebellum and to the contralateral superior colliculus. The conjunction of ocular and cervical proprioceptive information presumably assists in the co-ordination of simultaneous movements of the eyes and head.

### *Pupillary light reflex (Figure 17.4)*

Constriction of the pupils in response to light involves four sets of neurons, as follows:

1. The afferent limb commences in the ganglionic layer of the retina, which gives rise to the optic nerve. It enters both optic tracts and terminates in the **pretectal nucleus,** situated just rostral to the superior colliculus.
2. The pretectal nucleus is linked by internuncial neurons to both Edinger–Westphal (parasympathetic) nuclei; the contralateral nucleus is reached by way of the *posterior commissure.*
3. Preganglionic parasympathetic fibers enter the oculomotor nerve, leave the branch to the inferior oblique and synapse in the ciliary ganglion.

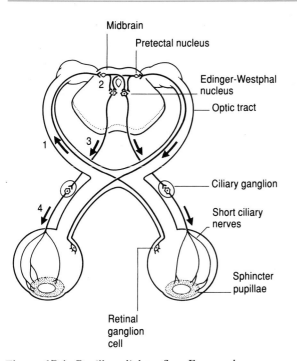

**Figure 17.4.** Pupillary light reflex. For numbers, see text.

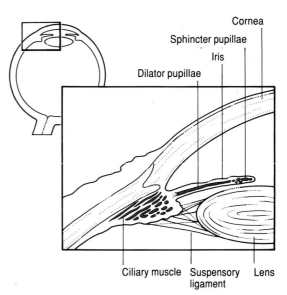

**Figure 17.5.** Intrinsic muscles of the eye.

4. Postganglionic fibers run in the short ciliary nerves and enter the iris to supply the sphincter pupillae.

## Accommodation: the near response

When the eyes view an object close up, the ciliary muscle contracts reflexly, thereby *relaxing* the suspensory ligament of the lens (*Figure 17.5*). Since the lens at rest is somewhat compressed (flattened) by tension exerted on the lens capsule by the suspensory ligament, the lens bulges passively when the ciliary muscle contracts. The thicker lens has the greater refractive power required to bring close-up objects into focus on the retina. The response of the lens is one of *accommodation*.

The *accommodation reflex*, as understood clinically, involves two other features. The sphincter pupillae contracts in order to eliminate passage of light through the peripheral, thinner part of the lens. At the same time, the visual axes of the two eyes converge, as a result of increased tone in the medial rectus muscles.

The three features described are also known as the *near response*.

## Pathway for the accommodation reflex

In order to execute the near response, a stereoscopic analysis of the object is carried out at the level of the visual association cortex. The afferent limb of the reflex passes from the retina to the occipital lobe via the lateral geniculate nucleus. The efferent limb passes from the occipital lobe to the midbrain, where some fibers activate the Edinger–Westphal nucleus and others activate *vergence cells* in the reticular formation. The vergence cells activate the nuclear groups serving the medial recti, with the effect of *fixating* the object onto the fovea centralis of each eye. The (con)vergence response is called the *fixation reflex*.

## Accommodation: the far response

Just as the state of the pupil depends upon the balance of sympathetic and parasympathetic activity, so does the state of the lens. At rest, both are in midposition. The resting focal length of the lens averages 1 meter (with considerable variation between individuals). This is because the ciliary muscle is tonically active. In order to bring a distant object into focus, the ciliary muscle must be inhibited, so that the suspensory ligament becomes taut and the lens flat. The sphincter of the pupil is inhibited as well.

The sympathetic system innervates all of the intrinsic muscles. It has a dual mode of action. It causes *contraction* of the dilator pupillae by way of *alpha* receptors on the muscle fibers, and it causes *relaxation* of the ciliary muscle and pupillary sphincter, by way of *beta* receptors. This dual effect constitutes the *far response*, and it is used to focus the eyes upon objects at a distance.

In stressed individuals, heightened sympathetic activity may interfere with the normal process of accommodation. For example, students taking an important written test may have difficulty in bringing the questions into proper focus.

### Notes on the sympathetic pathway to the eye

The great length of the sympathetic pathway is indicated in *Figure 17.6*.

1. *Central* fibers descending from the hypothalamus cross to the other side in the midbrain. In the pons and medulla they are joined by ipsilateral fibers descending from the reticular formation.
2. *Preganglionic* fibers emerge in the first thoracic ventral nerve root, and run up in the sympathetic chain to the superior cervical ganglion.
3. *Postganglionic* fibers run along the external and internal carotid arteries and their branches.

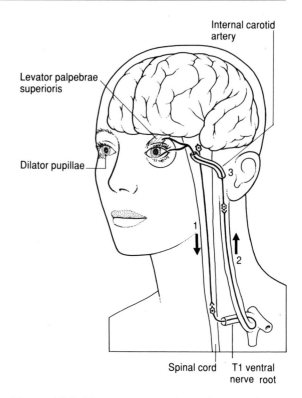

**Figure 17.6.** Three neuron pathway from the hypothalamus to the eye. Arrows indicate directions of impulse conduction. For numbers, see text.

---

### CLINICAL PANEL 17.1 • OCULAR PALSIES

One or more of the three ocular motor nerves may be paralyzed by disease within the brainstem (e.g. multiple sclerosis, vascular thrombosis), in the subarachnoid space (e.g. meningitis, aneurysm in the circle of Willis, or distortion by an expanding intracranial lesion), or in the cavernous sinus (e.g. thrombosis of the sinus, aneurysm of the internal carotid artery).

#### Oculomotor nerve

#### Complete third nerve palsy

The three characteristic signs of complete third nerve paralysis are shown in *Figure CP 17.1.1*. They are:

1. Complete ptosis of the eyelid (unopposed orbicularis oculi).

2. A fully dilated, non-reactive pupil (unopposed dilator pupillae).
3. A fully abducted eye (unopposed lateral rectus), which is also depressed (unopposed superior oblique).

#### Partial third nerve palsy

The pupils are *always* monitored when cases of head injury come to medical attention. Rapidly increasing intracranial pressure, resulting from an acute extradural or subdural hematoma (Chapter 4), often compresses the third nerve on the crest of the petrous temporal bone. The autonomic fibers are superficially placed and are the first to suffer, and the pupil dilates progressively on the affected side. *Pupillary dila-*

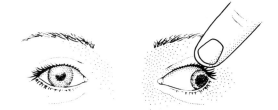

**Figure CP 17.1.1.** Complete third nerve paralysis. The closed eyelid has been raised by the examiner's finger.

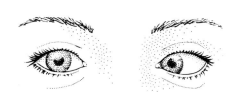

**Figure CP 17.1.2.** Complete left sixth nerve paralysis.

*tation is an urgent indication for surgical decompression of the brain.*

### Trochlear nerve

The fourth nerve is rarely paralyzed alone. The cardinal symptom is diplopia (double vision) on looking down, for example when going down stairs. This happens because the superior rectus normally assists the inferior oblique in pulling the eye downward, especially when the eye is in a medial position.

### Abducens nerve

The effect of a *complete* sixth nerve paralysis is shown in *Figure CP 17.1.2*. The eye is fully adducted by the unopposed pull of the medial rectus.

The abducens has the longest course in the subarachnoid space of any cranial nerve. It also bends sharply over the crest of the petrous temporal bone. A space-occupying lesion affecting *either* cerebral hemisphere may cause compression and paralysis of the nerve.

'Spontaneous' paralysis of the sixth nerve may be caused by an arterial aneurysm at the base of the brain or by hardening (atherosclerosis) of the internal carotid artery in the cavernous sinus.

### Ocular sympathetic supply

Any one of the three sequential sets of neurons depicted in *Figure 17.6* may be interrupted by local pathology.

1. The *central* set may be interrupted by a vascular lesion of the pons or medulla oblongata. The usual picture is one of Horner's syndrome (ptosis and miosis, as described in Chapter 9) and cranial nerve involvement on one side, together with motor weakness and/or sensory loss in the limbs on the contralateral side. The Horner's syndrome is associated with *anhidrosis*—absence of sweating—in the face and scalp on the same side, together with congestion of the nose (engorged turbinates).
2. The *preganglionic* set is most often interrupted by stony, cancerous deep cervical lymph nodes in the lower part of the neck. A Horner's syndrome is associated with anhidrosis of the face and scalp (and nasal congestion) on the same side.
3. The *postganglionic* set accompanying the *external* carotid artery is rarely damaged directly. The set accompanying the *internal* carotid artery may be interrupted as part of a jugular foramen syndrome (Chapter 14), or by pathology in the cavernous sinus. Horner's syndrome is accompanied by anhidrosis of the forehead and anterior scalp (territory of the supraorbital and supratrochlear arteries).

The *external* carotid sympathetic fibers accompany all of the branches of the external carotid artery. Those accompanying the facial artery supply the arterioles of the cheek and lips and are particularly responsive to emotional states. Those accompanying the maxillary artery supply the cavernous tissue covering the nasal conchae (turbinate bones).

Two sets of sympathetic fibers accompany the *internal* carotid artery. One set joins the ophthalmic division of the fifth nerve in the cavernous sinus, leaves it in the long and short ciliary nerves, and supplies the vessels and smooth muscles of the eyeball. The second set forms a plexus around the internal carotid artery and its branches including the ophthalmic artery. The ophthalmic artery gives off supratrochlear and supraorbital branches which carry sympathetic fibers to the skin of the forehead and scalp.

Interruption of the postganglionic fibers at the jugular foramen (see jugular foramen syndrome, Chapter 14) or in the cavernous sinus produces *anhidrosis* (loss of sweating) on the forehead and scalp.

## Ocular palsies

The effects of paralysis of the motor nerves to the eye are described in Panel 17.1.

## CONTROL OF EYE MOVEMENTS

The eyes normally move as a pair. This *conjugate* movement is of three fundamentally different kinds, as follows:

1. *Scanning.* The eyes flick from one visual target to another, in high-speed movements called *saccades.*
2. *Tracking.* In tracking, or *smooth pursuit,* the eyes follow an object of interest across the visual field.
3. *Compensation.* The gaze can be held on an object of interest during movements of the head. This is the vestibulo-ocular or *fixation* reflex, which depends upon displacement of endolymph in the kinetic labyrinth.

## Scanning

Four separate *gaze centers* in the brainstem pick out motoneurons appropriate to the direction of movement: leftward, rightward, upward, or downward. The centers are small nodes in the reticular formation. They contain *burst cells,* which discharge at 1000 Hz (impulses/second) and entrain the appropriate motoneurons momentarily at this rate.

The paired centers (left and right) for horizontal saccades are in the paramedian pontine reticular formation; hence the designation, PPRF. Each pulls the eyes to its own side (*Figure 17.7*). The midbrain contains a bilateral center for upward saccades located in the rostral end of the medial longitudinal fasciculus (MLF), at the level of the pretectal nucleus. It is called the *rostral interstitial nucleus* (riMLF). At the same level but a little ventral to this is a bilateral center for downward gaze.

*Automatic* scanning movements are activated by the superior colliculus, on receipt of visual information from the retina through the medial root of the optic tract. Examples of automatic scanning include the sideward glance toward an object attracting attention in the peripheral visual field,

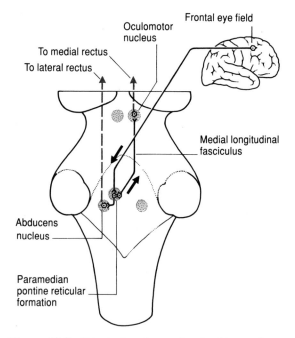

**Figure 17.7.** Principal pathways involved in a voluntary ocular saccade to the left.

and the saccadic movements used in reading. The projections cross the midline before proceeding to the gaze centers.

*Voluntary* scanning movements are initiated in the *frontal eye fields*, directly in front of the premotor cortex. From each frontal eye field, a projection descends in the anterior limb of the internal capsule. *Most* of the fibers cross over before terminating in the gaze centers.

As explained in Chapter 24, the ipsilateral superior colliculus is activated at the same time, to reinforce the excitation of the appropriate gaze center.

The projection from the frontal eye field is interrupted in about one-third of patients who suffer a stroke involving the internal capsule. The result is *paralysis of contraversive horizontal gaze*. 'Contraversive' refers to an inability to make a voluntary saccade away from the side of the lesion. The gaze paralysis vanishes within a week, even if the hemiplegia remains profound—presumably because of takeover by uncrossed fibers.

The frontal eye field appears to inhibit the ipsilateral collicular neurons during voluntary saccades, by way of a direct corticicollicular projection onto inhibitory internuncials. As well, it seems to have a permissive function for automatic saccades, by releasing the collicular neurons from a tonic inhibition that governs it in the intervals between saccades. The permissive pathway passes through the basal ganglia.

The best known afferents to the frontal eye field come from the parietal cortex, from cells concerned with *visual attention*. In monkeys, some cells in the posterior parietal cortex become active when an object of interest is seen. These cells project to the frontal eye field and are thought to facilitate eye movement in the direction of the object. In humans, *neglect* of the contralateral visual field is a well-known feature of damage to the posterior parietal lobe, especially on the right side (Chapter 23).

## Tracking

The neural mechanisms for tracking must be complex because of the following basic requirements: (a) intact visual pathways to monitor the position of the object throughout the movement; (b) neurons to signal the rate of movement of the object *(velocity detectors)*; (c) neurons to coordinate movements of the eyes and head *(neural integrator)*; and

(e) a system to monitor smooth execution of the tracking movement.

Monkey and cat experiments indicate the following. (a) Object position information is forwarded from the visual cortex to the posterior parietal cortex, and from there to the reticular formation of the pons. (b) Velocity detectors are present in the upper part of the pons, apparently receiving information direct from the retina via the medial root of the optic tract. (c) Head movement is signaled by the dynamic labyrinth, and is integrated with spatial and velocity information in the *nucleus prepositus hypoglossi*—a node of the reticular formation which is in fact closer to the abducens nucleus than to the hypoglossal nucleus. The nucleus prepositus projects to the paramedian pontine reticular formation (PPRF), which controls conjugate eye movements. The pathway to the neck muscles (for turning the head) may involve the superior colliculus. (d) Smooth execution of tracking movements is monitored by the flocculus of the cerebellum, which has two-way connections to the vestibular nucleus and pontine reticular formation.

## Compensation

The dynamic labyrinth and cerebellum cooperate to keep the eyes on target during movement of the head, as described in Chapter 15.

## REFERENCES

Goldberg, M.E. and Segraves, M.A. (1990) The role of the frontal eye field and its corticotectal projection in the generation of eye movements. In *Vision and the Brain* (Cohen, B. and Bodis-Wallner, I., eds), pp. 195–209. New York: Raven Press.

Keller, E.L. and Heinen, S.J. (1991) Generation of smooth pursuit eye movements: neuronal mechanisms and pathways. *Neurosci. Res.* **11**: 79–107.

Kommerell, G. (1984) Supranuclear and nuclear disorders of eye movement. In *Neuro-ophthalmology, Vol. 3* (Lessell, S. and van Dalen, J.T.W., eds), pp. 277–289. Amsterdam: Elsevier.

Miyazaki, S. (1985) Location of motoneurons in the oculomotor nucleus and the course of their axons in the oculomotor nerve. *Brain Res.* **348**: 57–63.

Oda, K. (1986) Motor innervation and acetylcholine receptor distribution of human extraocular muscle fibers. *J. Neurol. Sci.* **74**: 125–133.

Parkinson, D. (1988) Further observations on the sympathetic pathways to the pupil. *Anat. Rec.* **220**: 108–109.

# 18

# Reticular formation

**The reticular formation is a neuronal network permeating the tegmentum or core of the brainstem. It participates in a huge array of activities ranging across somatic, visceral and psychic domains.**

The reticular formation (RF) is phylogenetically a very old neural network, being a prominent feature of the reptilian brainstem. It originated as a slowly conducting, polysynaptic pathway intimately connected with olfactory and limbic regions. The progressive dominance of vision and hearing over olfaction led to lateralization of sensory and motor functions within the tectum of the midbrain. Direct spinotectal and tectospinal tracts bypassed the RF, which was largely relegated to automatic functions in relation to posture and to the autonomic system. In mammals, the tectum in turn has been relegated to minor status with the emergence of very fast pathways linking the cerebral cortex with the peripheral sensory and motor apparatus.

In the human brain, the RF continues to be of importance in relation to automatic and reflex activities, and it has retained its linkages to the limbic system.

## ORGANIZATION

### Topography

The term *reticular formation* refers only to the polysynaptic network in the brainstem, although the network continues rostrally into the thalamus and hypothalamus, and caudally into the propriospinal network of the spinal cord.

The characteristic RF neuron is *isodendritic*. The dendrites are long and branch at regular intervals. They have a predominantly transverse orientation and their interstices are penetrated by long pathways running to and from the thalamus and cerebral cortex.

The ground plan of the RF is shown in *Figure 18.1A*. In the midline is a series of **raphe nuclei** (pron. 'raffay' and derived from the Greek, *seam*). Next to this is the **magnocellular reticular formation** which, in the lower pons and upper medulla, becomes **gigantocellular** before blending with the **central reticular nucleus** of the medulla. Lateralmost is the **parvocellular reticular formation**, which extends into the midbrain. Finally, **paramedian** and **lateral reticular nuclei** in the medulla have two-way connections with the cerebellum; the latter also has connections with the spinal cord.

The parvocellular RF is a predominantly *afferent* system. It receives fibers from all of the sensory pathways, including the special senses:

- Olfactory fibers are received through the median forebrain bundle, which passes alongside the hypothalamus.
- Visual pathway fibers are received from the superior colliculus.
- Auditory pathway fibers are received from the superior olivary nucleus.
- Vestibular fibers are received from the medial vestibular nucleus.
- Somatic sensory fibers are received from the spinoreticular tracts.

Most parvocellular axons ramify extensively among the dendrites of the magnocellar RF. However, some synapse within the nuclei of cranial nerves and act as pattern generators (see later).

The magnocellular RF is a predominantly *efferent* system. The axons are relatively long. Some ascend to synapse in the midbrain RF or in the thalamus. Others have both ascending and descending branches contributing to the polysynaptic

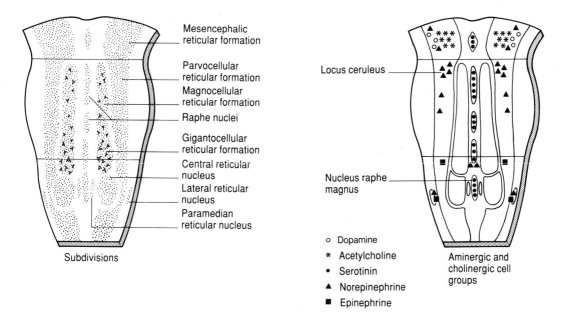

**Figure 18.1.** Reticular formation. The pons is marked off by the horizontal lines.

network. The magnocellular component receives corticoreticular fibers from the premotor cortex and gives rise to the pontine and medullary reticulospinal tracts.

### Aminergic neurons of the brainstem

Embedded in the reticular formation are sets of *aminergic neurons* (*Figure 18.1B*). They include one set producing *serotonin* (5-hydroxytryptamine) and three sets producing *catecholamines*, as listed below.

| Transmitter | Location |
|---|---|
| Serotonin | Raphe nuclei of midbrain, pons, medulla |
| Dopamine | Tegmentum of midbrain |
| Norepinephrine | Mainly pons (locus ceruleus) |
| Epinephrine | Medulla oblongata |

*The serotoninergic neurons have the largest territorial distribution of any set of CNS neurons.* In general, those of the midbrain project rostrally into the cerebral hemispheres; those of the pons ramify in the brainstem and cerebellum; and those of the medulla supply the spinal cord (*Figure 18.2A*). All parts of the CNS gray matter are permeated by serotonin-secreting axonal varicosities.

The *dopaminergic* neurons of the midbrain fall into two groups. Those of the substantia nigra are categorized with the basal ganglia. Dorsal to these are *mesolimbic* neurons categorized with the RF.

Their somas occupy the *ventral tegmental area (of Tsai)*. They project mainly to frontal and temporal areas of the cerebral cortex which are associated with the limbic system (*Figure 18.2B*).

The *noradrenergic* neurons are only marginally less prodigious than the serotoninergic ones. About 90% of the somas are pooled in the **locus ceruleus**, a 'violet spot' in the floor and side wall of the fourth ventricle at the upper end of the pons (*Figure 18.3*). Neurons of the locus ceruleus project in *all* directions, as indicated in *Figure 18.2C*.

*Epinephrine-secreting* neurons are relatively scarce and are confined to the medulla oblongata. Some project rostrally to the hypothalamus, others project caudally to synapse upon preganglionic sympathetic neurons.

In the cerebral cortex, the ionic and electrical effects of aminergic neuronal activity are quite variable. Firstly, more than one kind of postsynaptic receptor exists for each of the amines. Secondly, some aminergic neurons liberate a peptide substance as well, capable of modulating the transmitter action—usually by prolonging it. Thirdly, the larger cortical neurons receive many thousands of excitatory and inhibitory synapses from local circuit neurons and they have numerous different receptors. Activation of a single kind of aminergic receptor may have a large or small effect depending on the current excitatory state.

Although our understanding of the physiology and pharmacology of the monoamines is far from

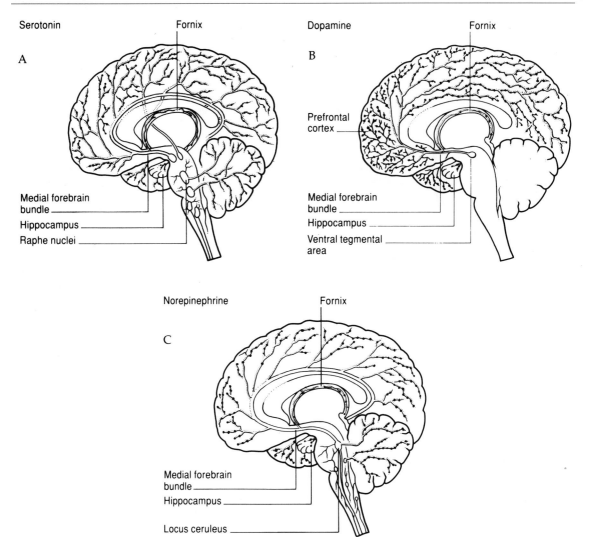

**Figure 18.2.** (A) Serotonergic neurons of the brainstem midline (raphe). (B) Dopaminergic projections from the ventral tegmental area of the midbrain. (C) Noradrenergic neurons of the pons and medulla oblongata.

complete, no one disputes their relevance to a wide range of *behavioral* functions. Monoamine transmitters/receptors are of particular interest to psychiatrists: for example, serotonin and norepinephrine have been implicated in endogenous depression (Panel 18.1) and dopamine in schizophrenia (Panel 18.2).

### Functional anatomy

The wide variety of functions served by different parts of the RF is indicated by the following list.

| RF element | Function |
| --- | --- |
| N. gigantocellularis | Posture, locomotion |
| Premotor cranial nerve nuclei | Patterned cranial nerve activities |
| Salivatory nuclei | Salivary secretion, lacrimation |
| Lateral pontine tegmentum | Bladder control |
| Parabrachial nucleus | Respiratory rhythm |
| Central nucleus of medulla oblongata | Vital centers (circulation, respiration) |
| Paramedian and lateral medullary nuclei | Convey somatic and visceral information to the cerebellum |
| Aminergic neurons | Sleeping and waking, attention and mood, sensory modulation |

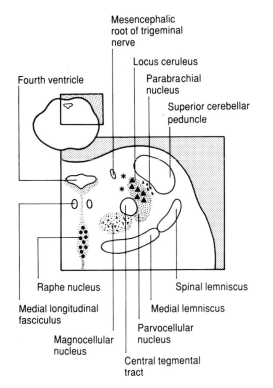

* Acetylcholine
• Serotonin
▲ Norepinephrine

**Figure 18.3.** Part of a transverse section through the upper part of the pons, showing elements of the reticular formation.

## Pattern generators

The contribution of N. gigantocellularis to posture and locomotion is described in Chapter 12.

Patterned activities involving *cranial nerves* include:

• Conjugate movements of the eyes controlled by nodal points (gaze centers) in the midbrain and pons feeding into the oculomotor, trochlear, and abducent nerves.
• Rhythmical chewing movements controlled by the supratrigeminal nucleus in the pons.
• Swallowing, vomiting, coughing, and sneezing, controlled by separate nodal points in the medulla feeding into the appropriate cranial nerves and into the respiratory centers.

The salivatory nuclei belong to the parvocellular RF of the pons and medulla oblongata. They contribute preganglionic fibers to the facial and glossopharyngeal nerves.

## Bladder control

The bladder control center is on the medial side of the locus ceruleus, with interconnections across the midline. The center exerts a tonic *inhibitory* action on the parasympathetic neurons in sacral segments 2, 3 and 4 of the spinal cord. The pontine center is inhibited in turn from a cortical zone within the precentral gyrus.

When the bladder is half full, vesical afferents in the pelvic splanchnic nerves relay the information through the spinoreticular tract to the pontine center, which responds by suppressing the parasympathetic activity that would otherwise occur through the sacrovesical reflex arc. At the same time, sympathetic activity in the lumbar splanchnic nerves (presumably influenced by the bladder center) assists in two distinct ways: bladder compliance is increased by $\beta_2$-receptor inhibition of the trabeculated detrusor musculature; and the tone of the smooth muscle at the bladder neck is increased by way of $\alpha$ receptors.

When the bladder is full and the time is opportune, the pontine center releases the sacral cord from inhibition. If the time is not opportune, the premotor cortex can defer voiding by reinforcing the inhibitory function of the pontine center.

## Respiratory control *(Figure 18.4)*

The respiratory cycle is regulated by *dorsal* and *ventral respiratory centers* located at the upper end of the medulla oblongata on each side. The dorsal respiratory center occupies the lateral side of the nucleus solitarius. The ventral center lies behind the nucleus ambiguus.

The dorsal respiratory center has an *inspiratory* function. It projects to the nuclei on the opposite side of the spinal cord supplying the diaphragm, intercostals, and accessory muscles of inspiration. It receives two major excitatory projections from *chemoreceptors*, as follows.

### MEDULLARY CHEMOSENSITIVE AREA
Close to the site of attachment of the glossopharyngeal nerve, the choroid plexus of the fourth ventricle pouts through the lateral aperture of the fourth ventricle to lie beside the medulla oblongata. Specifically at this location, RF cells at the medullary surface are exquisitely sensitive to the $H^+$ ion concentration in the neighboring cerebrospinal fluid. In effect, the chemosensitive area samples the $CO_2$ level in the blood supplying the brain. Any increase in $H^+$ ions stimulates the dorsal respiratory center through a direct synaptic linkage.

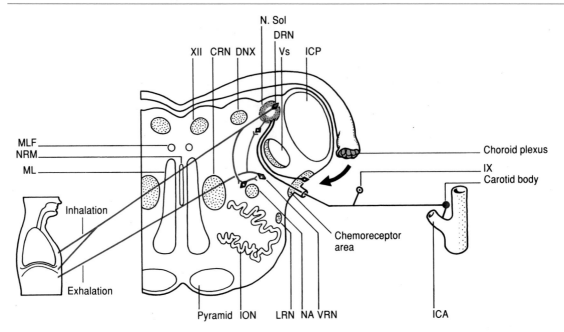

**Figure 18.4.** Upper part of medulla oblongata showing relationships of the respiratory nuclei. CRN, central reticular nucleus; DNX, dorsal nucleus of vagus; ICP, inferior cerebellar peduncle; ION, inferior olivary nucleus; IX, glossopharyngeal nerve; LRN, lateral reticular nucleus; ML, medial lemniscus; MLF, medial longitudinal fasciculus; NA, nucleus ambiguus; NRM, nucleus raphe magnus; N. sol., nucleus solitarius; VRN, ventral respiratory nucleus; Vs, spinal tract of trigeminal nerve; XII, hypoglossal nerve. Arrow indicates movement of cerebrospinal fluid.

## CLINICAL PANEL 18.1 • ENDOGENOUS DEPRESSION

Endogenous depression, as the name implies, is a state of depressed mood occurring without an adequate explanation in terms of external events. This distinguishes the condition from *reactive* depression brought on by an event such as bereavement or job loss.

Endogenous depression is characterized by at least several of the following features:

- Depressed general mood, with loss of interest in normal activities and outside events.
- Diminished energy, easy fatigue, loss of appetite and of sex drive, constipation.
- Impairment of self-image, with a feeling of personal inadequacy.
- Insomnia, usually with early waking.
- Aches and pains. Recurrent abdominal pains may simulate organ disease.
- Periods of agitation, with restlessness and perhaps suicidal tendency.

Endogenous depression affects about 4% of the adult population, and there is a genetic predisposition: about 20% of first-degree relatives have it too. Phases of depression may begin in childhood or adolescence.

Several lines of evidence implicate deficient function of noradrenergic neurons, serotonergic neurons, or both, in depressive disorders:

- Attention was first drawn to aminergic function by the chance observation that the use of reserpine in treatment of hypertension produced depression as a side effect. Reserpine depletes amine transmitter stores.
- In a significant number of depressed patients, metabolic products of norepinephrine and/or serotonin in the cerebrospinal fluid are reduced in amount.
- Drugs that prolong the availability of biogenic amines in the synaptic cleft are of

benefit to the great majority of depressed patients. Two classes of drugs are in common use: *monoamine oxidase inhibitors*, which increase the amine content of nerve endings by inhibiting amine degradation, as explained in Chapter 9; and *tricyclic antidepressants*, which inhibit the specific reuptake mechanism in the presynaptic membrane.

The above drugs take about 3 weeks to become effective, and it seems likely that receptor function becomes slowly altered on one or both sides of the synaptic cleft. Possibilities include *increased* postsynaptic receptor efficacy, and *decreased* presynaptic receptor efficacy. The presynaptic receptors are autoreceptors that normally limit the amount of transmitter that can be released (Chapter 9).

## CLINICAL PANEL 18.2 • SCHIZOPHRENIA

Schizophrenia occurs in about 1% of the population in all countries where the incidence has been studied. In about 10% of cases there is some evidence of a schizophrenic personality in one or more close relatives.

The mode of presentation is quite variable but the behavioral changes permit most patients to be categorized into two classes: those in whom positive symptoms predominate, and those in whom negative symptoms predominate.

*Positive* symptoms include hallucinations, delusions, and bizarre behavior. Hallucinations are typically auditory (the patient hears voices, and commonly converses with them aloud). Delusions often take a paranoid form, with a belief that one's thoughts and actions are being controlled by some outside agency. Bizarre behavior may include physical agression in response to the hallucinations or delusions.

*Negative* symptoms are those of withdrawal from society into a private world. The patient has little to say, and in conversation rambles from one inconsequential theme to another. There is a notable 'flattening of affect': a loss of emotional responsiveness. Personal hygiene is a matter of indifference.

Although patients with positive symptoms may cause great alarm, they respond much better to treatment than patients whose behavioral change is negative.

*Treatment* of schizophrenia is by means of one of the antipsychotic drugs (for example, chlorpromazine or haloperidol). These drugs are very effective in terminating bouts of bizarre behavior and in reducing the likelihood of recurrence. A side effect that all of the drugs have in common is a tendency to produce some of the physical symptoms of Parkinson's disease. Parkinson's disease is associated with progressive loss of dopaminergic neurons projecting from the substantia nigra to the striatum (caudate nucleus and putamen). For this reason, and because of the character of the behavioral changes, overactivity of the mesocortical/mesolimbic dopaminergic system is considered significant in relation to schizophrenia.

On closer examination, the relationship is not a simple one. Firstly, the antipsychotic drugs are of little value where negative symptoms dominate the clinical picture. Postmortem studies of such patients have revealed a significant amount of brain atrophy, notably in the parahippocampal gyrus of the dominant hemisphere. For these two reasons, psychotic disorders with negative symptoms may constitute a separate disease entity.

Secondly, overactivity of the dopaminergic system seems not to be a matter of overproduction of dopamine, but of increased synaptic effectiveness. This could come about through an increase in the number of postsynaptic receptors (making a given amount of transmitter more effective). Several postmortem neurochemical studies have supported this idea. Overactivity could also come about through a decrease in the number of presynaptic receptors, because these are autoreceptors (having a braking action on transmitter release).

CAROTID CHEMORECEPTORS

The pin-head *carotid body* is situated beside the stem of the internal carotid artery. A twig from the internal carotid ramifies within it, and the blood flow is so intense that the arteriovenous $PO_2$ changes by less than 1% during passage. The chemoreceptors are *glomus cells* to which branches of the sinus nerve (IX) are applied. The carotid chemoreceptors respond to either a fall in $PO_2$ or a rise in $PCO_2$. (The chemoreceptors of the aortic bodies seem to be relatively insignificant in humans.)

The ventral respiratory center is *expiratory* (in the main). During quiet breathing it functions as an oscillator, being engaged in reciprocal inhibition with the inspiratory center. During forced breathing it activates the abdominal and other muscles required to empty the lungs.

The simple connections shown in the Figure are a simplification. Animal experiments indicate that excitation of the neurons projecting to the spinal cord is mainly by way of internuncials contacted by the primary afferents. Some of these internuncials discharge to the dorsal respiratory center to initiate inspiration, others project to the ventral respiratory center to initiate expiration.

A third respiratory center, the *medial parabrachial nucleus,* is adjacent to the locus ceruleus. It seems to have a pacemaker function governing respiratory rate (cycles per minute).

## Cardiovascular control

Because of the prevalence of essential hypertension in late middle age, the neural and endocrine systems controling cardiac output and peripheral arterial resistance are subjects of major research effort. Particular attention is being given to the medially placed cells of the nucleus solitarius, which receive *baroreceptor afferents* from the carotid sinus and aortic arch. The baroreceptors are stretch receptors (a multitude of free nerve endings) in the adventitial coat of these vessels. Afferents from the carotid sinus travel in the glossopharyngeal nerve; afferents from the aortic arch travel in the vagus. The baroreceptor afferents are known as 'buffer nerves' because they act to correct any deviation of the arterial blood pressure from the norm.

The nucleus solitarius (N. sol.) responds to a rise in arterial pressure by slowing the heart (increased vagal activity) and by lowering peripheral arterial resistance (reduced sympathetic activity). The heart is slowed by an excitatory

projection from N. sol. to the cardioinhibitory center in the nucleus ambiguus (Chapter 13). The *barovagal reflex* involves a sequence of four neurons, the final one (on the wall of the heart) being inhibitory.

Animal experiments indicate that the *barosympathetic reflex* uses a sequence of six neurons. It involves a *pressor center* and a *depressor center*, both of these being located in the ventral region of the medulla oblongata. The pressor center has a tonic excitatory effect on the thoracolumbar sympathetic outflow through descending fibers, some of which secrete norepinephrine and others serotonin. The depressor center exerts a GABAergic braking action on the pressor center, and N. sol. reduces sympathetic activity by means of an excitatory (glutamate) projection to the depressor center.

## EXERCISE

Make a diagram of the shortest pathway from carotid sinus to peripheral arteriole. Represent the CNS by a rectangle and label the four cell groups inside and the two outside. Use the diagram to explain (a) why the pressor center is released when you get up out of bed, and (b) why the pressor center is rendered ineffective by a crush injury of the spinal cord at cervical level.

## Sleeping and wakefulness

The onset of sleep is accompanied by a change in the electrical group activity of neurons in the cerebral cortex, as revealed by electroencephalography (EEG). The rapid, low voltage pattern of the waking state is replaced by slow waves which have higher voltage because group activity is more synchronized. After about 90 minutes, S (synchronized) sleep is replaced by a D (desynchronized) sleep in which the EEG pattern resembles the waking state. During D sleep dreams take place and there are rapid eye movements (hence the term 'REM sleep'). Several S and D phases occur during a normal night's sleep.

Details of brainstem involvement in sleep phenomena are available in psychology texts. Some salient experimental evidence may be summarized:

- In animal experiments, destruction of the raphe neurons in the midbrain, or pharmacological prevention of serotonin synthesis, results in insomnia lasting for several days.

- Serotonin and norepinephrine neuronal activities fluctuate in parallel. Both are most active during attentive wakefulness, sluggish during S sleep, and virtually silent during REM sleep.
- Brainstem serotonin neurons form numerous surface varicosities on the walls of the third ventricle. Serotonin liberated into the cerebrospinal fluid seems to be metabolized by hypothalamic neurons to form a sleep-inducing substance.
- *Cholinergic* neurons close to the locus ceruleus are active during REM sleep, and they appear to cause the rapid eye movements by playing upon the ocular motor nuclei.

ASCENDING RETICULAR ACTIVATING SYSTEM (ARAS)
This term refers to the participation of RF neurons in *activation* of the cerebral cortex, as shown by a change in EEG records from high-amplitude, slow waves to low-amplitude, fast waves during spontaneous arousal from sleep. The strongest candidates for such a role seem to be the sets of cholinergic neurons close to the locus ceruleus (*Figure 18.3*). As well as supplying the above-mentioned fibers to the ocular motor nuclei, these cholinergic neurons project to nearly all of the nuclei of the *thalamus*, and they have an excitatory effect upon thalamic neurons projecting to the cerebral cortex.

The *hypothalamus* is an important controling center for various body rhythms, including sleep and wakefulness. A second candidate for cortical activation has been found here, namely the *tuberomammillary nucleus*. This nucleus contains histaminergic neurons having widespread projections to the cerebral cortex and brainstem (Chapter 20).

Following arousal, the waking-state EEG pattern seems to be sustained by the continued discharge of the brainstem and hypothalamic neurons mentioned; also by a third set of neurons, embedded in the basal forebrain immediately above the optic chiasma. The third set occupies the *basal nucleus of Meynert* (see Chapter 25) and projects fine, cholinergic axons to most parts of the cerebral cortex.

## Sensory modulation: gate control

Sensory transmission from primary to secondary afferent neurons (at the levels of the posterior gray horn and posterior column nuclei) and from secondary to tertiary (at the level of the thalamus), is subject to *gating*. The term *gating* refers to the degree of freedom of synaptic transmission from one set of neurons to the next.

*Tactile* sensory transmission is gated at the level of the posterior column nuclei. Pyramidal tract neurons in the postcentral gyrus may facilitate or inhibit sensory transmission at this level, as described in Chapter 12.

*Nociceptive* transmission from the trunk and limbs is gated in the posterior gray horn of the spinal cord. From the head and upper part of the neck, it is gated in the spinal trigeminal nucleus. A key structure in both areas of gray matter is the substantia gelatinosa, which is packed with small excitatory and inhibitory internuncial neurons. The excitatory internuncial transmitter is glutamate; the inhibitory one is GABA for some internuncials, enkephalin (an opiate pentapeptide) for others.

Finely myelinated ($A\delta$) polymodal nociceptive fibers synapse directly upon dendrites of lamina I and lamina V relay neurons of the lateral spinothalamic tract and of its trigeminal equivalent. The $A\delta$ fibers signal sharp, well-localized pain. Unmyelinated, C fiber nociceptive afferents have mainly indirect access to relay cells, via excitatory gelatinosa internuncials. The C fibers signal dull, poorly localized pain. Most of them contain substance P, which may be liberated as a cotransmitter with glutamate.

SEGMENTAL ANTINOCICEPTION
Large ($A\beta$) mechanoreceptive afferents from hair follicles synapse upon anterior spinothalamic relay cells (and their trigeminal equivalents). They give off collaterals to *inhibitory* (mainly GABA) gelatinosa cells which synapse in turn upon *lateral* spinothalamic relay cells (*Figure 18.5*). Some of the internuncials exert presynaptic inhibition as well, upon C fiber terminals, either by axo-axonic contacts (which are very difficult to find in experimental material), or by dendro-axonic contacts.

Gating of the spinothalamic response to C fiber activity can be induced by stimulating the mechanoreceptive afferents, thereby recruiting inhibitory gelatinosa cells. This simple circuit accounts for the relief afforded by 'rubbing the sore spot'. It also provides a rationale for the use of *transcutaneous electrical nerve stimulation* (TENS) by physical therapists, for pain relief in arthritis and other chronically painful conditions. The standard procedure in TENS is to apply a stimulating electrode to the skin at the same segmental level as the source of noxious C fiber activity, and to deliver a current sufficient to produce a pronounced buzzing sensation.

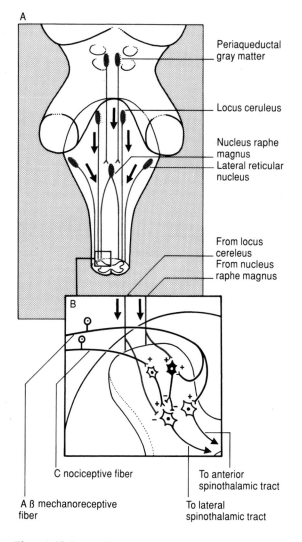

**Figure 18.5.** (A) Three antinociceptive pathways descending (arrows) from brainstem to spinal cord. (B) Enlargement from (A) showing excitatory (+) and inhibitory (−) inputs to spinothalamic transmission cells. Solid black = inhibitory internuncial.

SUPRASPINAL ANTINOCICEPTION

Three supraspinal pathways having antinociceptive functions descend from the reticular formation to the spinal cord and spinal trigeminal nucleus (*Figure 18.5*):

(1) From the nucleus raphe magnus (NRM) and adjacent gigantocellular RF, *raphespinal* fibers descend within Lissauer's tract, terminating in the substantia gelatinosa. In animals, electrical stimulation of NRM may produce total analgesia throughout the body, with little effect on tactile sensation. Many fibers of the raphespinal tract liberate *serotonin*, which excites enkephalinergic internuncials in the posterior gray horn and spinal trigeminal nucleus. The internuncials induce both pre- and postsynaptic inhibition on the relevant relay cells.

*Diffuse noxious inhibitory controls.* NRM is not somatotopically arranged, but it does receive inputs from spinoreticular and trigeminoreticular neurons responding to peripheral noxious stimulation. This anatomical connection accounts for what are called *diffuse noxious inhibitory controls. Painful stimulation of one part of the body may produce pain relief in all other parts.* The arrangement accounts well for the heterotopic relief of pain in acupuncture, where needles are used to excite nociceptive afferents in the most superficial musculature.

*Stimulus-induced analgesia.* NRM is intensely responsive to stimulation of the periaqueductal gray matter (PAG) of the midbrain. This connection has been used to advantage for patients suffering intractable pain: a fine stimulating electrode can be inserted into PAG and wired so that the patient can control the level of self-stimulation.

*Stress-induced analgesia.* At rest, the PAG projection to NRM is under tonic inhibition by inhibitory internuncials present within PAG. The internuncials are themselves inhibited by opiate peptides—notably by $\beta$-endorphin released from a small set of hypothalamic neurons projecting to PAG. In life-threatening situations, where injury may be the price to be paid for escape, PAG may be released (disinhibited) by the hypothalamus. This seems to be the mechanism whereby a bullet wound may be scarcely noticed in the heat of battle.

(2) The *locus ceruleus* (*Figure 18.5*) has an antinociceptive action when stimulated. Some *ceruleospinal* axons descend in the lateral funiculus and exert direct postsynaptic inhibition on spinothalamic relay cells.

(3) Some cells in the lateral reticular nucleus of the medulla oblongata can exert a powerful antinociceptive effect upon the posterior gray horn. Their mode of action is not well understood.

In addition to the segmental and supraspinal controls of nociceptive transmission from primary to secondary afferents, gating occurs within the thalamus (see Chapter 21). Furthermore, perception of the aversive (unpleasant) quality of pain seems to require participation of the anterior cingulate cortex, which is rich in opiate receptors (see Chapter 25).

## REFERENCES

Bentivoglio, M. and Steriade, M. (1990) Brainstem–diencephalic circuits as a structural substrate of the ascending reticular activation concept. In *The Diencephalon and Sleep* (Mancia, M. and Marini, G., eds), pp. 7–29. New York: Raven Press.

Bowsher, D. (1988) Recent anatomical contributions to the understanding of pain. *Clin. Anat.* **1:** 157–170.

Brody, M.J., Alper, R.H.,O'Neill, T.P. and Porter, J.P. (1986) Central neural control of the cardiovascular system. In *Handbook of Hypertension, Vol. 8: Pathophysiology of Hypertension-regulating Mechanisms* (Zanchetti, A. and Tarazi, R.C., eds), pp. 1–25. Amsterdam: Elsevier.

Chalmers, J. and Pilowski, P. (1991) Brainstem and bulbospinal systems in the control of blood pressure. *J. Hypertens.* **9:** 675–694.

De Keyser, J., Ebinger, G. and Vauquelin, G. (1989) Evidence for a widespread dopaminergic innervation of the human cerebral neocortex. *Neurosci. Lett.* **104:** 281–285.

Jensen, T.S. and Gebhart, G.F. (1988) General anatomy of antinociceptive systems. In *Basic Mechanisms of Headache* (Olesen, J. and Edvinsson, L., eds), pp. 189–198. Amsterdam: Elsevier.

Pearson, J., Goldstein, M., Markey, K. and Brandeis, L. (1983) Human brainstem catecholamine neuronal anatomy as indicated by immunocytochemistry with antibodies to tyrosine hydroxylase. *Neuroscience* **8:** 3–32.

Reis, D.J., Morrison, S. and Ruggiero, D.J. (1988) The C1 area of the brainstem in tonic and reflex control of blood pressure. *Hypertension* **11 (Suppl 1):** 1–8.

Sacher, E.J. (1985) Disorders of thought: the schizophrenic syndromes. In *Principles of Neural Science*, 2nd edn (Kandel, E.R. and Schwartz, J.H., eds), pp. 704–716. New York: Elsevier.

# 19

# Cerebellum

**CHAPTER SUMMARY**

Functional anatomy
Microscopic anatomy
Afferent pathways
Efferent pathways
*CLINICAL PANELS*
Midline lesions: trunk ataxia · Anterior lobe
 lesions: gait ataxia · Neocerebellar lesions:
 incoordination of voluntary movement

**The best-known function of the cerebellum is the co-ordination of movements. In pursuit of this function the cerebellum receives information both from the motor areas of the cerebral cortex and from the locomotor apparatus. Acting upon this information, it monitors motor performance so as to ensure smooth execution of movements of all kinds. Patients suffering from cerebellar disease are disabled because of uneven execution of habitual motor sequences and an inability to learn new ones. A recent focus of attention is upon the lateral region of the posterior lobe, which is outstandingly large in the human brain. Surprisingly, this region seems to be engaged in cognitive activities, especially in relation to language.**

Phylogenetically, the initial development of the cerebellum (in fishes) took place in relation to the vestibular labyrinth. With development of quadrupedal locomotion the anterior lobes (in particular) became richly connected to the spinal cord. Assumption of the erect posture and achievement of a whole new range of physical skills has been accompanied by the appearance of massive linkages between the posterior lobes and the cerebral cortex. In general, cerebellar connections with the labyrinth, spinal cord and cerebral cortex are arranged such that each cerebellar hemisphere is primarily concerned with the coordination of movements *on its own side*.

The gross anatomy of the cerebellum is described briefly in Chapter 3, where it may be reviewed at this time.

### Functional anatomy

Phylogenetic and functional aspects can be combined (to an approximation) by dividing the cerebellum into strips, as shown in *Figure 19.1*. The median strip contains the vermis, together with a paired **fastigial nucleus** in the white matter close to the nodule (*Figure 19.2*). This strip is the *vestibulocerebellum;* it has a two-way connection with the vestibular nucleus. It controls the responses of the nucleus to signals from the vestibular labyrinth.

A paramedian strip, the *spinocerebellum,* includes the paravermal region and the **nucleus globosus** and **nucleus emboliformis** in the white matter (*Figure 19.2*). The two nuclei are together called the *interposed nucleus.* The spinocerebellum is rich in spinocerebellar connections. It is involved in the control of posture and gait.

The remaining, lateral strip is much the largest and takes in the wrinkled **dentate nucleus** (*Figure*

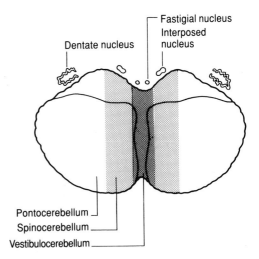

**Figure 19.1.** Zonation of cerebellum. The central nuclei are represented separately.

*19.2*). This strip is the *pontocerebellum,* because it receives a massive input from the contralateral nuclei pontis. It is also called the *neocerebellum* because the nuclei pontis convey information from large areas of the cerebral neocortex. The neocerebellum is uniquely large in the human brain.

## MICROSCOPIC ANATOMY

The structure of the cerebellar cortex is uniform throughout. From within outward, the cortex comprises **granular, piriform,** and **molecular** layers (*Figure 19.3*).

The *granular layer* contains myriads of *granule cells,* whose somas are about the size of erythrocytes. Their short dendrites receive so-called *mossy fibers* from all sources except the inferior olivary nucleus. Before reaching the cerebellar cortex the mossy fibers, which are excitatory in nature, give off collateral branches to the central nuclei.

**Figure 19.2.** Transverse section of lower pons and cerebellum showing the position of the central and vestibular nuclei.

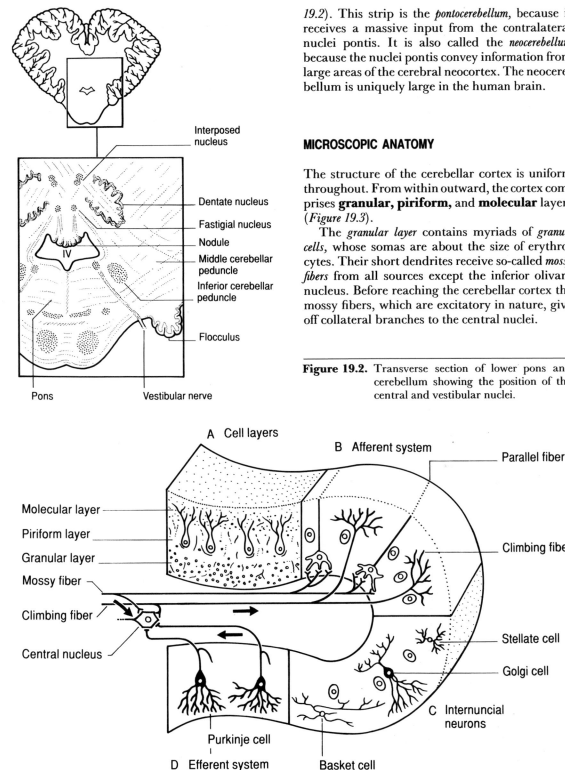

**Figure 19.3.** Cerebellar cortex. (A) Cell layers; (B) afferent system; (C) internuncial neurons; (D) efferent system.

The axons of the granule cells pass to the molecular layer where they divide in a T-shaped manner to form *parallel fibers*. The parallel fibers run parallel to the axes of the folia. They make excitatory contacts with Purkinje cells.

The granular layer also contains Golgi cells (see later).

The *piriform layer* consists of very large, **Purkinje cells**. The fan-shaped dendritic trees of the Purkinje cells are the largest dendritic trees in the entire nervous system. The fans are disposed at right angles to the parallel fibers.

The dendritic trees of Purkinje cells are penetrated by huge numbers of parallel fibers, each one making a single synapse upon the tip of a dendritic spine of about 400 Purkinje cells. Not surprisingly, stimulation of small numbers of granule cells by mossy fibers has a merely facilitatory effect upon Purkinje cells. Many thousands of parallel fibers must act simultaneously to bring the membrane potential to firing level.

Each dendritic tree also receives a single *climbing fiber* from the contralateral inferior olivary nucleus. This fiber divides at the dendritic branch-points and makes thousands of synaptic contacts with the bases of dendritic spines. A single threshold pulse applied to one climbing fiber elicits a short burst of action potentials from the client Purkinje cell. Climbing fiber effects on Purkinje cells are so powerful that, for some time after they cease firing, the synaptic effectiveness of bundles of parallel fibers is reduced. In this sense, the Purkinje cells *remember* that they have been excited by olivocerebellar fibers.

The axons of the Purkinje cells are the *only* axons to emerge from the cerebellar cortex. Remarkably, they are entirely inhibitory in their effects. Their principal targets are the central nuclei. They give off collateral branches as well, mainly to Golgi cells.

The *molecular layer* is almost entirely taken up with Purkinje dendrites, parallel fibers, supporting neuroglial cells, and blood vessels. However, two sets of inhibitory neurons are also found here, lying in the same plane as the Purkinje cell dendritic trees. Near the cortical surface are small, *stellate cells,* and close to the piriform layer are larger, *basket cells.* Both sets are contacted by parallel fibers, and they both synapse on Purkinje cells. The stellate cells synapse upon dendritic shafts whereas the basket cells form a 'basket' of synaptic contacts around the soma, as well as forming axo-axonic synapses upon the initial segment of the

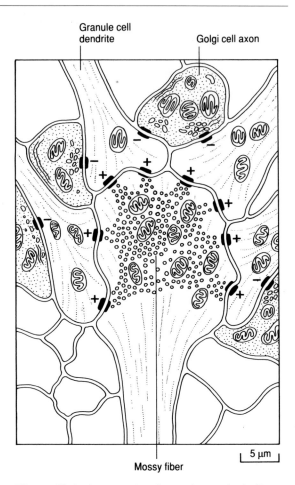

**Figure 19.4.** A synaptic glomerulus. +/− indicates excitation/inhibition.

axon. A single basket cell synapses upon some 250 Purkinje cells.

The final cell type in the cortex is the *Golgi cell,* whose dendrites are contacted by parallel fibers and whose axons divide extensively before synapsing upon the short dendrites of granule cells. The synaptic ensemble that includes a mossy fiber terminal, granule cell dendrites, and Golgi cell boutons, is known as a **glomerulus** (*Figure 19.4*).

### Spatial effects of mossy fiber activity (*Figure 19.5*)

As already noted, cerebellar afferents other than olivocerebellar ones form mossy fiber terminals after giving off excitatory collaterals to one of the central nuclei. The afferents excite groups of granule cells, which in turn facilitate many hundreds of

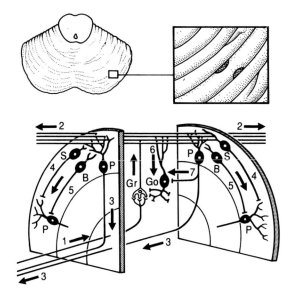

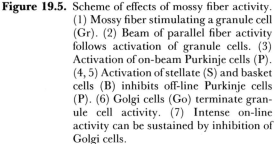

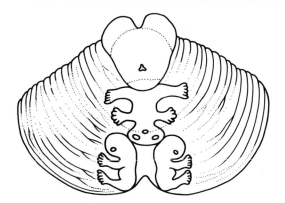

**Figure 19.6.** Upper surface of cerebellum showing position of somatotopic maps, based on animal experiments.

**Figure 19.5.** Scheme of effects of mossy fiber activity. (1) Mossy fiber stimulating a granule cell (Gr). (2) Beam of parallel fiber activity follows activation of granule cells. (3) Activation of on-beam Purkinje cells (P). (4, 5) Activation of stellate (S) and basket cells (B) inhibits off-line Purkinje cells (P). (6) Golgi cells (Go) terminate granule cell activity. (7) Intense on-line activity can be sustained by inhibition of Golgi cells.

Purkinje cells. Along most of the beam of excitation, known as a *microzone,* the Purkinje cells begin to fire, and to inhibit patches of cells in one of the deep nuclei. At the same time, weakly facilitated Purkinje cells along the edges of the microzone are shut off by stellate and basket cells. As a result, the beam of excitation is sharply focused. The excitation is terminated by Golgi cell inhibition of the granule cells that initiated it. Powerful excitation will last longer because highly active Purkinje cells inhibit underlying Golgi cells through their collateral branches.

### Representation of body parts

Representation of body parts in the human cerebellar cortex is currently under investigation by means of positron emission tomography. These investigations, along with some evidence from clinical cases, indicate the presence of somatotopic maps in the anterior and posterior lobes (*Figure 19.6*).

The maps have been worked out in some detail in laboratory animals during movements. The maps for movement match up with maps of skin, eye, ear, and visceral representation worked out by stimulation of body parts.

See also Higher Brain Functions, later.

### *Afferent pathways*

From the muscles and skin of the trunk and limbs, afferent information travels in the posterior spinocerebellar and the cuneocerebellar tract and enters the inferior cerebellar peduncle on the same side. Comparable information from the territory served by the trigeminal nerve enters all three cerebellar peduncles.

Afferents from spinal reflex arcs run in the anterior spinocerebellar tract, which reaches the upper pons before looping into the superior cerebellar peduncle.

Special sense pathways comprise tectocerebellar fibers entering the superior peduncle from the ipsilateral midbrain colliculi, and vestibulocerebellar fibers from the ipsilateral vestibular nucleus.

Two massive pathways enter from the contralateral brainstem. The pontocerebellar tract enters through the middle peduncle, and the olivocerebellar tract enters through the inferior peduncle.

Reticulocerebellar fibers enter the inferior peduncle from the paramedian and lateral reticular nuclei of the medulla oblongata.

Finally, aminergic fibers enter all three peduncles from noradrenergic and serotonergic cell groups in the brainstem. Under experimental conditions, both kinds of neurons appear to facilitate excitatory transmision in mossy and climbing fiber terminals.

## Olivocerebellar tract

The sensorimotor cortex projects in an orderly, somatotopic manner onto the ipsilateral inferior and accessory olivary nuclei. The order is preserved in the olivary projections onto the body maps in the contralateral cerebellar cortex (from principal nucleus to the posterior map, from the accessory nuclei to the anterior map). Under resting conditions in animal experiments, groups of olivary neurons discharge synchronously at 5–10 Hz (impulses/second). The synchrony is probably due to the observed presence of electrical synapses (gap junctions) between dendrites of neighboring neurons. In the cerebellar cortex, the response of Purkinje cells takes the form of *complex spikes* (multiple action potentials in response to single pulses), because of the spatiotemporal effects of climbing fiber activity along the dozens of branches of the dendritic tree.

When an animal has been trained to perform a motor task, increased discharge of Purkinje cells during task performance takes the form of *simple* spikes produced by bundles of active parallel fibers. If an unexpected obstacle is introduced into the task (e.g. momentary braking of a lever that the animal is operating), bursts of complex spikes occur each time the obstacle is encountered. As the animal learns to overcome the obstacle so that the task is completed in the set time, the spike bursts dwindle in number and finally disappear. This is just one of several experimental indicators that the olive has a significant *teaching* function in the acquisition of new motor skills.

The olive receives direct ipsilateral projections from the premotor and motor areas of the cerebral cortex, and from the visual association cortex, providing an apparently suitable substrate for its activities. As well, it is in touch with the outside world through the spino-olivary tract (Chapter 11).

In theory, the red nucleus of the midbrain could function as a *novelty detector* because it receives collaterals both from cortical fibers descending to the olive and from cerebellar output fibers ascending to the thalamus. Much the largest output from the red nucleus is to the ipsilateral olive, which it appears to inhibit. Upon detection of a mismatch between a movement intended and a movement organized, the red nucleus could release the appropriate cell groups in the olive until the two are harmonized.

## Efferent pathways (Figure 19.7)

From the *vestibulocerebellum* (fastigial nucleus), axons project to the vestibular nuclei of both sides, through the inferior cerebellar peduncles. The contralateral projection crosses over within the cerebellar white matter.

Vestibulocerebellar outputs to the medial and superior vestibular nuclei control movements of the eyes (Chapter 14). A separate output to the lateral vestibular (Deiters') nucleus of the same side controls the balancing function of the vestibulospinal tract. Some Purkinje fibers bypass the fastigial nucleus and exert tonic inhibition on Deiters' nucleus.

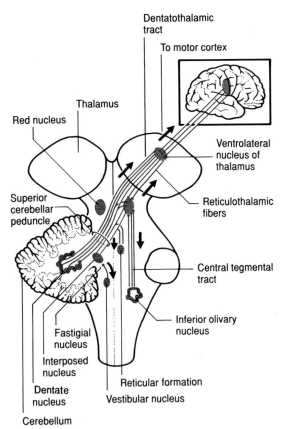

**Figure 19.7.** Principal cerebellar efferents. Arrows indicate directions of impulse conduction.

From the *spinocerebellum* (interposed nucleus), axons emerge in the superior cerebellar peduncle. They terminate mainly in the contralateral reticular formation and red nucleus. Those descending to the pontomedullary reticular formation regulate the functions of the reticulospinal tracts in relation to posture and locomotion. Those ascending to the red nucleus may be involved in motor learning, because the output of the human red nucleus is almost entirely to the inferior olivary nucleus on that side.

From the *neocerebellum*, the massive *dentatothalamic tract* forms the bulk of the superior cerebellar peduncle. It decussates with its opposite number in the lower midbrain and later gives collaterals to the red nucleus before synapsing in the ventral lateral nucleus of the thalamus. The onward projection from the thalamus is to the motor cortex.

### The cerebellum and higher brain functions

Positron emission tomography (PET) provides information about regional changes in blood flow and oxygen consumption. 'Movement maps' such as those in *Figure 19.6* are derived from simple repetitive movements such as opening and closing a fist. A striking feature of movement maps is *how small and how medial they are*. Prior to PET, it was assumed that the lateral expansion of the human posterior lobe was necessary for manual dexterity. Instead, it now appears that the lateral expansion is associated with linguistic and other cognitive functions, having an anatomical base in linkages with the lateral prefrontal cortex of the cerebral hemisphere. Lateral activity seems to be greatest during speech, with a right-sided predominance consistent with a possible linkage (via the thalamus) with the motor speech area of the dominant, left frontal cortex (Chapter 23). Something more than mere motor control is involved, because lateral cerebellar activity is greater during functional naming, e.g. 'dig', 'travel', than during object identification, e.g. 'shovel', 'airplane'.

### Clinical disorders of the cerebellum

Diseases involving the cerebellum usually involve more than one lobe and/or more than one of the three sagittal strips. However, characteristic clinical pictures have been described in association with lesions of the vermis (Panel 19.1), of the anterior lobe (Panel 19.2), and of the neocerebellum (Panel 19.3).

### Posturography

*Posturography* is the instrumental recording of the erect posture. The subject stands on a platform and spontaneous body sway is detected by strain gauges beneath the corners of the platform. Linkage of the strain-guage data to a computer can yield a graphic record of anteroposterior and side-to-side sway, first with the eyes open and then with the eyes closed. This is *static posturography*, and it helps to distinguish among different causes of ataxia.

*Dynamic posturography* provides information on the effects of an abrupt 4° backward tilt of the supporting platform. For this phase of the examination surface EMG electrodes are applied over the

---

**CLINICAL PANEL 19.1 ● MIDLINE LESIONS: TRUNCAL ATAXIA**

Lesions of the vermis occur most often in children, in the form of *medulloblastomas* in the roof of the fourth ventricle. These tumors expand rapidly and produce signs of raised intracranial pressure: headache, vomiting, drowsiness, papilledema. In the recumbent position there may be no abnormality of motor co-ordination in the limbs. Nystagmus can usually be elicited on visual tracking of the examiner's finger from side to side. A dramatic feature of these cases is the inability to stand upright without support — a state of *truncal ataxia*. This tumor, which is highly sensitive to radiotherapy, is clearly attacking the neuronal pathway from the vermal cortex through the fastigial nucleus to the nucleus of the vestibular nerve. The nystagmus reflects malfunction of the medial vestibular nucleus on being deprived of its normal regulatory input. The ataxia reflects malfunction of the lateral vestibular nucleus and consequently of the vestibulospinal tract. Deficient antigravity function in this uncrossed pathway causes the child to fall to the more affected side on attempting to stand or walk.

---

### CLINICAL PANEL 19.2 • ANTERIOR LOBE LESIONS: GAIT ATAXIA

Disease of the anterior lobe is most often observed in chronic alcoholics. Postmortem studies reveal pronounced shrinkage of the cortex of the anterior lobe, with up to 10% loss of granule cells, 20% loss of Purkinje cells, and 30% reduction in the thickness of the molecular layer. The lower limbs are most affected, and a staggering, drunken gait is evident even when the patient is sober. Some degree of correction may be exercised by voluntary control. Instability of station with the feet together, and failure to 'toe the line' on walking, are present even when the eyes are open. As the disease progresses, a peripheral sensory neuropathy may be added, giving rise to signs of sensory ataxia (Chapter 11) as well.

---

### CLINICAL PANEL 19.3 • NEOCEREBELLAR LESIONS: INCOORDINATION OF VOLUNTARY MOVEMENTS

Disease of the neocerebellar cortex, dentate nucleus or superior cerebellar peduncle leads to incoordination of voluntary movements, particularly in the upper limb. When fine purposive movements are attempted (e.g. grasping a glass, using a key) an *intention tremor* develops: the hand and forearm quiver as the target is approached, owing to faulty muscle synergies around the elbow and wrist. The hand may travel past the target ('overshoot'). Because cerebellar guidance is lost, the normal smooth trajectory of reaching movements may be replaced by stepped flexions, abductions, etc. ('decomposition of movement').

Rapid alternating movements performed under command, such as pronation/supination, become quite irregular. The 'finger-to-nose' and 'heel-to-knee' tests are performed with equal clumsiness whether the eyes are open or closed—in contrast to performance in posterior column disease (Chapter 11).

Speech is impaired both with regard to phonation and to articulation. Phonation (production of vowel sounds) is uneven and often tremulous owing to loss of smoothness of contraction of the diaphragm and intercostals. The terms 'explosive' and 'scanning' have been applied to this feature. Articulation is slurred because of faulty timing of impulses in the nerves supplying the lips, mandible, tongue, palate, and the infrahyoid muscles.

Signs of neocerebellar disorder sometimes originate in the *midbrain* or *pons* rather than in the cerebellum itself. The lesion responsible (usually vascular) interrupts one or other corticopontocerebellar pathway. If the corticopontine component is interrupted, ataxia will appear in the contralateral limbs. If the pontocerebellar component is interrupted, the ataxia will be ipsilateral.

---

calf muscles (ankle plantarflexors) and over the tibialis anterior (an ankle dorsiflexor). The normal response to the backward tilt is threefold: (a) a monosynaptic, spinal, stretch reflex contraction of the calf muscles after 45 msec; (b) a polysynaptic stretch reflex contraction of the calf muscles after 95 msec; and (c) a *long-loop*, reflex contraction of the ankle dorsiflexors after 120 msec. The ascending limb of the long loop is via the tibial-sciatic nerve and the posterior column-medial lemniscal pathway to the somatosensory cortex; the descending limb is via the corticospinal tract and the sciatic-peroneal nerve. Dynamic posturography helps to distinguish among a wide variety of disorders affecting different levels of the CNS and PNS.

### EXERCISES

BRAINSTEM LESIONS
Using the brainstem sections in Chapter 13 as the main frame of reference, work out the minimal size

of lesion that would account for the neurological deficits listed below. Express locations as, for example, right ventral pons, left medial medulla.

**1** (*a*) Spastic weakness of the left arm and leg
   (*b*) Cerebellar ataxia in the right arm and leg.
**2** (*a*) Spastic weakness of the left arm and leg
   (*b*) Loss of joint sense and vibration sense in the left leg
   (*c*) Wasting of the right side of the tongue.
**3** (*a*) Horner's syndrome on the right
   (*b*) Loss of pinprick perception on the right side of the face
   (*c*) Hoarseness.
**4** (*a*) Inability to wrinkle the forehead or to bare the teeth on the left side
   (*b*) Inability to abduct the left eye.
**5** (*a*) Visible wasting of the right masseter muscle
   (*b*) Loss of pinprick perception on the right side of the face
   (*c*) Loss of pinprick perception on the left leg.
**6** (*a*) A dilated pupil on the right, together with ptosis and a divergent squint
   (*b*) Motor weakness of the limbs and lower face on the left side.

## REFERENCES

Diener, H.-C. and Dichgans, J. (1992) Pathophysiology of cerebellar ataxia. *Movement Disorders* **7**: 95–109.

Ebner, T.J. and Bloedel, J.R. (1987) Climbing fiber afferent system: intrinsic properties and role in cerebellar information processing. In *New Concepts in Cerebellar Neurobiology* (King, J.S., ed.), pp. 371–386. New York: Alan R. Liss.

Fox, P.T., Raichle, M.E. and Thach, W.T. (1985) Functional mapping of the human cerebellum with positron emission tomography. *Proc. Natl. Acad. Sci. USA* **82**: 7462–7466.

Gilbert, P.F.C. and Thach, W.T. (1977) Purkinje cell activity during motor learning. *Brain Res.* **128**: 309–328.

Houk, J.C. and Gibson, A.R. (1987) Sensorimotor processing through the cerebellum. In *New Concepts in Cerebellar Neurobiology* (King, J.S., ed.), pp. 387–416. New York: Alan R.Liss.

Kennedy, P.R. (1979) The rubro-olivo-cerebellar teaching circuit. *Med. Hypoth.* **5**: 799–807.

Leiner, H.C., Leiner, A.L. and Dow, R.S. (1991) The human cerebro-cerebellar system: its computing, cognitive, and language skills. *Behav. Brain Res.* **44**: 113–128.

# 20

# Hypothalamus

The hypothalamus is phylogenetically a very ancient part of the brain. It evolved as part of the limbic system, which is concerned with survival of the individual and of the species. It provides the interface between the nervous and endocrine systems. Most of its functions are expressed through the pituitary gland and through both divisions of the autonomic nervous system.

The hypothalamus occupies the side walls and floor of the third ventricle. It is a bilateral, paired structure. Despite its small size—it weighs only 4 grammes—it has major functions in homeostasis and survival. Its homeostatic functions include control of the body temperature and the circulation of the blood. Its survival functions include regulation of food and water intake, the sleep–wake cycle, sexual behavior patterns, and defense mechanisms against attack.

## Boundaries

The boundaries of the hypothalamus are as follows (see *Figures 20.1* and *20.2*):

*Superior:* the **hypothalamic sulcus** separating it from the thalamus.
*Inferior:* the **optic chiasm, tuber cinereum** and **mamillary bodies.** The tuber cinereum shows a small swelling, the **median eminence,** immediately behind the **infundibulum** ('funnel') atop the pituitary stalk.
*Anterior:* the lamina terminalis.
*Posterior:* the tegmentum of the midbrain.
*Medial:* the third ventricle.
*Lateral:* the internal capsule.

## Subdivisions and nuclei

In the sagittal plane, it is customary to divide the hypothalamus into three regions: *anterior (supraoptic), middle (tuberal)* and *posterior (mamillary).* The descriptive use of 'regions' has been convenient for

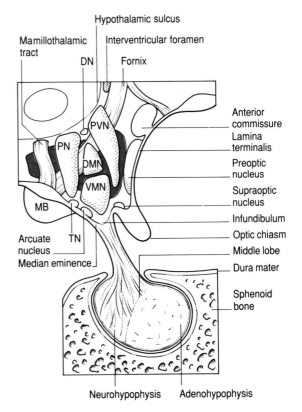

**Figure 20.1.** Hypothalamic nuclei and hypophysis, viewed from the right side. DN, dorsal nucleus; DMN, dorsomedial nucleus; LN, lateral nucleus (in red); MB, mamillary body; PN, posterior nucleus; PVN, periventricular nucleus; TN, tuberomamillary nucleus; VMN, ventromedial nucleus. The lateral hypothalamic nucleus is shown in red.

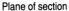

Plane of section

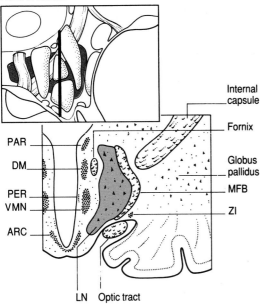

Internal capsule

Fornix

PAR

DM

Globus pallidus

MFB

PER

VMN

ZI

ARC

LN   Optic tract

**Figure 20.2.** Hypothalamic nuclei, and related neural pathways, in a coronal section. ARC, arcuate nucleus; DM, dorsomedial nucleus; LN, lateral nucleus; MFB, medial forebrain bundle; PAR, paraventricular nucleus; PER, periventricular nucleus; VMN, ventromedial nucleus; ZI, zona incerta.

animal experiments involving placement of lesions. Named nuclei in the three regions are listed in Table 20.1.

**Table 20.1.** Hypothalamic nuclei

| Anterior | Intermediate | Posterior |
|---|---|---|
| Preoptic | Arcuate (infundibular) | Mamillary |
| Supraoptic | Tuberal | Posterior |
| Suprachiasmatic | Lateral | |
| Paraventricular | Dorsal | |
| Anterior | Dorsomedial | |
| | Ventromedial | |
| | Posterior | |
| | Periventricular | |

In the coronal plane, the hypothalamus can be divided into lateral, medial, and periventricular regions. The full length of the lateral region is occupied by the lateral hypothalamic nucleus.

## Hypothalamic control of the pituitary gland

The arterial supply of the pituitary gland comes from hypophysial branches of the internal carotid artery (*Figure 20.3*). One set of branches supplies a capillary bed in the wall of the infundibulum. These capillaries drain into *portal vessels* which pass into the adenohypophysis. There they break up to form a second capillary bed which bathes the endocrine cells and drains into the cavernous sinus.

The neurohypophysis receives a direct supply from another set of hypophyseal arteries. The capillaries drain into the cavernous sinus, which delivers the secretions of the anterior and posterior lobes into the general circulation.

Secretions of the pituitary gland are controlled by two sets of *neuroendocrine cells*. Neuroendocrine cells are true neurons in having dendrites and axons and in conducting nerve impulses. They are also true endocrine cells because they liberate their

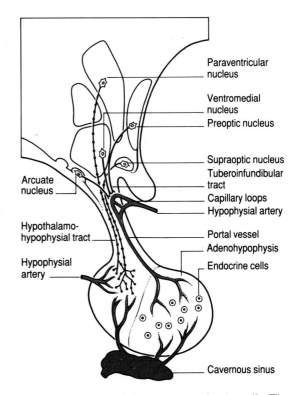

Paraventricular nucleus

Ventromedial nucleus

Preoptic nucleus

Supraoptic nucleus

Tuberoinfundibular tract

Capillary loops

Hypophysial artery

Portal vessel

Adenohypophysis

Endocrine cells

Arcuate nucleus

Hypothalamo-hypophysial tract

Hypophysial artery

Cavernous sinus

**Figure 20.3.** Hypothalamic neuroendocrine cells. The blood supply to the hypophysis, including the endocrine cells of the adenohypophysis, is also shown (arrows indicate direction of blood flow).

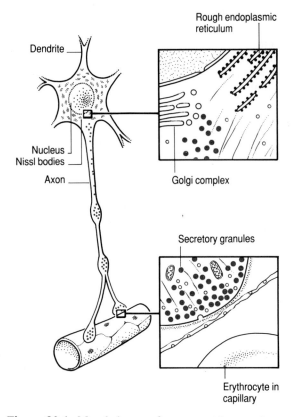

**Figure 20.4.** Morphology of a peptide-secreting neuroendocrine cell.

secretions into capillary beds (*Figure 20.4*). With one exception (mentioned below), the secretions are peptides, synthesized in clumps of granular endoplasmic reticulum and packaged in Golgi complexes. The peptides are attached to long-chain polypeptides called *neurophysins*. The capillaries concerned are outside the blood–brain barrier, and are fenestrated.

The somas of the neuroendocrine cells occupy the *hypophysiotropic area* in the lower half of the preoptic and tuberal regions. Contributory nuclei are the preoptic, supraoptic, paraventricular, ventromedial, and arcuate (infundibular). Two classes of neurons can be identified: parvocellular (small) neurons reaching the median eminence, and magnocellular (large) neurons reaching the posterior lobe of the pituitary gland.

### The parvocellular neuroendocrine system

*Parvocellular* neurons of the hypophysiotropic area give rise to the *tuberoinfundibular tract*, which

reaches the infundibular capillary bed. Action potentials traveling along these neurons result in calcium-dependent exocytosis of *releasing hormones* from some and *inhibiting hormones* from others, for transport to the adenohypophysis in the portal vessels. The cell types of the adenohypophysis are stimulated/inhibited in accordance with *Table 20.2*. In the left hand column, the only non-peptide parvocellular hormone is the prolactin-inhibiting hormone, which is *dopamine*, secreted from the arcuate (infundibular) nucleus.

**Table 20.2** Hypothalamic parvocellular releasing/inhibiting hormones (RH/IH)

| RH/IH | | Anterior lobe hormone |
|---|---|---|
| Corticotropin RH | | ACTH |
| Thyrotropin RH | | Thyrotropin |
| Growth hormone RH | | Growth hormone |
| Growth hormone IH | | Growth hormone |
| Prolactin RH | | Prolactin |
| Prolactin IH | | Prolactin |
| Gonadotropic hormone RH | | FSH/LH |

The releasing/inhibiting hormones are not wholly specific: they have major effects on a single cell type, and minor effects on one or two others.

Multiple controls exist for parvocellular neurons of the hypophysiotropic area. The controls include: depolarization by afferents entering from the limbic system and from the reticular formation; hyperpolarization by local-circuit GABA neurons, some of which are sensitive to circulating hormones; and inhibition of transmitter release by opiate-releasing internuncials, which are numerous in the intermediate region of the hypothalamus. The picture is further complicated by the fact that opiates and other modulatory peptides may be released into the portal vessels and activate receptors on the endocrine cells of the adenohypophysis.

### Magnocellular neurons of the neuroendocrine system

*Magnocellular* neurons in the supraoptic and paraventricular nuclei give rise to the *hypothalamohypophysial tract,* which descends to the posterior lobe (*Figure 20.3*). Minor contributions to the tract are received from opiatergic and other peptidergic neurons in the periventricular region of the hypothalamus, and from aminergic neurons of the brainstem.

---

### CLINICAL PANEL 20.1 • HYPOTHALAMIC DISORDERS

The most dramatic disorder of hypothalamic function is *diabetes insipidus*, which is brought about by interruption of the hypothalamohypophyseal pathway—sometimes by tumors in the region, sometimes by head injury. The patient drinks upwards of 10 liters of water per day, and excretes a similar amount of urine. Historically, the term *insipidus* refers to the absence of taste sensation from the urine, in contrast to *diabetes mellitus*, in which the urine is sweet-tasting *(mellitus)* owing to its sugar content.

Hypophysectomy (surgical removal of the pituitary gland) can be performed in the treatment of other diseases, without causing more than temporary diabetes insipidus, provided the pituitary stalk is sectioned at a low level. Within a short period, sufficient ADH is secreted into the capillary bed of the median eminence to ensure adequate water conservation.

A wide variety of hypothalamic dysfunctions have been reported in the clinical literature. Causes are also varied, and include tumors, congenital malformations, and head injury. Clinical manifestations include gross obesity, disturbances of autonomic control, excessive sleepiness, and memory loss.

---

Two hormones are secreted by separate neurons located in both the supraoptic and paraventricular nuclei: antidiuretic hormone (vasopressin) and oxytocin. Axonal swellings containing the secretory granules for these hormones make up nearly half the volume of the neurohypophysis. The largest swellings, called *Herring bodies*, may be as large as erythrocytes. The Herring bodies are thought to provide a local source of granules for release from smaller, terminal swellings into the capillary bed.

### Antidiuretic hormone

Antidiuretic hormone (ADH) continuously stimulates water uptake by the distal convoluted tubules and collecting ducts of the kidneys. The chief regulator of electrical activity in the ADH-secreting neurons is the osmotic pressure of the blood. A rise of as little as 1% in the osmotic pressure causes the plasma to be diluted to normal levels by means of increased water uptake. The neurons are themselves sensitive to osmolar changes, but they are facilitated by inputs from osmolar and volume detectors elsewhere, notably a small **organum vasculosum** behind the lamina terminalis.

Some ADH neurons also synthesize corticotropin releasing hormone, the two hormones being released together from collateral branches, into the capillary pool of the infundibulum. It is of interest that ADH neuronal activity is increased when the body is stressed, and that the output of ACTH is boosted by the presence of ADH in the adenohypophysis.

Withdrawal of ADH secretion results in *diabetes insipidus* (see Panel 20.1).

### Oxytocin

The principal function of oxytocin is to participate in a *neurohumoral reflex* when an infant is suckling at the breast. The afferent limb of this reflex is provided by impulses traveling from the nipple to the hypothalamus via the spinoreticular tract. Oxytocin is liberated by magnocellular neurons in response to suckling. Having entered the general circulation, it causes the expression of milk by stimulating myoepithelial cells surrounding the lactiferous ducts of the breast.

Oxytocin also has a mild stimulating action on uterine muscle during labor. The afferent stimulus in this case originates in the genital tract once labor gets under way.

### *Other hypothalamic connections and functions*

### Autonomic centers

In animals, stimulation of the anterior hypothalamic area produces parasympathetic effects: slowing of the heart, constriction of the pupil, salivary secretion and intestinal peristalsis. On the other hand, stimulation of the posterior hypothalamic area produces sympathetic effects: increase in heart rate and blood pressure, pupillary dilatation, and intestinal stasis. Axons from both areas project to autonomic nuclei in the brainstem and spinal cord. In the midbrain and pons, this projection occupies a small *posterior longitudinal fasciculus* in the central gray matter.

## Temperature regulation

The hypothalamus contains *thermosensitive neurons* which initiate appropriate responses to changes in the core temperature of the body. Activity of these neurons is reinforced by thermal information received (via the spinoreticular tract) from thermosensitive neurons supplying the skin (Chapter 8).

A slight change in the core temperature can usually be corrected by directing blood flow into or away from the skin, as appropriate. The requisite control of the sympathetic nervous system resides in the region of the posterior nucleus of the hypothalamus, which sends axons all the way to the lateral horn of the spinal cord.

Hypothalamic control of the sympathetic system diminishes with age. For this reason, the elderly are particularly prone to develop *hypothermia* in cold weather.

*Hyperthermia* is characteristic of *fevers*. Infectious agents (bacteria, viruses, parasites) cause tissue macrophages to liberate *endogenous pyrogen* — a protein that causes the hypothalamic 'thermostat' to be reset to a higher value. The chief mechanisms used to raise the body temperature to the new set point are cutaneous vasoconstriction and shivering.

## Drinking

The chief center controling the intake of water appears to be a ribbon of cells alongside the lateral nucleus known as the **zona incerta** (*Figure 20.2*). Stimulation of this region may produce excessive drinking; lesions may result in refusal to drink, with consequent severe dehydration.

## Eating

Eating habits have obvious social and cultural components, causing dietary practise to vary widely between individuals and between communities. The hypothalamus provides a baseline for caloric and nutrient intake, in the form of interplay between the lateral and ventromedial nuclei. Together, they constitute the *appestat* (appetite set point). Stimulation of a lateral hypothalamic *feeding center* causes a cat or rat to eat excessively, whereas destruction of this center results in refusal to eat. Conversely, stimulation of a ventromedial *satiety center* inhibits the urge to eat, and bilateral ventromedial lesions result in persistent overeating and gross obesity. The satiety center is normally very sensitive to glucose levels in the blood.

## Rage and fear

The lateral and ventromedial nuclei are concerned with *mood* as well as food. Cats that are overweight in consequence of ventromedial lesions tend to be highly aggressive. Conversely, animals rendered underweight by ventromedial stimulation tend to be unduly docile. (See also the amygdala, in Chapter 25.)

## Sleeping and waking

A small *suprachiasmatic nucleus* embedded in the upper surface of the optic chiasma receives a direct retinal input in mammals including monkeys. In laboratory animals, lesions of this nucleus disrupt the normal diurnal variation of various body rhythms.

Lesions of the posterior hypothalamic area may cause hypersomnolence or even coma. This area contains the *tuberomamillary nucleus* (*Figure 20.1*), housing hundreds of *histaminergic neurons*, which project widely to the gray matter of the brain and spinal cord. Some of the fibers run rostrally within the medial forebrain bundle, in company with two other sets of aminergic fibers: dopaminergic from the midbrain and noradrenergic from the pons (Chapter 18). Histaminergic fibers destined for the cerebral cortex fan out below the genu of the corpus callosum. They branch within the superficial layers of the frontal cortex, and run back to supply the cortex of the parietal, occipital and temporal lobes.

In animals, there is abundant physiological evidence in support of an *arousal function* for the histaminergic system.

## Memory

The mamillary bodies belong to a limbic circuit involving the fornix, which sends fibers to it, and the mamillothalamic tract which projects to the anterior nucleus of the thalamus. This circuit may have a function in relation to memory (Chapter 25).

## REFERENCES

Akil, H. and Watson, S.J. (1987) Neuropeptides in brain and pituitary: overview. In *Psychopharmacology: The Third Generation of Progress* (Meltzer, H.Y., ed.), pp. 367–371. New York: Raven Press.

Gordon, C.J. (1986) Integration and central processing in temperature control. *Ann. Rev. Physiol.* **48**: 595–612.

Hatton, G.L. (1990) Emerging concepts of structure–function dynamics in adult brain: the hypothalamo-neurohypophysial system. *Progr. Neurobiol.* **34**: 337–504.

Kordon, C. (1985) Neural mechanisms involved in pituitary control. *Neurochem. Int.* **7**: 917–925.

Lutten, P.G.M., ter Horst, T.J. and Steffens, A.B. (1986) The hypothalamus: intrinsic connections and outflow pathways to the endocrine system in relation to the control of feeding and metabolism. *Progr. Neurobiol.* 28: 1–54.

Schwartz, J-C., Arrang, J-M., Garbarg, M., Pollard, H. and Ruat, M. (1991) Histaminergic transmission in the mammalian brain. *Physiol. Rev.* **71**: 1–51.

The thalamus, with which this chapter is mainly concerned, is the largest nuclear mass in the entire nervous system. It is a prominent feature in MRI scans in each of the three planes in which slices are taken. The afferent and efferent connections of the nine main nuclear groups are listed; these are so diverse that the thalamus cannot be said to have a unitary function.

## THE THALAMUS

As noted in Chapter 2, the two thalami lie at the very center of the brain. Their medial surfaces face one another across the third ventricle and their lateral surfaces are in contact with the posterior limb of the internal capsule. The upper surface of each occupies the floor of the lateral ventricle and the lower surface receives the somatic sensory pathways as well as an upward continuum of the reticular formation.

### Thalamic nuclei

The Y-shaped **internal medullary lamina** of white matter divides the thalamus into three large cell groups: *mediodorsal, anterior,* and *lateral* (*Figure 21.1A*). The lateral group comprises dorsal and ventral nuclear tiers. At the back of the thalamus are the medial and lateral geniculate nuclei. The **external medullary lamina** separates the thalamus from the shell-like *reticular nucleus*.

The thalamic nuclei may be categorized into three functional groups: specific or relay nuclei, association nuclei, and non-specific nuclei.

### Specific nuclei

The specific or relay nuclei are reciprocally connected to specific motor or sensory areas of the cerebral cortex. They comprise the nuclei of the

ventral tier and the geniculate nuclei. Their afferent and efferent connections are indicated in *Figure 21.1B*.

The **ventral anterior nucleus** (VA) receives afferents from the globus pallidus, and it projects to the prefrontal cortex.

The anterior part of the **ventral lateral nucleus** (VL) receives afferents from the globus pallidus and projects to the supplementary motor area. The posterior part of VL is the principal target of the contralateral superior cerebellar peduncle, which originates in the central nuclei contained in the cerebellar white matter. The posterior VL projects to the motor cortex.

*Note:* VL appears to provide a linkage between the dentate nucleus of the cerebellum and premotor areas of the cerebral hemisphere, notably in connection with speech (Chapter 23).

The **ventral posterior nucleus** (VP) receives all of the fibers of the medial, spinal, and trigeminal lemnisci (*Figure 21.2*). It projects to the somatic sensory cortex (SI). A smaller projection is sent to the second somatic sensory area (SII) at the foot of the postcentral gyrus (see Chapter 23).

The VP is somatotopically arranged, as indicated in *Figure 21.3*. The portion of the nucleus devoted to the face and head is called the *ventroposteromedial* nucleus (VPM), that for the trunk and limbs the *ventroposterolateral* nucleus (VPL). Modality segregation is a feature of both nuclei, with proprioceptive neurons most anterior, tactile neurons in the mid-region, and nociceptive neurons at

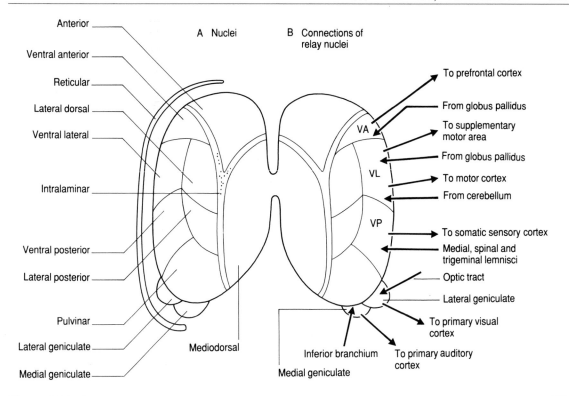

**Figure 21.1.** Schematic illustration of the two thalami, viewed from above. VA, ventral anterior nucleus; VL, ventral lateral nucleus; VP, ventral posterior nucleus.

the back. The nociceptive region is sometimes called the *posterior nucleus.*

There is no evidence in the VP of an antinociceptive mechanism comparable to that found in the substantia gelatinosa region of the spinal cord and spinal trigeminal nucleus. An unexplained disorder, the *thalamic syndrome,* may follow a vascular lesion that disconnects the posterior thalamic nucleus from the somatic sensory cortex. In this condition a period of complete sensory loss may occur on the contralateral side of the body, to be replaced by bouts of severe pain occurring either spontaneously or in response to tactile stimuli.

The **medial geniculate nucleus** *(medial geniculate body)* is the thalamic nucleus for hearing. It receives the inferior brachium, and it projects to the primary auditory cortex.

The **lateral geniculate nucleus** *(lateral geniculate body)* is the principal thalamic nucleus for vision. It receives retinal inputs from both eyes, and it projects to the primary visual cortex. The visual pathways are described in Chapter 22.

### Association nuclei

The association nuclei are reciprocally connected to the association areas of the cerebral cortex.

The **anterior nucleus** receives the mamillothalamic tract and projects to the cingulate cortex. It is involved in a limbic circuit and seems to have a function in relation to memory (Chapter 25).

The **anterior dorsal nucleus** properly belongs with the anterior nucleus, being only partially separated from it by the internal medullary lamina.

The **mediodorsal nucleus** receives inputs from the olfactory and limbic systems and is reciprocally connected with the entire prefrontal cortex. It has poorly understood functions in relation to cognition (thinking), judgement, and mood.

The **lateral posterior nucleus** and the **pulvinar** belong to a single nuclear complex. They project to the entire visual association cortex and

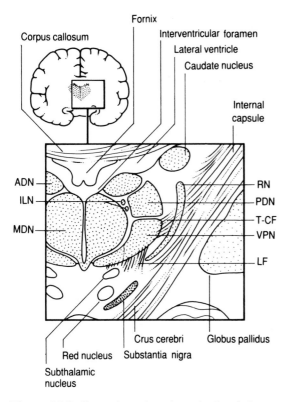

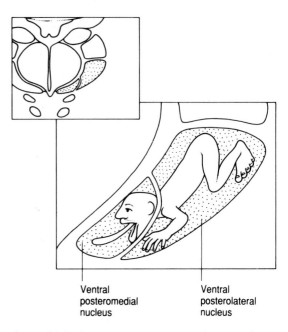

**Figure 21.3.** Somatic sensory map in the ventral posterior thalamic nucleus. (Redrawn and modified from Ohye (1990) with permission.)

**Figure 21.2.** Coronal section through the thalamus and related structures. ADN, anterior dorsal nucleus; ILN, intralaminar nucleus; LF, lemniscal fibers; MDN, mediodorsal nucleus; PDN, posterior dorsal nucleus; RN, reticular nucleus; T-CF, thalamocortical fibers.

to the entire parietal association cortex. The only known afferent source of consequence (apart from the cortex to which it is distributed) is the superior colliculus. An 'extrageniculate visual pathway' runs from the optic tract to the visual association cortex by way of the superior colliculus and the pulvinar. It seems to have the function of drawing attention to objects of interest in the peripheral field of vision, but it is not itself a source of conscious visual perception.

**Non-specific nuclei**

The non-specific nuclei include the intralaminar and reticular nuclei.

The **intralaminar nuclei** are contained within the internal medullary lamina of white matter. They can be regarded as a rostral continuation of

the reticular formation of the midbrain (see Ascending Reticular Activating System in Chapter 18). They project widely to the cerebral cortex, as well as to the corpus striatum.

The **reticular nucleus** surrounds the front and lateral side of the thalamus. All of the thalamocortical projections pass through the reticular nucleus and give collateral branches to it. The nucleus reciprocates by sending a matching, *inhibitory* (GABAergic) supply to the corresponding thalamic nucleus—both to the projection neurons and to a set of GABAergic internuncials within the nucleus.

**Synaptic interplay in the ventral thalamus**

*Figure 21.4* shows synaptic relationships in the ventral posterior nucleus. *Specific afferents* (the medial, spinal and trigeminal lemnisci) synapse upon the inhibitory internuncials as well as on the thalamocortical neurons. A feature (of uncertain significance) in all of the ventral tier nuclei is an abundance of inhibitory, dendrodendritic synapses between the internuncials and the projection cells.

Some *non-specific afferents* from the midbrain reticular formation synapse in the reticular nucleus. Others pass to the intralaminar nuclei and to the nucleus of Meynert in the basal forebrain (Chapter 25).

In animal experiments (cat), thalamocortical neurons are inhibited by the reticular nucleus during sleep, exhibiting only intermittent short bursts of activity. During wakefulness, thalamocortical neurons fire continuously, apparently because of *disinhibition:* the reticular nucleus is still active, but its effect seems to be shifted to the inhibitory internuncials.

Not represented in *Figure 21.4* are *aminergic afferents* passing to the ventral and intralaminar nuclei, from the midbrain raphe *(serotonin)* and locus ceruleus *(norepinephrine)*. The proven value of tricyclic antidepressants in the therapy of chronic pain may be related to drug-induced prolongation of aminergic effects on thalamocortical neurons.

## Overview of the thalamus

The word 'thalamus' is the Greek for a meeting place. Current research suggests that the word is a misnomer, because the nine principal nuclei of the thalamus are essentially independent of one another, with the solitary exception of the reticular nucleus.

## Thalamic peduncles

The reciprocal connections between the thalamus and the cerebral cortex travel in four **thalamic peduncles,** as shown in *Figure 21.5*. The **anterior thalamic peduncle** passes through the anterior limb of the internal capsule to reach the prefrontal cortex and cingulate gyrus. The **superior thalamic peduncle** passes through the posterior limb of the internal capsule to reach the premotor, motor, and somatic sensory cortex. The **posterior thalamic peduncle** passes through the retrolentiform part of the internal capsule to reach the occipital lobe and the posterior parts of the parietal and temporal lobes. The **inferior thalamic peduncle** passes below the lentiform nucleus to reach the anterior temporal and orbital cortex. Each of the four fans becomes incorporated into the corona radiata.

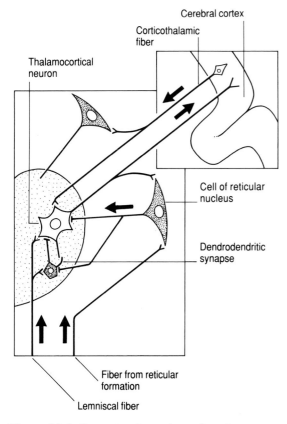

**Figure 21.4.** Synaptic relationships of a relay neuron in the ventral posterior nucleus of the thalamus. Arrows indicate directions of impulse transmission. Inhibitory neurons are shown in black.

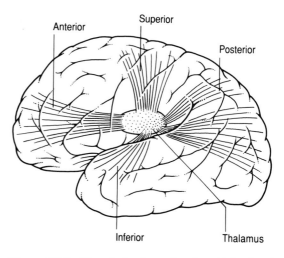

**Figure 21.5.** The thalamic peduncles (right hemisphere).

## EPITHALAMUS

The epithalamus includes the pineal gland, habenula, and stria medullaris. The latter two are included with the limbic system in Chapter 25.

### *Pineal gland*

The pineal gland synthesizes *melatonin,* an amine hormone having an obscure relation to gonadal function. Melatonin is derived from serotonin, the requisite enzymes being unique to this gland.

From the third decade onward, calcareous deposits ('pineal sand') accumulate within astrocytes in the pineal. Calcification is often detectable in plain radiographs of the head. A shift of the gland may denote a space-occupying lesion within the skull. However, a normal pineal may lie slightly to the left because the right cerebral hemisphere is usually a little wider than the left at this level.

## REFERENCES

Jones, E.G. (1985) *The Thalamus.* New York: Plenum Press.

Kultas-Ilinsky, K. and Ilinsky, I.A. (1986) Neuronal and synaptic organization of the motor nuclei of mammalian thalamus. In *Current Topics in Research on Synapses, Vol.3,* pp. 77–145. New York: Alan R. Liss

Lenz, F.A. (1992) Ascending modulation of thalamic function and pain. In *Advances in Pain Research and Therapy* (Sicuteri, F. *et al,* eds), pp. 177–196. New York: Raven Press.

Ohye, C. (1990) Thalamus. In *The Human Nervous System* (Paxinos, G., ed.), pp. 439–468. San Diego: Academic Press.

Steriade, M. and Llinas, R.R. (1988) The functional states of the thalamus and the associated neuronal interplay. *Physiol. Rev.* **68:** 649–742.

# 22

# Visual system

**The visual system is of outstanding importance in clinical neurology. It extends from the retina of the eye to the occipital lobe of the brain. Its great length makes it especially vulnerable to demyelinating diseases such as multiple sclerosis; to tumors of the brain or pituitary gland; to vascular lesions in the territory of the middle or posterior cerebral artery; and to head injuries.**

The visual system comprises the retinas, the visual pathways from the retinas to the brainstem and visual cortex, and the cortical areas devoted to higher visual functions. The retinas and visual pathways are described in this chapter. Higher visual functions are described in Chapter 23.

## RETINA

The retina is formed by an outgrowth from the diencephalon called the **optic vesicle.** The optic vesicle is invaginated by the lens and becomes the two-layered **optic cup.**

The outer layer of the optic cup becomes the **pigment layer** of the mature retina. The inner, **nervous layer** of the cup gives rise to the retinal neurons.

*Figure 22.1* shows the general relationships in the developing retina. The nervous layer contains three sets of neurons: **photoreceptors,** which become applied to the pigment layer when the **intraretinal space** is resorbed; **bipolar neurons;** and **ganglion cells** which form the optic nerve and project to the thalamus and midbrain. (The fibers of the optic nerve grow along the walls of a fissure which invaginates the under surface of the optic cup.)

Note that the retina is *inverted:* light must pass through the layers of optic nerve fibers, ganglion cells, and bipolar neurons to reach the photoreceptors. At the point of most acute vision, the **fovea centralis,** the inner layers lean away all around a cental pit (fovea), and light strikes the photoreceptors directly. In the mature eye, the fovea is about 1.5 mm in diameter and occupies the center of the **macula lutea** ('yellow spot'). The fovea is the

point of most acute vision and lies in the *visual axis* — a line passing from the center of the *visual field* of the eye, through the center of the lens, to the fovea (*Figure 22.2*). To *fixate* or *foveate* an object is to gaze directly at it so that light reflected from its center registers on the fovea.

The visual fields of the two eyes overlap across two-thirds of the total visual field. Outside this *binocular field* is a *monocular crescent* on each side (*Figure 22.3*). During passage through the lens, the image of the visual field is *reversed,* with the result that, for example, objects in the left part of the binocular visual field register on the right half of

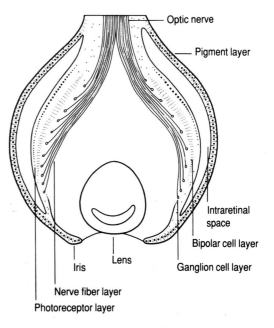

**Figure 22.1.** Embryonic retina.

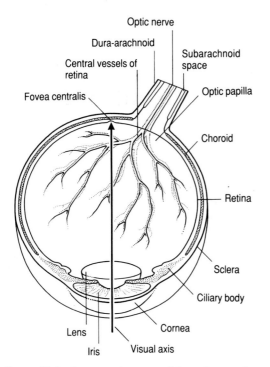

**Figure 22.2.** Horizontal section of the right eye, showing the visual axis.

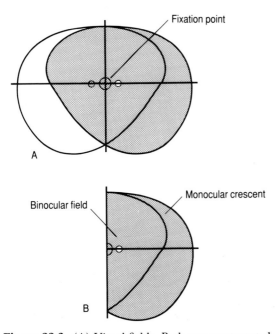

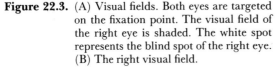

**Figure 22.3.** (A) Visual fields. Both eyes are targeted on the fixation point. The visual field of the right eye is shaded. The white spot represents the blind spot of the right eye. (B) The right visual field.

each retina and objects in the lower part of the visual field register on the upper half.

From a clinical standpoint, it is essential to appreciate that vision is a crossed sensation. The visual field on one side of the visual axis registers on the visual cortex of the other side. In effect, the right visual cortex 'sees' the left visual field. Only half of the visual information crosses in the optic chiasma, for the simple reason that the other half has already crossed the midline in space.

Visual defects caused by interruption of the visual pathway are always described *from the patient's point of view*, i.e. in terms of the visual fields, and not in terms of retinal topography.

### Structure of the retina

The retina contains three sets of neurons arranged in series: **photoreceptors, bipolar neurons,** and **ganglion cells.** As well, it contains two sets of neurons arranged transversely: **horizontal cells,** and **amacrine cells** (*Figure 22.4*).

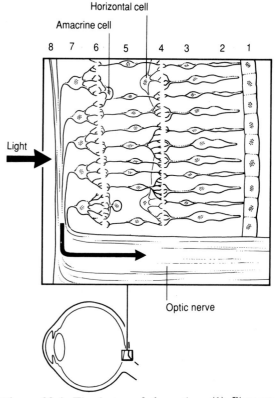

**Figure 22.4.** The layers of the retina. (1) Pigment layer; (2) photoreceptor layer; (3) outer nuclear layer; (4) outer plexiform layer; (5) inner nuclear layer; (6) inner plexiform layer; (7) ganglion cell layer; (8) nerve fiber layer.

Action potentials are generated by the ganglion cells, providing the requisite speed for conduction to the thalamus and midbrain. For the other cell types, distances are very short and passive electrical change (electrotonus) is sufficient for intercellular communication, whether by gap-junctional contact or transmitter release.

## Photoreceptors

The photoreceptor neurons comprise **rods** and **cones.** Rods function only in dim light and are not sensitive to color. They are absent from the fovea. Cones respond to bright light, are sensitive to color and shape, and are most numerous in the fovea.

Each photoreceptor has an outer and an inner segment and a synaptic end-foot. In the outer segment the plasma membrane is folded to form hundreds of membranous discs which incorporate visual pigment formed in the inner segment. The synaptic end-foot makes contact with bipolar neurons and horizontal cell processes in the *outer plexiform layer.*

A surprising feature of the photoreceptors is that they are *hyperpolarized* by light. During darkness Na$^+$ channels are opened, creating sufficient positive electrotonus to cause leakage of transmitter from the end-feet. Illumination causes the Na$^+$ channels to close.

## Cone and rod bipolar neurons

### Cone bipolar neurons
Cone bipolar neurons are of two types. ON bipolars are switched on (depolarized) by light, being inhibited by transmitter released in the dark. They converge onto ON ganglion cells. OFF bipolars have the reverse response and converge onto OFF ganglion cells (*Figure 22.5*).

### Rod bipolar neurons
Rod bipolar neurons are all hyperpolarized by light. They activate ON and OFF ganglion cells *indirectly,* by way of amacrine cells.

## Horizontal cells

The dendrites of horizontal cells are in contact with photoreceptors. The peripheral dendritic branches give rise to axon-like processes which make inhibitory contacts with bipolar neurons.

The function of horizontal cells is to inhibit bipolar neurons, of similar kind, outside the immediate zone of excitation. The excited bipolars

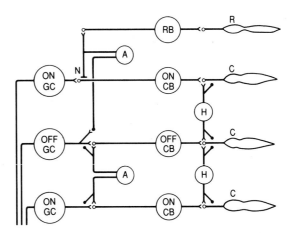

**Figure 22.5.** Retinal circuit diagram. (Adapted from Massey and Redburn (1987).) A, amacrine cell; C, cone; CB, cone bipolar neuron; GC, ganglion cell; H, horizontal cell; N, nexus (gap junction); R, rod; RB, rod bipolar.

and ganglion cells are said to be *on-line,* the inhibited ones are *off-line.*

## Amacrine cells

Amacrine cells have no axons. Their appearance is octopus-like, the dendrites all emerging from one side of the cell. Dendritic branches come into contact with bipolar neurons and ganglion cells.

More than a dozen different morphological types of amacrine cells have been identified, as well as several different transmitters including acetylcholine, dopamine, and serotonin. Possible functions include contrast enhancement and movement detection. For the rods, they convert large numbers of rods from OFF to ON with respect to ganglion cells.

## Ganglion cells

The ganglion cells receive synaptic contacts from bipolar neurons in the *inner plexiform layer.* The typical response of ganglion cells to bipolar activity is 'center-surround'. An ON ganglion cell is excited by a spot of light, and inhibited by a surrounding annulus (ring) of light. The inhibition is caused by horizontal cells. OFF ganglion cells give the reverse response.

### Coding for color
There are three types of cone with respect to spectral sensitivity. One is sensitive to red, one to

green, and one to blue. Groups of each type are connected to ON or OFF ganglion cells.

The characteristic response of ganglion cells is one of *color opponency:*

- Ganglion cells that are on-line for green are off-line for red.
- Ganglion cells that are on-line for red are off-line for green.
- Ganglion cells that are on-line for blue are off-line for *yellow*, i.e. for green and red cones acting together.

### Coding for black and white

White light is a mixture of green, red, and blue. In bright conditions it is encoded by the three corresponding cones, all of them converging onto common ganglion cells. Both ON and OFF ganglion cells are involved in black-and-white vision, just as in color vision.

In very dim conditions, e.g. starlight, only rod photoreceptors are active, and objects appear in varying shades of gray. The rods are subject to the same rules as cones, showing center-surround antagonism between white and black, and being connected to ON or OFF ganglion cells.

## CENTRAL VISUAL PATHWAYS

### *Optic nerve, optic tract*

The optic nerve is formed by the axons of the retinal ganglion cells. The axons acquire myelin sheaths as they leave the optic disc.

The number of ganglion cells varies remarkably between individuals, from 800 000 to 1.5 million. Since every ganglion cell contributes to the optic nerve, the number of axons in the optic nerve is correspondingly variable.

The retinal ganglion cells are homologous with the projection neurons of the spinal cord. The optic nerve is homologous with spinal cord white matter, and is *not* a peripheral nerve. As explained in Chapter 7, peripheral nerves, whether cranial or spinal, contain Schwann cells and collagenous sheaths, and are capable of regeneration. The optic nerve contains neuroglial cells of central type (astrocytes and oligodendrocytes) and is not capable of regeneration in mammals. As well, the nerve is invested with meninges containing an extension of the subarachnoid space—a feature largely responsible for the changed appearance of the fundus oculi when the intracranial pressure is raised (Chapter 6).

---

### CLINICAL PANEL 22.1 • LESIONS OF THE VISUAL PATHWAYS

The following points arise in testing the visual pathways:

- The patient may be unaware of quite extensive blindness—sometimes even of a hemianopia
- Large visual defects can often be detected by simple *confrontation*, as follows. The patient covers one eye at a time, and focuses on the examiner's nose. The examiner, seated opposite, looks the patient in the eye while bringing one or other hand into view from various directions, with the index finger wiggling.
- In a blind area, the patient does not see blackness; the patient does not see *anything*. (We are normally unaware of the 'blind spot' created by the optic nerve head, even with one eye closed.)
- Visual defects are described from the patient's viewpoint, in terms of the visual fields.

Possible sites of injury to the visual pathways are shown in *Figure CP 22.1.1*. The effects produced correspond to the numbers in the following list.

| Lesions | Field defects |
|---|---|
| 1 Partial optic nerve | Ipsilateral scotoma[a] |
| 2 Complete optic nerve | Blindness in that eye |
| 3 Optic chiasm | Bitemporal hemianopia |
| 4 Optic tract | Homonymous[b] hemianopia |
| 5 Meyer's loop | Homonymous upper quadrant anopia |
| 6 Optic radiation | Homonymous hemianopia |
| 7 Visual cortex | Homonymous hemianopia |
| 8 Macular cortex (bilateral) | Central scotomas |

[a] *A scotoma is a patch of blindness.*
[b] *Matching.*

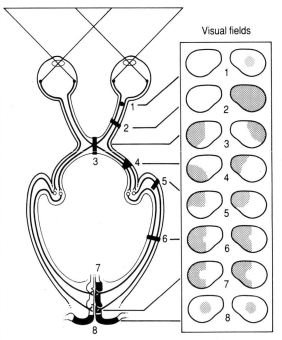

**Figure CP 22.1.1.** Visual field defects following various lesions of the visual pathways.

### Notes on the numbered lesions

1. Eccentric lesions of the optic nerve produce scotomas in the nasal or temporal field of the affected eye. When a young adult presents with a scotoma, multiple sclerosis must always be suspected.

3. Compression of the middle of the chiasm is most often caused by an adenoma (benign tumor) of the pituitary gland.
4. Lesions of the optic tract are rare. Although homonymous (matching) visual fields are affected, the outer, exposed half of the tract tends to be more affected than the inner half, and the hemianopia is then described as *incongruous*.
5. Meyer's loop may be selectively caught by a tumor in the temporal lobe.
6. Lesions involving the optic radiation include tumors arising in the temporal, parietal, or occipital lobe. The visual fields of both eyes tend to be affected to an equal extent *(congruously)*. Tumors impinging on the radiation from below produce an upper quadrantic defect at first whereas tumors impinging from above produce a lower quadrantic defect. The stem of the radiation occupies the retrolentiform part of the internal capsule and is often compromised for some days by edema, following hemorrhage from a branch of the middle cerebral artery (classical stroke, Chapter 27).
7. Thrombosis of the posterior cerebral artery produces a homonymous hemianopia. The notches in field chart no. 7 represent *macular sparing*. Sparing of the macular hemifields is inconstant.
8. Bilateral central scotomas are most often caused by a backward fall with occipital concussion.

At the optic chiasm, fibers from the nasal hemiretina enter the contralateral optic tract whereas those from the temporal hemiretina remain uncrossed and enter the ipsilateral tract.

The optic tract winds around the midbrain and divides into a medial and a lateral root.

### Medial root of optic tract

The medial root contains 10% of the optic nerve fibers. It enters the side of the midbrain. It contains up to six distinct sets of fibers, three of them targeting the superior colliculus:

1. Some fibers enter the superior colliculus and provide the afferent limb of the visual grasp reflex (Chapter 17).
2. Other fibers entering the superior colliculus provide for automatic scanning, e.g. in reading this page.
3. Some fibers are relayed from the superior colliculus to the pulvinar of the thalamus; they belong to the extra-geniculate visual pathway to the visual association cortex (Chapter 21).
4. Some fibers enter the pretectal nucleus and serve the pupillary light reflex (Chapter 17).
5. Some fibers enter the parvocellular reticular formation, where they have an arousal function (Chapter 18).
6. Some medial root axons *probably* enter the human suprachiasmatic nucleus in the hypothalamus. Such a connection has been invoked to account for the beneficial effect of bright artificial light, for several hours per day, in the treatment of wintertime depression.

### Lateral root of the optic tract and lateral geniculate nucleus

The lateral root of the optic tract terminates in the lateral geniculate nucleus (body) of the thalamus (LGN).

LGN shows six cellular laminae, three of which are devoted to crossed fibers and three to uncrossed fibers. The two deepest laminae (one for crossed and one for uncrossed fibers) are magnocellular and receive axons from ganglion cells

---

**Figure 22.6.** Left optic radiation visualized from the left side.

**Figure 22.7.** A dissection of the visual pathways, viewed from below. (Photograph reproduced from *The Human Brain*, by N. Gluhbegovic and T.W. Williams, by kind permission of the authors and of J.B. Lippincott, Inc.)

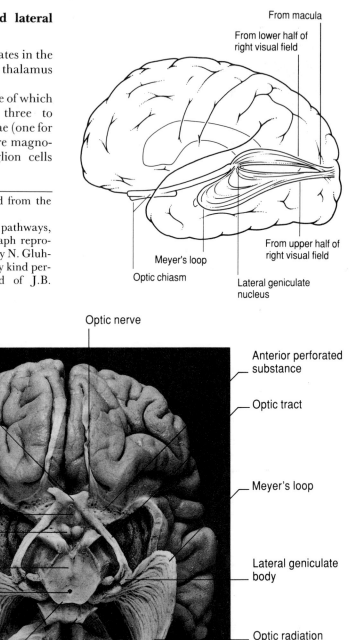

From macula

From lower half of right visual field

From upper half of right visual field

Meyer's loop

Optic chiasm

Lateral geniculate nucleus

Optic chiasm

Optic nerve

Anterior perforated substance

Optic tract

Meyer's loop

Infundibulum

Mamillary body

Tegmentum of midbrain

Aqueduct

Lateral geniculate body

Optic radiation

Calcarine sulcus

Primary visual cortex

Superior colliculus

Splenium

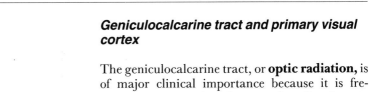

### Geniculocalcarine tract and primary visual cortex

The geniculocalcarine tract, or **optic radiation,** is of major clinical importance because it is frequently compromised by vascular disorders or tumors in the posterior part of the cerebral hemisphere. It travels from the lateral geniculate nucleus to the primary visual cortex.

The anatomy of the optic radiation is shown in *Figures 22.6–22.8*. Fibers destined for the lower half of the primary visual cortex sweep forward into the temporal lobe, as *Meyer's loop*, before turning back to accompany those traveling to the upper half. The tract enters the retrolentiform part of the internal capsule and continues in the white matter underlying the lateral temporal cortex. It runs alongside the posterior horn of the lateral ventricle before turning medially to enter the occipital cortex.

The **primary visual cortex** occupies the walls of the calcarine sulcus along its entire length (the sulcus is 10 mm deep). It emerges onto the medial surface of the hemisphere for 5 mm both above and below the sulcus, and onto the occipital pole of the brain for 10 mm. Its total area is about 25 cm$^2$. In the freshly cut brain it is easily identified by a thin band of white matter (the **visual stria** of Gennari) within the gray matter—hence an alternative term, *striate cortex*. The left and right eyes are represented in the cortex in alternating stripes called *ocular dominance columns* (see Chapter 23).

RETINOTOPIC MAP

The contralateral visual field is represented upside down. The plane of the calcarine sulcus represents the horizontal meridian. Retinal representation is posteroanterior, with a greatly magnified foveal representation in the posterior half and the monocular crescent close to the corpus callosum.

The clinical effects of various lesions of the visual pathway are described in Panel 22.1.

The visual cortex and higher visual areas are described in Chapter 23.

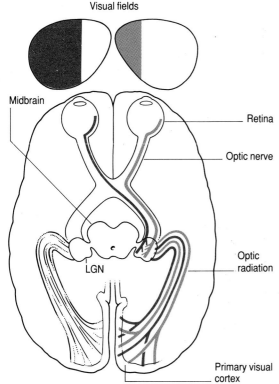

**Figure 22.8.** Diagram of the visual pathways. The two visual fields are represented separately, without the normal overlap.

(known as Y cells) having large receptive fields and being concerned with detection of movement. The other four receive the axons of X cells, which are concerned with visual detail and with color.

The circuitry of LGN resembles that of other thalamic relay nuclei, and includes inhibitory (GABA) terminals derived from internuncial neurons and from the thalamic reticular nucleus. (The portion of the reticular nucleus serving LGN is called the *perigeniculate nucleus*.) Corticogeniculate axons arise in the primary visual cortex and synapse upon distal dendrites of relay cells as well as upon inhibitory internuncials. Cortical synapses on relay cells are twice as numerous as those derived from retinal ganglion cells. Cortical stimulation usually enhances the response of relay cells to a given retinal input. A likely, but unproven function could be that of selective enhancement of particular features of the visual scene, e.g. when searching for an object of known shape or color.

### REFERENCES

Bynke, H. (1984) The visual fields. In *Neuro-ophthalmology, Vol. 3* (Lessell, S. and van Dalen, J.T.W., eds), pp. 348–357. Amsterdam: Elsevier.

Curcio, C.A. and Kimberly, A.A. (1990) Topography of ganglion cells in human retina. *J. Comp. Neurol.* **300:** 5–25.

Frisen, L. (1980) The neurology of visual acuity. *Brain* **103:** 639–670.

Karten, H.J., Keyser, K.T. and Brecha, N.C. (1990) Biochemical and morphological heterogeneity of retinal ganglion cells. In *Vision and the Brain* (Cohen, B. and Bodis-Wollner, I., eds), pp. 19–33. New York: Raven Press.

Koch, C. (1987) The action of the corticofugal pathway on thalamic nuclei: a hypothesis. *Neuroscience* **23:** 399–406.

Massey, S.C. and Redburn, D.A. (1987) Transmitter circuits in the vertebral retina. *Prog. Neurobiol.* **28:** 55–96.

# 23

# Cerebral cortex

The cerebral cortex is the part of the body that makes us truly human. Its structure is enormously complex, and the assignment of functions to different parts is made difficult by the multiplicity of interconnections. Interpretation of the effects of pathological lesions presents a dual problem because lesions are seldom sharply circumscribed, and some effects can be produced at a distance by disconnection of linkages with other areas.

Although damage often leads to permanent disability, the cortex does exhibit a degree of 'plasticity' which is very relevant to the field of rehabilitation.

After completing this chapter, the reader is advised to give a first reading to Chapter 26, where many of the observations recur in the context of cerebrovascular disease.

The cerebral cortex varies in thickness from 2 to 4 mm, being thinnest in the primary sensory areas and thickest in the motor and association areas. More than half is hidden from view in the walls of the sulci. The cortex contains about 50 billion neurons; about ten times that number of supporting, neuroglial cells; and a dense capillary bed.

The cortex has both a *laminar* and a *columnar* structure. The general cytoarchitecture varies in detail from one region to another, permitting the cortex to be mapped into dozens of histologically different 'areas'. Although considerable progress has been achieved in relating individual 'areas' to specific functions, they are merely nodal points having widespread connections with other parts of the brain.

## STRUCTURAL ASPECTS

### Laminar organization

A laminar (layered) arrangement of neurons is apparent in sections taken from any part of the cortex. Phylogenetically old elements, including the limbic cortex in the medial temporal lobe, are trilaminar whereas six cellular laminae are seen in the *neocortex* covering the remainder of the brain.

### Cellular laminae of the neocortex *(Figure 23.1A)*

I  The **molecular layer** contains the most distal dendritic branches of the pyramidal cells, and the most distal branches of axons projecting from the intralaminar nuclei of the thalamus.

II The **outer granular layer** contains small pyramidal and stellate cells.

III The **outer pyramidal layer** contains medium-sized pyramidal cells projecting to other parts of the cortex.

IV The **inner granular layer** contains stellate cells receiving afferents from the thalamic relay nuclei. Stellate cells are especially numerous in the primary somatic, primary visual, and primary auditory cortex. The term *granular cortex* is applied to these areas. In contrast, the primary motor cortex contains relatively few stellate cells in lamina IV and is called *agranular*.

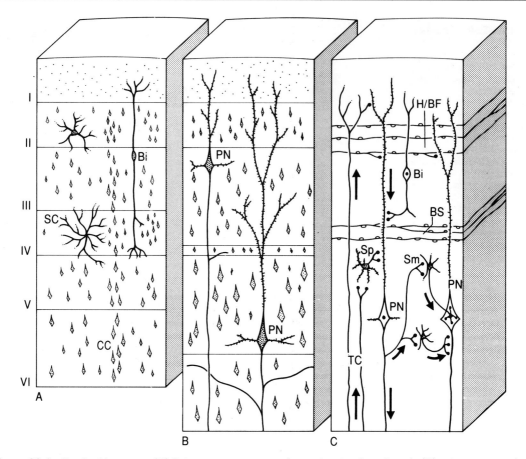

**Figure 23.1.** Cerebral isocortex. (A) Primary sensory cortex (somatic, visual, auditory); (B) primary motor (area 4); (C) elementary circuits. Bi, bipolar neuron; BS, afferents from brainstem; CC, cell column; H/BF, afferents from hypothalamus and basal forebrain; PN, pyramidal neuron; SC, stellate cell; Sm, smooth stellate cell; Sp, spiny stellate cell; TC, thalamocortical afferents.

V The **inner pyramidal layer** contains large pyramidal cells projecting to the corpus striatum, brainstem, and spinal cord.

VI The **fusiform layer** contains modified pyramidal cells projecting to the thalamus.

### *Columnar organization* (Figure 23.1A)

In the somatic sensory cortex, the neurons were discovered (in monkeys) to be arranged functionally in terms of *columns* 300–500 μm in diameter extending radially through all laminae. Within each column, all of the cells are modality-specific. For example, a given column may respond to movement of a particular joint but not to stimulation of the overlying skin. Subsequent research has shown that cell columns comprising several

hundred neurons are the functional units or *modules* of the cortex. Some modules are activated by specific thalamocortical inputs, others by corticocortical inputs from the same hemisphere, others again by inputs from the opposite hemisphere. Aggregates of modules create a *cortical mosaic*.

### *Cell types* (Figure 23.1B, C)

The three principal morphological cell types are pyramidal cells, spiny stellate cells, and smooth stellate cells.

*Pyramidal cells* have cell bodies ranging in height from 20–30 μm in laminae II and III to more than twice that height in lamina V. Tallest of all, at 80–100 μm, are the *giant cells of Betz* in the motor cortex. The *apical* and *basal* dendrites of pyramidal cells branch freely and are studded with spines. The axon gives off recurrent branches before leaving the gray matter. All pyramidal cells are excitatory, and use glutamate or closely related aspartate as transmitter.

*Spiny stellate cells* have spiny dendrites and in general are excitatory. They receive most of the afferent input from the thalamus and from other areas of the cortex, and they synapse upon pyramidal cells.

*Smooth stellate cells* have non-spiny dendrites and in general are inhibitory. They receive recurrent collateral branches from pyramidal cells and they synapse upon other pyramidal cells. Inhibitory, GABA-secreting neurons make up about 25% of all neurons in the cerebral cortex. Some synapse upon the bases of dendritic spines, some synapse upon the somas, and some synapse upon initial axonal segments. As is the case in the cerebellar cortex (Chapter 19), the GABA neurons exert a focusing action by silencing weakly active cell columns.

*Bipolar cells* are found mainly in the outer laminae. Most contain one or more peptides, such as VIP (vasoactive intestinal polypeptide), CCK (cholecystokinin), or somatostatin. Peptides are also co-liberated with GABA from many smooth stellate cells.

Human cortical neurons can be captured in fragments of biopsies taken for other purposes. They can be kept alive for several hours and examined for responses to transmitters and transmitter analogues. It appears that a single pyramidal cell may have as many as ten different kinds of receptor scattered over its surface. It also appears that the response of the neuron to a particular transmitter is not completely predictable being modified by concurrent effects of other transmitters.

### Afferents

Afferents to a given region of the cortex are derived from five sources:
1. Long and short *association fibers* from other parts of the ipsilateral hemisphere.
2. *Commissural fibers* from the matching region of the opposite hemisphere.
3. *Thalamocortical fibers* from the appropriate specific or association nucleus.
4. *Non-specific thalamocortical fibers* from the intralaminar nuclei.

5. *Neuraxial fibers* from the hypothalamus and brainstem. Nuclei and transmitters are as follows:

> tuberoinfundibular (hypothalamus): histamine
> tegmentum (midbrain): dopamine
> raphe nucleus (midbrain): serotonin
> locus ceruleus (pons): norepinephrine

### Targets of pyramidal neurons

* *Association fibers* are composed of axons of small pyramidal cells that loop from one part of the cortex to another within a hemisphere. Short association fibers interconnect neighboring gyri. Long association fibers, including the *superior* and *inferior longitudinal fasciculi* and the *arcuate fasciculus*, link different lobes of the brain. The *cingulum* underlying the cingulate cortex contains short and long association fibers and belongs to the limbic system (Chapter 25).
* *Commissural fibers* are composed of axons of medium-sized pyramidal cells that link corresponding areas of cortex on the two sides of the brain. The corpus callosum is much the largest of the commissures. Other commissures are the anterior, posterior, habenular, and hippocampal.
* *Projection fibers* are axons of large pyramidal cells that project to the basal ganglia, brainstem, and spinal cord.

## CORTICAL AREAS

The most widely used reference map is that of Brodmann, who divided the cortex into 47 areas on the basis of cytoarchitectural differences. Most of these areas are shown in *Figure 23.2*.

### Sensory areas

#### Somatic sensory cortex (areas 3, 1, 2)

The somatic sensory or *somesthetic* cortex occupies the entire postcentral gyrus including its anterior and posterior surfaces. Representation of contralateral body parts is inverted and the hand, lips and tongue have disproportionately large representations. Separate body maps can be constructed for different modalities of sensation. Thus, slowly adapting cutaneous receptors relay to area 3, rapidly adapting ones to area 1, and

Lateral surface

Medial surface

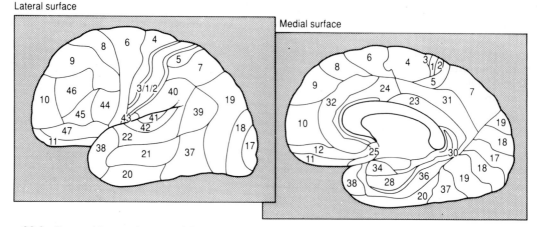

**Figure 23.2.** Cytoarchitectural areas of Brodmann. (Redrawn, and slightly modified, from Zilles (1990), with permission.)

articular receptors to area 2. A fourth area (called 3a), in the floor of the central sulcus, receives information relayed from muscle spindles.

In addition to thalamic afferents from the ventral posterior nucleus, the somesthetic cortex receives commissural fibers from its opposite number through the corpus callosum, and short association fibers from the motor cortex. Many of the fibers from the motor cortex are collaterals of corticospinal fibers traveling to the anterior horn of the spinal cord, and they may contribute to the *sense of weight* when an object is lifted.

Efferents from the somesthetic cortex pass to the motor cortex, to the opposite somesthetic cortex, and to area 5 of the posterior parietal cortex. In addition, *projection fibers* descend to sensory relay nuclei, namely the ventral posterior nucleus of the thalamus, the posterior column nuclei, and the posterior gray horn of the spinal cord.

On the medial surface of the parietal operculum is a small *secondary somatic sensory area* (SII), whose function is obscure. It receives more *nociceptive* relays from the thalamus than does the primary sensory area (SI).

Area 5 is called the *supplementary sensory area* by some workers, and the *somesthetic association area* by others. In animal experiments, individual cortical modules have peripheral receptive fields covering several body segments. Many modules are *multimodal*, responding to both cutaneous and proprioceptive stimuli. Multimodal cell columns seem to provide the neccessary basis for *stereognosis*—the ability to identify a three-dimensional object held in the hand.

PLASTICITY OF THE SOMATIC SENSORY CORTEX

In monkeys, cortical sensory representations of the individual digits of the hand can be defined very exactly by recording the electrical response of cortical cell columns to tactile stimulation of each digit in turn.

The digital maps can be altered by peripheral sensory experience, as the following experiments indicate:

- The median nerve supplies the ventral surface of the outer three digits of the hand whereas the radial nerve supplies their dorsal surfaces. If the median nerve is crushed, the representation of the dorsal surface on the digital map increases at the expense of the ventral representation. The increase begins within hours and progresses slowly over a period of weeks. With regeneration of the median nerve, the cortical map reverts to normal.
- If the middle digit is removed, the corresponding cortical area is unresponsive for a few hours, then becomes progressively (over weeks) taken over by expansion of the representations of the second and fourth digits.
- If the pad skin of a digit is chronically stimulated, e.g. by having to press a rotating sanded disc in order to release pellets of food, representation of the pad may increase to twice its original size over a period of weeks, reverting to normal after the experiment is discontinued.

These experiments show that somatic sensory maps are *plastic*, being modified by peripheral events. A purely anatomical explanation (for example, sprouting of nerve branches within the CNS, or peripherally) is not appropriate for the earliest changes, which begin within hours. Instead, they can be accounted for on the basis of sensory competition.

SENSORY COMPETITION

Sensory maps made at the level of the posterior gray horn, posterior column nuclei, thalamus, and somesthetic cortex all show evidence of anatomical overlap. For example, the thalamocortical projection for the digit 3 overlaps the projections for digits 2 and 4. Within the zone of overlap, cortical columns are shared by afferents from two adjacent digits. As already explained, smooth stellate cells exert lateral inhibition upon weakly stimulated columns. Under experimental conditions (in cats), the number of columns responding to a particular thalamocortical input can be increased by local infusion of a GABA antagonist drug, which suppresses lateral inhibition. The effect of removal of a peripheral sensory field may be comparable: if one set of thalamocortical neurons falls silent due to loss of sensory input, it no longer exerts lateral inhibition and cortical columns within its territory are taken over by neighboring, active sets. (*Note:* In monkeys, complete sensory deafferentation of an arm is followed after several *years* by takeover of the entire cortical arm representation by the adjacent lower face. The most likely (but untested) basis of explanation may be the occurrence of sprouting of trigeminothalamic terminals into the nearby arm representation in the ventral posterolateral nucleus of the thalamus.)

## Visual cortex

The visual cortex comprises the *primary visual cortex* (area 17) and the *visual association cortex* (areas 18 and 19).

PRIMARY VISUAL CORTEX

As noted in Chapter 22, the primary visual cortex is the target of the geniculocalcarine tract, which relays information from the ipsilateral halves of both retinas, and therefore from the contralateral visual field. The myelinated fibers enter the cortex and create the visual stria (of Gennari). They terminate by synapsing upon spiny stellate cells of the highly granular lamina IV. The spiny stellate cells belong to *ocular dominance columns*, so named because alternating columns are dominated by inputs from the left and right eyes (*Figure 23.3*). In a surface view of the visual cortex, the columnar

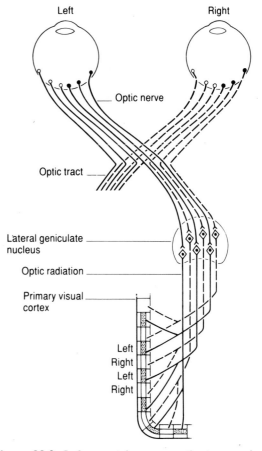

**Figure 23.3.** Left-eye, right-eye contributions to the ocular dominance columns in the primary visual cortex.

arrangement takes the form of whorls, resembling finger prints. The geniculocalcarine projection is so ordered that matching points from the two retinas are registered side by side in contiguous columns. This arrangement is ideal for binocular vision because cells at the edge of a column respond to inputs from both eyes.

Under experimental conditions (monkeys), spiny stellate cells of the primary visual cortex give either 'concentric' (center-surround) or 'simple' responses. 'Simple' cells respond to slits of light of a particular orientation, and the effect seems to be produced by cells receiving convergent afferents from a row of 'concentric' cells. Pyramidal cells may be 'complex', responding to bars (broad slits) of a particular orientation, or 'hypercomplex', responding to L-shapes. Again, the different responses can be explained on the basis of convergence.

VISUAL ASSOCIATION CORTEX

Afferents to areas 18 and 19 are mainly from area 17 but include some direct thalamic projections from the lateral geniculate nucleus and the pulvinar. Groups of cell columns are concerned with *feature extraction:* some respond to geometrical shapes, some respond to movement in a particular direction, some respond to color, and some are involved in stereopsis (depth perception). Many cell columns have large receptive fields, some of which straddle the physiological blind spot (optic nerve head) and may be responsible for 'covering up' the blind spot during monocular vision.

Outputs from the visual association cortex are mainly *dorsal* and *ventral* (*Figure 23.4*). Dorsal outputs pass to the posterior parietal cortex (area 7); they are mainly concerned with stereopsis and movement. Ventral outputs pass to the *inferotemporal cortex* (areas 20, 21); they are concerned with analysis of form and color.

The inferotemporal cortex is regarded as the highest visual area. It is interconnected with the lateral prefrontal cortex. Electrical stimulation of area 21 (in patients undergoing temporal lobe surgery) may evoke lifelike visual hallucinations. Behind it, at the occipitotemporal junction (area 37), the cortex contains modules specifically devoted to the recognition of *faces*. Failure of this function (*prosopagnosia*) may occur as an early and heart-breaking sign of Alzheimer's disease (Chapter 25): overnight, the patient may no longer recognize family members.

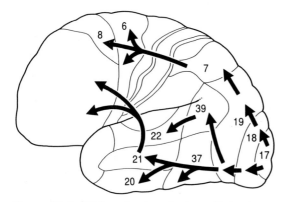

**Figure 23.4.** Higher visual projections. Projections to and from area 7 are concerned with stereopsis and movement. Projections to and from area 20/21 are concerned with detail and color. Projections to and from area 39 are concerned with symbols including letters and numbers.

PLASTICITY OF THE PRIMARY VISUAL CORTEX

The basic pattern and balance of ocular dominance columns is preserved in animals reared in complete darkness. On the other hand, if one eye is sealed from birth the stripes in area 17 for that eye become abnormally narrow, and those for the open eye abnormally broad. The effect can be explained on the basis of *synaptic competition.* During a critical period (6th postnatal week in monkeys), the right-eye left-eye projections from the lateral geniculate nucleus overlap extensively. As the cortex matures the redundant axonal arbors (multiple branches) are withdrawn and the column edges become sharply defined. If one eye is deprived of sensory experience from birth, the corresponding geniculocalcarine neurons branch less extensively and those from the 'experienced' eye do not withdraw.

## Auditory cortex

The *primary auditory cortex* occupies the anterior transverse temporal gyrus (of Heschl) and corresponds to areas 41 and 42. (Some workers would not include the whole of area 42.) Both occupy the upper surface of the superior temporal gyrus. The *auditory association cortex* corresponds to area 22.

Columnar organization in the primary auditory cortex takes the form of *isofrequency stripes,* each stripe responding to a particular tonal frequency. Higher frequencies activate lateral stripes in Heschl's gyrus, lower frequencies activate medial stripes. Because of crossover at all levels of the central auditory pathway in the brainstem (Chapter 15), *each ear is represented bilaterally.* In experimental recordings, the primary cortex responds equally well from both ears in response to *monaural* stimulation but the contralateral cortex is more responsive during simultaneous *binaural* stimulation.

The auditory association cortex includes Wernicke's area for language perception (see under Language, later). Visual and auditory data are brought together in the cortex bordering the superior temporal sulcus (junction of areas 21 and 22 in *Figure 23.2*).

Excision of the entire auditory cortex (in the course of removal of a tumor) has no obvious effect on auditory perception. The only significant defect is loss of *stereoacousis:* on testing, the patient has difficulty in appreciating the direction and the distance of a source of sound.

## Motor areas

### Primary motor cortex

The primary motor cortex (area 4) is a strip of agranular cortex within the precentral gyrus. It gives rise to about 80% of the corticospinal (pyramidal) tract. The remaining 20% originate in the premotor and supplementary motor areas and from the parietal cortex, as illustrated in Chapter 12. There is an inverted somatotopic representation of contralateral body parts, with relatively large areas devoted to the hand and tongue. The hand areas of the motor and somatic sensory cortex occupy the corresponding walls of the central sulcus. Direct stimulation of the human motor cortex indicates that individual modules are concerned with specific movements (such as abduction of a joint) rather than for specific cell columns in the spinal cord.

The course and terminations of the pyramidal tract are described in Chapters 12, 13 and 15.

SOURCES OF AFFERENTS TO THE MOTOR CORTEX
- Somatosensory cortex, including positive feedback from muscle spindles.
- Cerebellum, via ventral lateral nucleus of thalamus.
- Premotor cortex.
- Supplementary motor area.

PLASTICITY IN THE MOTOR CORTEX
In monkeys and in lower mammals, small lesions of the motor cortex produce an initial paralysis of the corresponding body part, followed within a few days (sometimes within hours) by progressive recovery. The recovery is attributable to a change of allegiance of cell columns close to the lesion, which take on the missing motor function. Instead of inflicting a lesion, it is possible to enlarge the motor territory of a patch of cortex merely by injecting a GABA antagonist drug locally into the cortex. Expansion of motor territories at spinal cord level is already provided for by extensive overlap of projections from area 4 to the motor cell columns in the ventral gray horn.

### Supplementary motor area and premotor cortex

The *supplementary motor area* (SMA) corresponds to area 6 on the medial surface of the hemisphere.

Afferents are received from the prefrontal cortex, from the basal ganglia (via thalamus) and from the contralateral SMA. Efferents project mainly to the primary motor cortex; a few join the corticospinal tract.

FUNCTIONAL OBSERVATIONS ON SMA (*FIGURE 23.5*)
- SMA shows increased activity *before* movement commences, as well as during movement. It therefore seems to be involved in motor planning.
- SMA is always active during speech whereas the premotor cortex is not.
- Unilateral lesions of SMA are associated with akinesia (difficulty in initiating movement) on the opposite side.
- Bilateral lesions are accompanied by total akinesia, including akinesia for speech initiation.

SMA is believed to be activated by internally generated movement intentions, originating in the prefrontal cortex in the absence of direct sensory cues. Appropriate motor programs are run via the motor cortex under the guidance of the basal ganglia, which project to SMA by way of the thalamus (Chapter 24).

The *premotor cortex* (PMC) corresponds to area 6 on the lateral surface of the hemisphere. It is six times larger than the primary motor cortex. Afferents are received from:

- Prefrontal cortex
- Basal ganglia, via the ventral lateral nucleus of thalamus
- Posterior parietal cortex (area 7)
- Contralateral PMC.

Efferents project to the motor cortex and to the nuclei of the reticular formation giving rise to the reticulospinal tracts. The PMC gives a small contribution to the corticospinal tract.

FUNCTIONAL OBSERVATIONS ON PMC (*FIGURE 23.6*)
- In normal subjects the PMC shows increased activity (indicated by increased blood flow) when motor routines are run in response to visual, auditory or somatic sensory cues, e.g. reaching for an object, obeying a spoken command, identifying something by manipulation.
- A lesion confined to the PMC on one side is associated with weakness of contralateral postural control of the shoulder and hip. Recovery

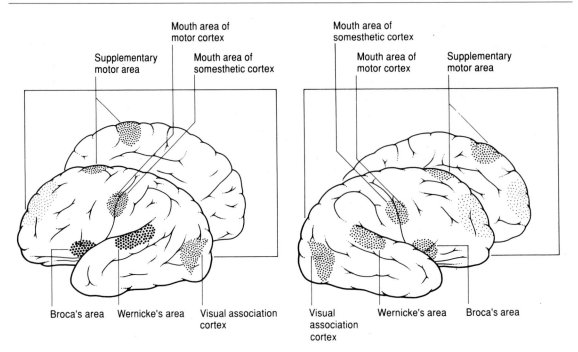

**Figure 23.5.** Areas of increased blood flow during speech. $^{133}$Xenon was injected into the carotid system and detected by sensors applied to the scalp. Activity at the occipital pole in the exclusive territory of the posterior cerebral artery is not detectable by the method. (Adapted from Lassen *et al.* (1978) *Sci. Am.* **239:** 62–66.)

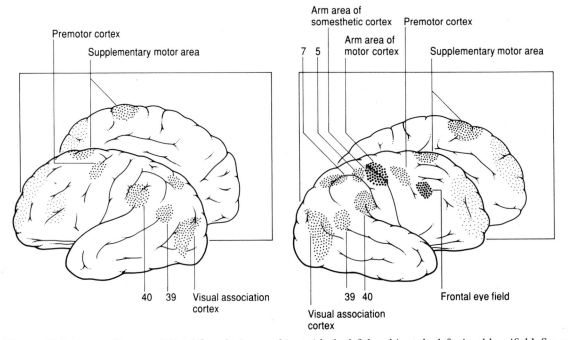

**Figure 23.6.** Areas of increased blood flow during reaching with the left hand into the left visual hemifield. Same technique as in *Figure 23.5*. Nos. 5, 3, 39, 40 refer to Brodmann's areas in *Figure 23.2*. (Adapted from Roland *et al.* (1989) *J. Neurophysiol.* **43:** 137–150.)

is usually rapid (within days) and is attributed to takeover by the opposite PMC, through uncrossed reticulospinal fibers.

PMC is believed to contain a large vocabulary of motor programs, which can be retrieved by appropriate sensory cues and run via the motor cortex.
. SMA and PMC are always activated bilaterally, even when the movement produced is strictly unilateral. The simplest explanation is that of *information transfer* from one hemisphere to the other, through the corpus callosum. In support of this idea, novel manipulations learned for the right hand are relatively quickly mastered afterward by the left hand—but not if the corpus callosum has been interrupted by disease or by surgery (so-called 'split brain').

**Frontal eye field** (*FIGURE 23.6*)

The frontal eye field (FEF) is mainly located in area 8, directly in front of the premotor cortex, but there is some overlap onto the precentral gyrus. The FEF is responsible (under control by the prefrontal cortex) for voluntary saccadic eye movements (Chapter 17). Both clinical and experimental (monkey) observations indicate that:

- The FEFs are tonically active, bilaterally.
- Increased activity in the midregion of the FEF on one side causes a horizontal saccade toward the contralateral visual hemispace (a *contraversive* saccade).

- Increased activity in the upper region on one side produces an obliquely downward contraversive saccade. Bilateral upper region activation causes both eyes to look straight down.
- Increased lower region activity has corresponding effects with respect to upward gaze.

### Prefrontal cortex

The prefrontal cortex has two-way connections with all parts of the isocortex except the primary motor and sensory areas, with its fellow through the genu of the corpus callosum, and with the mediodorsal nucleus of the thalamus. It is uniquely large in the human brain and is concerned with the highest brain functions including abstract thinking, decision making, anticipating the effects of particular courses of action, and social behavior. Any or all of these may be compromised by frontal lobe disease (Panel 23.1).

## HEMISPHERIC ASYMMETRIES

The two cerebral hemispheres are *asymmetrical* in certain respects. The most notable asymmetries are in respect of language and complex motor activities, but there are other, more subtle differences that come under the general heading of *cognitive style*.

---

### CLINICAL PANEL 23.1 • FRONTAL LOBE DYSFUNCTION

*General symptoms* of frontal lobe disease include loss of short-term memory, lack of foresight (failure to anticipate the consequences of a course of action), and distractibility (poor concentration). These symptoms often signal the onset of Alzheimer's disease (Chapter 25). *Local symptoms* may be added to the general picture, if the disease process is predominantly in the dorsolateral or orbital parts of the prefrontal cortex.

Large *dorsolateral lesions* are associated with hypokinesia and apathy, with indifference to surrounding events. The picture resembles that of the 'withdrawn' type of schizophrenia, and it

is of interest that in 'withdrawn' schizophrenic patients cortical blood flow may not show the anticipated increase in the dorsolateral region, in response to appropriate psychological tests.

Large *orbitofrontal lesions* are associated with hyperkinesia, with increased instinctual drives in relation to food and sexual behavior, and often with rather puerile jocularity. Hyperkinetic frontal lobe disorders have been treated in the past by means of *leukotomy*—a surgical procedure in which the white matter above the orbital cortex was severed through a supraorbital incision.

## *Language*

In 90% of subjects the left hemisphere is dominant for language. In 5% the right hemisphere is dominant, and in 5% the two hemispheres have an equal share. There is no hemispheric bias for language with respect to left or right handedness.

### Language areas

Although several areas of the cortex, notably in the frontal lobe, are active during speech, two areas are specifically devoted to this function.

#### BROCA'S AREA *(FIGURE 23.5)*

The French pathologist Pierre Broca assigned a motor speech function to the inferior frontal gyrus of the left side in 1861. The principal premotor area for speech is in fact area 44 of Brodmann, at the posterior end of the inferior frontal gyrus (*Figure 23.2*). The main output of area 44 is to cell columns in the face and tongue areas of the motor cortex. Lesions involving Broca's area are associated with *expressive aphasia* (see Panel 23.2). Area 44 is also linked to the supplementary motor area, which seems to be concerned with initiation of speech.

#### WERNICKE'S AREA *(FIGURE 23.5)*

The German neurologist Karl Wernicke made extensive contributions to language processing in the late nineteenth century. He designated the posterior part of area 22 in the superior temporal gyrus of the left hemisphere as a sensory area concerned with understanding the spoken word. The upper surface of this area is called the *temporal plane (Figure 23.7)*. In two-thirds of the population the temporal plane is distinctly longer on the left side, the lateral fissure being necessarily longer as well. Lesions involving Wernicke's area are associated with *receptive aphasia* (see Panel 23.2).

Wernicke's area is linked to Broca's area by the **arcuate fasciculus**, which curves around the posterior end of the lateral fissure within the white matter deep to the supramarginal gyrus.

#### RIGHT HEMISPHERE CONTRIBUTION

During normal conversation there is some increase in blood flow in areas of the right hemisphere matching those of the left (*Figure 23.5*). These areas are believed to be concerned with melodic aspects of speech—the cadences, emphases, and nuances, collectively called *prosody*. Disturbances of the melodic function are called *aprosodias* (Panel 23.2).

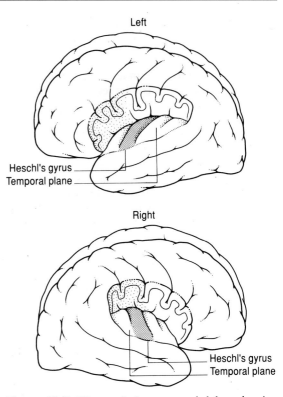

**Figure 23.7.** Views of the temporal lobe, showing Heschl's gyrus and the temporal plane.

#### ANGULAR GYRUS

The angular gyrus (area 39) belongs descriptively to the inferior parietal lobule. The *left* angular gyrus receives a projection from the inferior part of area 19 (the lingual gyrus), and itself projects to the temporal plane. It is commonly included as a part of Wernicke's area.

The angular gyrus seems to contain a neural lexicon of words, syllables, and numerical or other symbols, which can be retrieved by visual inputs— or even by visual imagery—and forwarded in the form of impulse trains to area 22. During reading, it is engaged in the conversion of syllables ('graphemes') into the corresponding sound equivalents ('phonemes').

### Modular organization of language

In alert subjects, electrical studies of the cortex exposed during neurosurgical procedures indicate the presence of a vast cortical mosaic for language. The mosaic extends along the entire length of the frontoparietal operculum above the lateral sulcus and of the temporal operculum below the sulcus.

## CLINICAL PANEL 23.2 • THE APHASIAS

*Aphasia* is a disturbance of language function caused by a lesion of the brain. The usual cause is a *stroke* produced by vascular occlusion in the anterior cortical territory of the left middle cerebral artery. (Vascular lesions of the forebrain are described in Chapter 26.)

### Expressive aphasia

Patients having a lesion that includes Broca's area suffer from *expressive aphasia*. These patients have difficulty in expressing what they want to say. Speech is slow, labored, and characteristically 'telegraphic' in style. The important nouns and verbs are spoken but prepositions and conjunctions are omitted. The patient comprehends what other people are saying and is well aware of being unable to speak fluently. There is usually an associated *agraphia* (inability to express thoughts in writing).

If the lesion involves a substantial amount of the cortical territory of the middle cerebral artery, there will be a motor weakness of the right lower face and right arm. Because the lips are affected, the patient will also have *dysarthria* (difficulty in speech articulation) in the form of slurring of certain syllables.

### Receptive aphasia

A lesion in Wernicke's area is accompanied by a deficit of *auditory comprehension*. As well as having difficulty in understanding the speech of others, the patient loses the ability to monitor his or her own conversation, and usually has difficulty in retrieving correct descriptive names. Speech fluency is normal but two kinds of abnormality occur in the use of nouns:

- *Verbal paraphrasia* (use of words usually of allied meaning): instead of 'use a knife', 'use a fork'.
- *Phonemic paraphrasia* (use of made-up but similar-sounding syllables): instead of 'knife and fork', 'bife and dork'.

The most striking feature of Wernicke's aphasia is that, despite garbling to the point of being unintelligible, the patient may be quite unaware of making mistakes.

### Aprosodia

Lesions of the *right* hemisphere may affect speech in subtle ways. Lesions that include area 44 tend to change the patient's speech to a dull monotone. On the other hand, lesions that involve area 22 may lead to *listening* errors—for example, being unable to detect inflections of speech, the patient may not know whether a particular remark is intended as a statement or as a question.

### Note on developmental dyslexia

Developmental dyslexia affects 3–4% of literate populations. The characteristic feature is a specific and pronounced reading difficulty in children who are the match of their peers in other respects. It is more frequent in boys, and in left-handers. Studies of sagittal MRI slices have shown that the temporal planes of dyslexic children tend to be relatively symmetrical. It is a matter of debate whether the symmetry reflects hypoplasia of the left temporal plane or a more bilaterally distributed function.

---

The frontoparietal operculum is predominantly concerned with the motor functions of speaking and writing, and the temporal operculum with the sensory functions of hearing and reading.

Language modules can be classified in various ways, in relation to function. For example, some are active only when the subject speaks in a foreign language; some are active during writing and others during reading; some are active only for one semantic class of nouns (such as the names of various fruits) and others only for verbs; and some are active only when words are being retrieved from memory.

### Cognitive style

Hemispheric specializations in relation to information processing have been revealed by various forms of visual, auditory and tactile tests. Results show that the left hemisphere is superior in processing information that is susceptible to *sequential analysis* of its parts whereas the right is superior in respect of *shapes* and of *spatial relationships*. Accordingly, the left hemisphere is described as being *analytical* and the right as being *holistic*. The right is also *musical:* there is a relative increase in blood flow in the right auditory association area when listening to music, versus a left-sided increase for words.

### Parietal lobe (Figure 23.8)

The parietal lobe—especially the *right* one—is of prime importance for appreciation of spatial relationships. There is also evidence that the parietal lobe—especially the *left* one—is concerned with initiation of movement.

### Posterior parietal lobe and covert attention

Clinically, the term *posterior parietal lobe* refers to area 7, which forms the bulk of the superior parietal lobule. Area 7 receives the dorsal visual

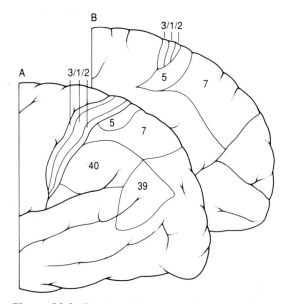

**Figure 23.8.** Brodmann's areas in the parietal lobe. (A) Lateral view; (B) medial view. 3/1/2, Somesthetic cortex; 5, somesthetic association area; 7, posterior parietal cortex; 39, angular gyrus; 40, supramarginal gyrus.

outputs of the visual association cortex, concerned with stereopsis and movement. It also receives inputs from the extrageniculate visual pathway, via the pulvinar (Chapter 21), and a substantial limbic input from the anterior cingulate gyrus. It projects via the superior longitudinal fasciculus to the ipsilateral frontal eye field and premotor cortex.

In monkeys, cell columns in area 7 are activated when a significant object (e.g. fruit) appears in the contralateral visual hemifield. The active columns increase the resting firing rate of cell columns in the frontal eye field and premotor cortex, without producing movement. The effect is called *covert attention,* or *covert orientation.* It becomes *overt* when the animal responds with a saccade with or without a reaching movement directed toward the object. (The scales may be tipped by an additional input from the prefrontal cortex.) Following a lesion to area 7, the motor responses to significant targets occur late, and are inaccurate.

In human volunteers, patches of increased cortical metabolism occur in area 7 and area 24 (anterior cingulate cortex) in response to objects of interest (or to any moving object) in the contralateral hemifield. The right hemisphere is more responsive than the left, and lesions of the right parietal lobe are more often accompanied by contralateral visual neglect (Panel 23.3).

### Inferior parietal lobule and the body schema

Clinically, the term *inferior parietal lobule* refers to area 40, which includes the supramarginal gyrus. Area 40 receives visual information from area 7 and tactile information from area 5; also a limbic input from the posterior cingulate cortex (area 23).

The term *body schema* refers to an awareness of the existence and spatial relationships of body parts, based on previous (stored) and current sensory experience. The reality of body schema has been established by the astonishing condition known as *anosognosia* (Greek, 'unawareness of disease') in which a patient who has suffered a massive stroke involving the parietal lobe as well as the descending motor pathways, denies ownership of the contralateral, hemiplegic side of the body. A relatively common disorder is that of *hemineglect,* where the contralateral side is ignored but can be used if attention is drawn to it (see Panel 23.3). Hemineglect is much commoner with a *right* parietal lobe lesion than a left one.

## CLINICAL PANEL 23.3 • PARIETAL LOBE DYSFUNCTION

Damage to one or more parts of the parietal lobe may result from vascular occlusion within the territory of the middle cerebral artery, or from a tumor.

### Somesthetic cortex

The somesthetic cortex (Brodmann's areas 3, 1, and 2) is most often compromised by rupture of a striate branch of the middle cerebral artery (*classical stroke*, Chapter 26). 'Cortical-type' sensory loss is shown by reduction in sensory acuity on the opposite side of the body (raised sensory threshold, poor point localization, poor two-point discrimination, loss of vibration sense and of position sense).

### Sensory association cortex

Area 5 may be damaged from behind, by a tumor or vascular lesion. The classical picture is that of a patient with normal sensory acuity who cannot identify an object such as a key on palpation alone. This sign is called *astereognosis*.

### Posterior parietal cortex

Lesions confined to area 7 are rare. They are associated with delayed and inaccurate saccading toward objects presented to the contralateral visual hemifield. Reaching movements into contralateral space are also inaccurate (the patient tends to knock things over).

### Supramarginal gyrus

Lesions affecting area 40 are usually vascular (middle cerebral artery) and are usually concomitant with contralateral hemiplegia with or without hemianopia. However, the blood supply to this area is sometimes selectively occluded.

The charasteristic result of damage to the supramarginal gyrus is *hemineglect*. The patient ignores the opposite side of the body unless attention is specifically drawn to it. A male patient will shave only the ipsilateral side of the face; a female patient will comb her hair only on the ipsilateral side. The patient will acknowledge a tactile stimulus to the contralateral side when tested alone; simultaneous testing of both sides will only be acknowledged ipsilaterally (*sensory extinction*).

Aspects of posterior parietal lobe function are affected as well. The patient tends to ignore the contralateral visual hemispace, even if the visual pathways are intact, and there is *visual extinction* (contralaterally) to simultaneous bilateral stimuli.

Hemineglect is at least five times commoner following lesions on the *right* side, regardless of handedness.

### Angular gyrus

An isolated vascular lesion of the *left* angular gyrus (very rare) usually produces *alexia* (complete inability to read) and *agraphia* (inability to write), because letters on the page are suddenly without any meaning. If the temporal plane has survived, patients can still name words spelt aloud to them. For *ideomotor apraxia*, see main text.

## Parietal lobe and movement initiation

There are several sites for movement initiation in different behavioral contexts. The present context is the performance of learned movements of some complexity: examples would include turning a door knob, combing one's hair, blowing out a match, and clapping. It is logical to anticipate a starting point within the dominant hemisphere,

because they can all be performed in reponse to verbal command (oral or written). This notion receives support from the observation that, if the corpus callosum has been severed surgically, the patient can perform a learned movement on command using the right hand, but not on attempting it with the *left* hand.

Failure to perform a learned movement on request is called *ideomotor apraxia*. It has been

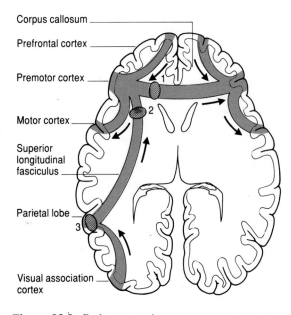

Corpus callosum

Prefrontal cortex

Premotor cortex

Motor cortex

Superior
longitudinal
fasciculus

Parietal lobe

Visual association
cortex

**Figure 23.9.** Pathways serving motor responses to sensory cues. (Adapted from Kertesz and Ferro (1984) *Brain* **107**: 921–933.) The premotor cortex is under higher control by the prefrontal cortex. For the numbers, see text.

repeatedly observed immediately following vascular lesions at the sites shown in *Figure 23.9*. Lesions at site 1 effectively sever the corpus callosum and produce ipsilateral limb apraxia (left lesion, left limb). Lesions at either site 2 (superior longitudinal fasciculus) or site 3 (angular gyrus) may produce *bilateral* limb apraxia. In practice, right-limb apraxia may be impossible to assess because of associated right hemiplegia or sensory aphasia.

Ideomotor apraxia can be accounted for if the dominant parietal lobe is considered to contain a

repertoire of learned movement programs which, on retrieval, elicit appropriate responses by the premotor cortex on one or both sides under directives from the prefrontal cortex. (The basal ganglia would be involved as well, as described in Chapter 24.)

Ideomotor apraxia is a transient phenomenon. Because parietal blood flow increases almost equally on both sides during reaching movements (*Figure 23.6*), the right hemisphere seems to be able to asssume a full role for the left arm when no longer overshadowed.

## REFERENCES

Cumming, W.J.K. (1988) The neurobiology of the body schema. *Br. J. Psychiat.* **153** (Suppl. 2): 7–11.

Fuster, J.M. (1989) *The Prefrontal Cortex.* New York: Raven Press.

Goodale, M.A. (1988) Hemispheric differences in motor control. *Behav. Brain Res.* **30**: 203–214.

Henderson, V.W. (1986) Anatomy of posterior pathways in reading: a reassessment. *Brain and Language* **29**: 119–133.

Kaas, J. H. (1991) Plasticity of sensory and motor maps in adult mammals. *Ann. Rev. Neurosci.* **14**: 137–167.

McCormick, D.A. and Williamson, A. (1989) Convergence and divergence of transmitter action in human cerebral cortex. *Proc. Natl. Acad. Sci. USA* **86**: 8098–8102.

Ojemann, G.A. (1991) Cortical organization of language. *J. Neurosci.* **11**: 2231–2287.

Weintraub, S. and Mesulam, M.-M. (1989) Neglect: hemispheric specialization, behavioral components and anatomical correlates. In *Handbook of Neuropsychology, Vol. 2* (Boller, F. and Grafman, J., eds), pp. 357–374. Amsterdam: Elsevier.

Zilles, K. (1990) Cortex. In *The Human Nervous System* (Paxinos, G., ed.), pp. 757–802. San Diego: Academic Press.

CHAPTER SUMMARY

Basic circuits
Information from clinical disorders
*CLINICAL PANELS*
Hypokinesia: Parkinson's disease · Hyperkinesia

# 24

# Basal ganglia

**The basal ganglia comprise a group of nuclei close to the base of the brain which participate in the control of movements. The mode of operation of the basal ganglia is only partially understood; it is a focus for intensive research because of the clinical consequences of malfunctions. This chapter offers some clues about the functional anatomy of the basal ganglia in health and disease.**

The term 'basal ganglia' originally encompassed all of the nuclear masses located at the base of the cerebral hemisphere. These nuclei are functionally diverse, and the term is now used to designate areas of the basal forebrain and midbrain known to be involved in the control of movement (*Figure 24.1*):

● The *striatum* (mainly the caudate nucleus and the putamen of the lentiform nucleus, but also including the nucleus accumbens which belongs to the limbic system).
● The *pallidum* (globus pallidus), which comprises a lateral part (GPL) and a medial part (GPM). GPM has a midbrain extension known as the *pars reticulata* of the substantia nigra (SNpr).
● The *subthalamic nucleus* (STN).
● The main, pigmented component of substantia nigra known as the *pars compacta* (SNpc).

Thalamic nuclei specifically devoted to basal gangliar function are the ventral anterior nucleus (VA) and the anterior part of the ventrolateral nucleus (VL). The mediodorsal nucleus is involved in a cognitive pathway (see later).

## Basic circuits

*Figure 24.2* is a diagram showing some major connections of the basal ganglia. The striatum receives excitatory (glutamate) inputs from the cerebral cortex. It houses excitatory, cholinergic internuncial neurons, as well as some GABA internuncials (*Figure 24.3*). Two sets of projection neurons emerge from the striatum. Both are inhibitory, combining GABA with either substance P or enkephalin. One set synapses in GPL, the other in GPM. From both segments of the pallidum another, purely GABAergic projection emerges:

from GPL to STN, and from GPM to the thalamus. STN sends an *excitatory* (glutamate) projection to GPM.

The monosynaptic pathway from the striatum to GPM (labeled 1 in *Figure 24.2*) is called the *direct route* to GPM. The alternative, trisynaptic pathway (labeled 2, 3, 4) is the *indirect route*.

The pathway from the thalamus back to the cerebral cortex is excitatory (glutamate).

**The substantia nigra, pars compacta** (SNpc) extends from the level of STN to the upper border of the pons. It contains about 400 000 neurons, nearly all of which project to the striatum in the *nigrostriatal pathway*. Each nigral neuron forms more than a million varicosities (beads) which make synaptic contact with the dendrites of the GABAergic neurons (*Figure 24.3*). The transmitter is dopamine. The predominant effect of dopaminergic activity in the striatum is inhibitory, especially upon the enkephalin-containing GABA cells projecting to GPL.

**The substantia nigra, pars reticulata** (SNpr) lies directly ventral to SNpc. Like its parent cell group (GPM), SNpr contains only pure GABA neurons. Some of them synapse in the superior colliculus, others in the mesencephalic reticular formation.

At least four distinct 'loops' pass from the cortex through the basal ganglia with a return to the cortex:

1. A sensorimotor loop, concerned with learned movements.
2. An associational loop, concerned with cognition.
3. A limbic loop, concerned with emotional aspects of movement.
4. An oculomotor loop, concerned with the frontal eye field.

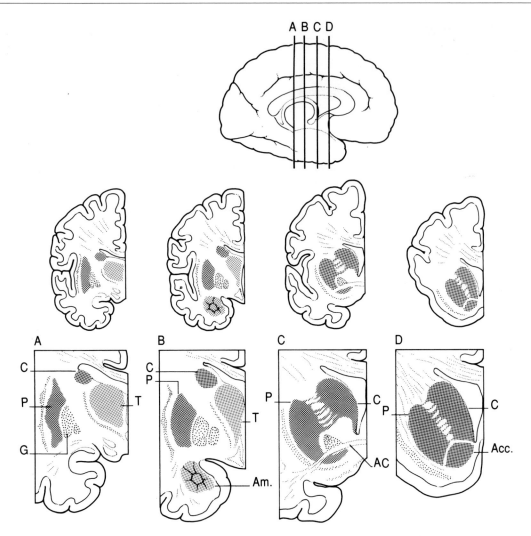

**Figure 24.1.** Four coronal sections of the brain, viewed from behind. Ventral parts enlarged below. Acc., nucleus accumbens; AC, anterior commissure; Am., amygdala; C, caudate nucleus; G, globus pallidus; P, putamen; T, thalamus.

### Sensorimotor loop *(Figure 24.4)*

The sensorimotor loop passes through the putamen, GPM and thalamic VL nucleus, returning to the supplementary motor area. It is somatotopically organized in the three nuclear groups, the leg being represented laterally, the arm centrally, and the face medially. The pathway from GPM to VL is split: one fiber group, the **lenticular fasciculus,** pierces the internal capsule; the other, the **ansa lenticularis,** loops below the edge of the internal capsule. The two groups unite as the **thalamic fasciculus** *(Figure 24.5)*. The thalamic fasciculus also contains cerebello-thalamic fibers ascending from the central cerebellar nuclei of the opposite side. Within the VL nucleus, the pallidal fibers terminate anterior to the cerebellar fibers.

The additional, side loop (indirect route) formed by GPL and STN is also somatotopically organized. The pathway from GPL to STN is called the **subthalamic fasciculus** *(Figure 24.5)*.

### Spontaneous and induced activity

The nigrostriatal pathway is spontaneously active at all times. In the resting state, its activity is sufficient to silence the striatum almost completely *(Figure 24.4A)*. Both sets of pallidal neurons are also spontaneously active at levels sufficient to silence the VL thalamus and STN.

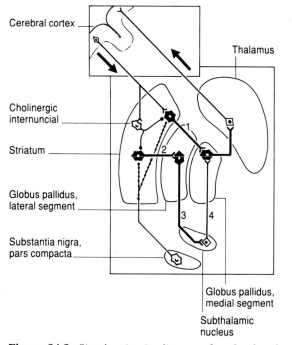

Cerebral cortex

Thalamus

Cholinergic internuncial

Striatum

Globus pallidus, lateral segment

Substantia nigra, pars compacta

Globus pallidus, medial segment

Subthalamic nucleus

**Figure 24.2.** Simple circuit diagram for the basal ganglia. Neurons shown in black secrete GABA. For numbers, see text.

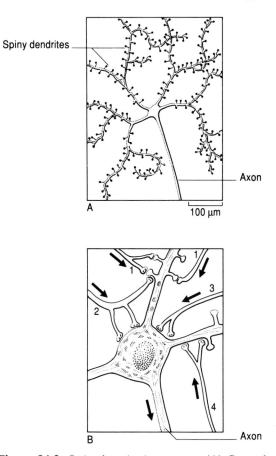

Spiny dendrites

Axon

A                                  100 μm

B                                  Axon

**Figure 24.3.** Striatal projection neuron. (A) General appearance; (B) enlargement showing synaptic contacts. 1, Corticostriate; 2, cholinergic internuncial; 3, GABAergic internuncial; 4, nigrostriatal. (Adapted from Smith and Bolam (1990).)

During movement, groups of direct-route pallidal neurons (in the appropriate somatotopic areas) become active, and the corresponding cells in the pallidum are inhibited. The result is *disinhibition* of the appropriate areas of VL, with onward excitation of the supplementary motor area (SMA) and the motor cortex (*Figure 24.4B*). However, STN is also stimulated by way of a direct projection from the motor cortex. Depending on the level of activity in GPL, STN can modulate the discharge pattern of GPM.

Discharges in the putamen, and downstream to VL, are related to the *direction* of the movement being undertaken. For example, one group is active during flexion of the shoulder, an adjacent group in abduction, and so on. Although movements can be produced on the opposite side of the body by direct electrical stimulation of the putamen, the basal ganglia do not normally initiate movements. They *are* active during all kinds of movement, whether fast or slow. They seem to be involved in scaling the strength of muscle contractions and, in collaboration with SMA, in organizing the requisite sequences of excitation of cell columns in the motor cortex. They come into action *after* the corticospinal tract has already been activated by other 'premotor' areas including the cerebellum. Because patients with Parkinson's disease have so much difficulty in performing internally generated movement sequences (see later), it has been speculated that the putamen provides a reservoir of learned motor programs which it is able to assemble in appropriate sequence for the movements decided upon, and to transmit the coded information to SMA.

## Associational loop

The caudate nucleus receives inputs from all of the association areas of the cortex. The output of the caudate passes through the pallidum and the VA nucleus of the thalamus. The VA nucleus projects to the prefrontal cortex. The cortical connections of the caudate suggest that it participates in *planning ahead*, particularly with respect to complex motor intentions.

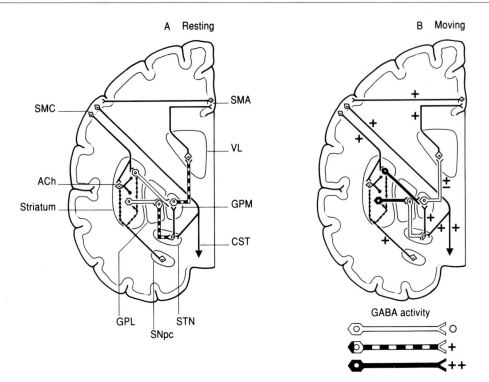

**Figure 24.4.** Activity in the sensorimotor loop. (A) at rest; (B) during movement. +,++, etc. represent levels of neural activity. CST, corticospinal tract; GPL, GPM, lateral and medial parts of globus pallidus; SMA, supplementary motor area; SMC, sensorimotor cortex; SNpc, substantia nigra, pars compacta; STN, subthalamic nucleus; VL, ventral lateral nucleus of thalamus.

## Limbic loop

The limbic loop passes from the cingulate gyrus and amygdala through the nucleus accumbens and the ventral part of the pallidum, returning via the mediodorsal thalamic nucleus to the premotor cortex and SMA. The nucleus accumbens is part of the limbic system, and this loop is likely to be involved in giving motor expression to emotions, for example through smiling or gesturing, or adoption of aggressive or submissive postures.

## Oculomotor loop

The oculomotor loop commences in the frontal eye field (area 8) and posterior parietal cortex (area 7). It passes through the caudate nucleus and the substantia nigra, pars reticulata (SNpr). It returns via the VA nucleus of the thalamus to the frontal eye field and prefrontal cortex. SNpr sends an inhibitory (GABA) projection to the superior colliculus, where it synapses upon the cells controlling

automatic saccades. When the eyes are at rest, SNpr is tonically active.

Whenever a deliberate saccade is made toward an object of interest, the appropriate gaze center is activated by the direct projection from the frontal eye field. The oculomotor loop is activated at the same time and the superior colliculus is disinhibited (just as the VL nucleus is disinhibited when the sensorimotor loop is activated). The superior colliculus then discharges to reinforce the activity of the direct pathway. Maximum speed (80 km/h) is achieved instantly.

### *Information from clinical disorders*

Some clues about basal gangliar function have been provided by two kinds of motor disorder. One kind, known as *hypokinesia* (reduced movement), is typified by Parkinson's disease. The other kind, *hyperkinesia* (excessive movement), is characterized by large-scale involuntary movements.

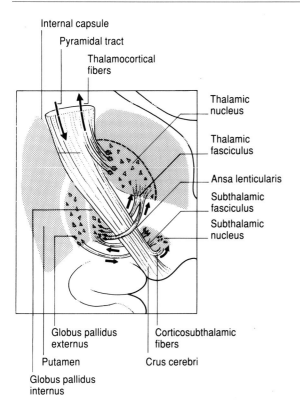

Figure 24.5. Schematic coronal view corresponding to *Figure 24.1A,* showing some connections.

Internal capsule
Pyramidal tract
Thalamocortical fibers
Thalamic nucleus
Thalamic fasciculus
Ansa lenticularis
Subthalamic fasciculus
Subthalamic nucleus
Globus pallidus externus
Corticosubthalamic fibers
Putamen
Crus cerebri
Globus pallidus internus

## Hypokinesia

The cardinal clinical features of Parkinson's disease are bradykinesia, rigidity, tremor, and impairment of postural reflexes (Panel 24.1). The cardinal *pathological* feature is loss of neurons from the substantia nigra. At least 80% of SNpc neurons have already been lost before symptoms appear. (There is significant loss of SNpr neurons as well.) During the earlier stages of neuronal loss, compensation occurs through two mechanisms: increased production of dopamine by the surviving neurons, and increased production of dopamine receptors by the target neurons in the striatum.

Experimental models of Parkinson's disease, in monkeys, indicate that the indirect pathway to the thalamus, in particular, escapes from tonic inhibition by dopamine and causes progressive silencing of the VL nucleus of thalamus (*Figure 24.6A*).

Figure 24.6. Basal ganglia: clinical disorders. (Based on Albin *et al.* (1989).) (A) Parkinson's disease; (B)choreoathetosis; (C) ballism. GPL, globus pallidus, lateral segment; GPM, globus pallidus, medial segment; SMA, supplementary motor area; SMC, sensorimotor cortex; SN, substantia nigra; STN, subthalamic nucleus; VL, ventral lateral nucleus of thalamus.

Parkinson's disease

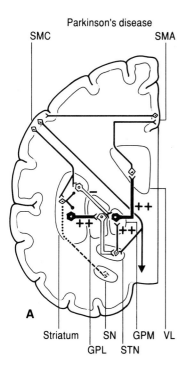

SMC     SMA

A

Striatum   SN   GPM   VL
GPL   STN

Choreoathetosis

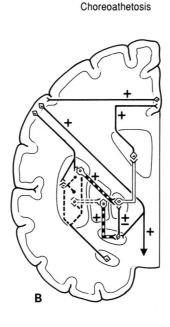

B

Ballism

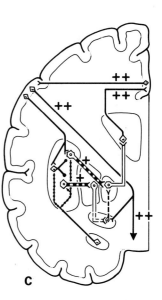

C

---

### CLINICAL PANEL 24.1 • HYPOKINESIA: PARKINSON'S DISEASE

Parkinson's disease affects about 1% of people over 50 years of age in all countries. Four symptoms/signs are characteristic, although not all are expressed in every patient:

1. *Bradykinesia* (Greek, slowness of movement). Movements are slow and laborious. Patients report that routine activities, such as getting out of a chair or opening a door, require deliberate planning and consciously guided execution. Sometimes a willed movement fails to get under way *(akinesia)*, or 'freezes' before completion. 'Casual', fidgety movements tend to be absent.

2. *Rigidity*. Rigidity affects all of the somatic musculature simultaneously, but a predilection for flexors imposes a stooped posture. Passive flexion and extension of the joints are resisted through the full range of movement. The term 'lead pipe rigidity' is used to distinguish it from the 'claspknife rigidity' of the spastic state that accompanies upper motor neuron lesions.

3. *Tremor*. Tremor at 3–6 Hz is usual and may be the cardinal feature. Typically, it involves muscle groups at rest, fading during voluntary movement and during sleep. (Cerebellar tremor, in contrast, is usually absent at rest and is brought out by voluntary movement.) Rhythmic head-nodding and rhythmic movements of the fingers and hands may be obvious. During passive movement of the joints, a subtle underlying tremor may give rise to ratchety 'cogwheeling'.

4. *Impairment of postural reflexes*. Patients go off balance easily, and tend to fall stiffly ('like a telegraph pole') in response to a mild accidental push. Strictly speaking, the underlying fault is an impairment of anticipatory postural adjustments (see main text).

Two other features should be mentioned.

*Oculomotor dyskinesia.* Under test conditions, saccadic movements of the eyes toward selected targets are found to be both delayed and slow.

Although not a cardinal feature of the condition, *dementia*, in the form of progressive deterioration of intellectual powers, is often observed after several years.

---

In consequence, SMA is no longer able to relay motor programs from the basal ganglia to area 4 in the normal manner. This may account for the *bradykinesia* encountered in clinical cases.

Patients may be able to perform motor tasks quickly in response to visual cues—for example, to trace a complex pattern using a finger, or to stride along a sequence of white squares. Theoretically, this facility could be accounted for by the use of a neural loop passing from the visual cortex to the cerebellum via the nuclei pontis, with a return to the motor cortex via the thalamus.

Difficulty in *initiating* movements, or failure to do so *(akinesia)*, is explained by an underscaling of the 'initial agonist burst', seen in electromyographic records taken from the appropriate prime movers (agonists).

*Rigidity* in Parkinson's disease is caused by an exaggerated response to the normal proprioceptive inflow from the muscles. Historically, it has been abolished by section of dorsal nerve roots, thus proving its peripheral sensory origin. It can also be abolished by placing a lesion in the VL nucleus of the thalamus, and it can be further exaggerated by electrical stimulation of the globus pallidus.

It is a matter of current debate whether $\alpha$ motoneurons are hyperexcitable through loss of an inhibitory descending influence (from SNpr), or whether the striatum is abnormally responsive to muscle afferent activity relayed to the somatosensory cortex and fed into the sensorimotor loop.

*Tremor* is associated with rhythmic bursting activity of cells in the striatum, pallidum and VL nucleus of thalamus, and in anterior horn cells of the spinal cord. Because bursting activity can be abolished by rigid fixation of the tremulous body part, the explanation would seem to lie in release of spinal reflex arcs from tonic inhibition (perhaps from SNpr), with the effect of setting up a flip-flop reciprocal inhibition of opposing muscle groups.

*Loss of postural reflexes* is in reality a reduction of anticipatory postural responses to perturbation. Normally, a push to the upper part of the body elicits immediate contraction of lower limb muscles appropriate for the maintenance of equilibrium.

*Oculomotor hypokinesia* can be explained on the basis of faulty disinhibition of the superior colliculus.

*Dementia* has been correlated with dopamine depletion of the caudate nucleus, which participates in the 'associational loop', including the prefrontal cortex. However, the dementia resembles that of Alzheimer's disease, and could be at least partly due to loss of cholinergic neurons from the basal forebrain (see Chapter 25).

## Treatment

Medical treatment of Parkinson's disease is by means of *levodopa*, a dopamine precursor which penetrates the blood–brain barrier and is converted to dopamine by the surviving cells of the substantia nigra. Levodopa is often very effective in alleviating bradykinesia and rigidity, but it has little effect on tremor. On the other hand, anticholinergic drugs may be useful for tremor. The effectiveness of levodopa diminishes with the continued loss of nigral neurons, requiring the use of a dopamine agonist drug instead, to act directly upon the receptors in the striatum.

---

### CLINICAL PANEL 24.2 ● HYPERKINESIA

Hyperkinetic states are characterized by spontaneous (involuntary) muscle contractions. They are most often seen in children, in association with *cerebral palsy*. A relatively rare, but well-known disorder associated with involuntary movements is *Huntington's chorea*. *Hemiballism* is a movement disorder that follows a vascular lesion of the subthalamic nucleus on one side.

#### Cerebral palsy

Cerebral palsy is an umbrella term covering a variety of motor disorders arising from damage to the brain in the perinatal period. The incidence is about 4 per 1000 live births in all countries. The most frequent association is with *prematurity* at the time of birth, with consequent risk of anoxia due to immaturity of the lungs. Other frequent links are with *brain hemorrhages* (pre-, intra-, or postnatal), and *hypoxia* before or during labor. During the early postnatal months affected children are usually 'floppy' (atonic). One or more of the following symptoms can usually be observed by the end of the first postnatal year:

- *Spasticity*, whether in the form of hemiplegia (one side), diplegia (legs only) or quadriplegia (all four limbs). The pyramidal tract is compromised, although the conduction rate in the tract develops normally.

- *Ataxia*, due to cerebellar damage.
- *Choreoathetosis*, due to basal gangliar damage (see main text). *Chorea* refers to spontaneous twitching of various muscle groups in a more or less random manner, which interferes with voluntary movements. *Athetosis* refers to writhing movements which may be so severe as to prevent sitting or standing. Waxing and waning of muscle tone commonly causes the head to roll about.

#### Huntington's chorea

Huntington's chorea is an autosomal (chromosome 4) dominant, inherited disease which occurs in 50% of the offspring of affected families. Onset of symptoms is usually delayed until the forties. The clinical history is one of chronic, progressive chorea, often with athetoid movements superimposed. Sooner or later, a progressive dementia sets in.

#### Hemiballism

Hemiballism (or *hemiballismus*) is marked by the abrupt onset of more or less wild, flailing movements of one arm (sometimes of the leg as well, on the opposite side). The appearances suggest that the motor system to the affected region has gone completely out of control.

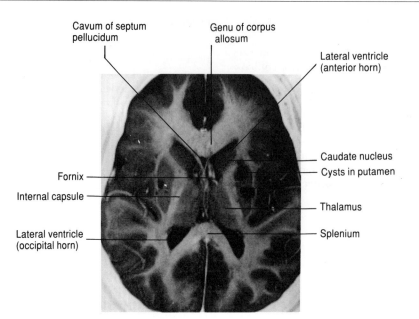

**Figure 24.7.** Horizontal MRI 'slice' at the level of the corpus striatum, from a 2-year-old girl suffering from severe choreoathetosis as a result of intrauterine infection (toxoplasmosis). The putamen on both sides is partly replaced by cysts. (Photograph kindly provided by Dr Paul Finn, Department of Radiology, New England Deaconess Hospital, Boston.)

## Hyperkinesia

Several hyperkinetic states are associated with diseases of the basal ganglia (Panel 24.2). The distinction drawn in the Panel between choreoathetosis and ballism is artificial in the sense that ballistic movements may appear in the course of choreoathetoid disorders, and choreoathetoid writhings may precede frank ballismus following infarction of the subthalamic nucleus.

Hyperkinetic states can be explained in terms of reduced STN activity. With choreoathetosis (*Figures 24.6B, 24.7*), moderate reduction of STN activity following a striatal lesion leads to incomplete disinhibition of VL (with consequent downstream effects mediated by the pyramidal tract). With ballism (*Figure 24.6C*), the relevant part of VL (upper limb representation as a rule) is completely disinhibited and the corresponding parts of SMA and motor cortex are out of control as a result.

## REFERENCES

Albin, R.L., Young, A.B. and Penney, J.B. (1989) The functional anatomy of basal ganglia disorders. *Trends Neurosci.* **12**: 366–375.

Alheid, G.F., Heimer, L. and Switzer, R.C. (1990) Basal ganglia. In *The Human Nervous System* (Paxinos, G., ed.), pp. 483–582. San Diego: Academic Press.

DeLong, M.R. (1990) Primate models of movement disorders of basal ganglia origin. *Trends Neurosci.* **13**: 281–289.

Goldman-Rakic, P.S. and Selemon, L.D. (1990) New frontiers in basal ganglia research. *Trends Neurosci.* **13**: 241–244.

Lee, R.G. (1987) Physiology of the basal ganglia and pathophysiology of Parkinson's disease. *Can. J. Neurol. Sci.* **14**: 373–380.

Smith, A.D. and Bolam, J.P. (1990) The neural network of the basal ganglia as revealed by the study of synaptic connections of identified neurones. *Trends Neurosci.* **13**: 259–271.

# 25

# Olfactory and limbic systems

The limbic system developed phylogenetically in close association with the olfactory system. Cortical and subcortical limbic areas are prominent features of the brain in primitive mammals, where they are intimately concerned with mechanisms of attack and defense, procreation, and feeding. The principal effector elements of the limbic system are the hypothalamus and the reticular formation. Studies in higher mammals have shown important relationships between limbic elements and memory.

## OLFACTORY SYSTEM

The olfactory system is unique in four respects:

1. The somas of the primary afferent neurons occupy a surface epithelium.
2. The axons of the primary afferents enter the cerebral cortex directly; second-order afferents are not interposed.
3. The primary afferent neurons undergo continuous turnover, being replaced from stem cells.
4. The pathway to the highest cortical centers (in the frontal lobe) is entirely ipsilateral.

The olfactory system comprises the olfactory epithelium and olfactory nerves; the olfactory bulb and tract; and several patches of olfactory cortex.

### Olfactory epithelium *(Figure 25.1)*

The olfactory epithelium occupies the upper one-fifth of the lateral and septal walls of the nasal

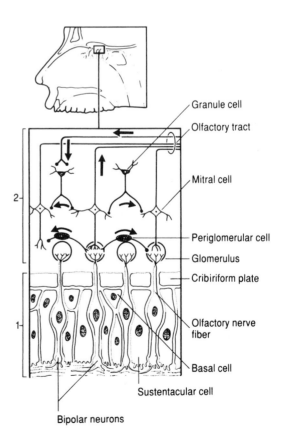

Granule cell
Olfactory tract
Mitral cell
Periglomerular cell
Glomerulus
Cribiriform plate
Olfactory nerve fiber
Basal cell
Sustentacular cell
Bipolar neurons

**Figure 25.1.** Connections of (1) olfactory epithelium and (2) olfactory bulb. The second glomerulus from the left is 'on line' (see text).

cavity. The epithelium contains three cell types:

1. **Olfactory neurons.** These are bipolar neurons, each with a dendrite extending to the epithelial surface and an unmyelinated axon contributing to the olfactory nerve. The dendrites are capped by immotile cilia containing molecular receptor sites. The axons run upward through the cribriform ('sieve-like') plate of the ethmoid bone and enter the olfactory bulb. The axons (some 3 million on each side) are grouped into *fila* (bundles) by investing Schwann cells. The collective fila constitute the olfactory nerve.
2. **Sustentacular cells** are interspersed among the bipolar neurons.
3. **Basal cells** lie between the other two cell types. Their function is to form fresh bipolar neurons. In monkeys, bipolar neurons survive for about a month. Turnover has yet to be demonstrated in humans, where progressive loss of total numbers in the epithelium may account for a general reduction in olfactory sensitivity with age.

### Olfactory bulb (Figure 25.1)

The **olfactory bulb** consists of three-layered, allocortex surrounding the commencement of the olfactory tract. The chief cortical neurons are some 50 000 **mitral cells,** which receive the olfactory nerve fibers and give rise to the olfactory tract.

Contact between olfactory fibers and mitral cell dendrites takes place in some 2000 **glomeruli,** which are sites of innumerable synapses and have a glial investment. Glomeruli which are 'on-line' (active) inhibit neighboring, 'off-line' glomeruli through the mediation of GABAergic **periglomerular cells** (cf. the horizontal cells of the retina). Mitral cell activity is also sharpened at a deeper level by **granule cells,** which are devoid of axons (cf. the amacrine cells of the retina). The granule cells receive excitatory dendrodendritic contacts from active mitral cells and they suppress neighboring mitral cells through inhibitory (GABA) dendrodendritic contacts.

### Central connections (Figure 25.2)

Mitral-cell axons run centrally in the **olfactory tract.** Collateral branches are given off to the **anterior olfactory nucleus,** which consists of scattered multipolar neurons within the tract. The

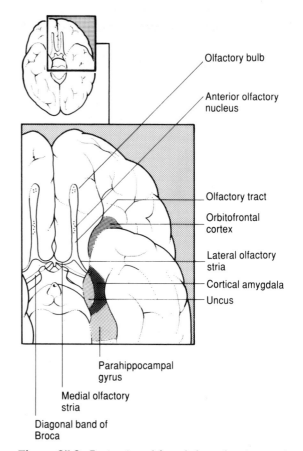

**Figure 25.2.** Brain viewed from below, showing cortical olfactory areas.

nucleus sends axons to the contralateral olfactory bulb via the anterior commissure. The crossed axons inhibit mitral cell activity in the contralateral bulb (by exciting granule cells there). The result is a relative enhancement of the more active bulb, providing a directional cue to the source of olfactory stimulation.

The olfactory tract divides into **lateral** and **medial olfactory striae.** The lateral olfactory stria terminates in the *piriform cortex* of the anterior temporal lobe. The human piriform cortex includes the cortical part of the amygdala, the uncus, and the anterior end of the parahippocampal gyrus. The highest center for olfactory discrimination is the posterior part of the orbitofrontal cortex, which receives connections from the piriform cortex via the mediodorsal nucleus of the thalamus.

The medial olfactory stria is linked to the septal area by the **diagonal band** of Broca (see under Limbic System).

---

**CLINICAL PANEL 25.1 • OLFACTORY DISTURBANCE**

A routine test of olfactory function is to ask the patient to identify strong-smelling substances such as coffee and chocolate through each nostril in turn. Loss of smell, or *anosmia*, may not be detected by the patient without testing if it is unilateral. If it is bilateral, the complaint may be one of loss of taste because the flavor of foodstuffs depends on the olfactory qualities of volatile elements; in such cases the four primary taste sensations (sweet, sour, salty, bitter) are preserved. Unilateral anosmia may be caused by a *meningioma* compressing the olfactory bulb or tract, or by a head injury with fracture of the anterior cranial fossa. Anosmia may be a clue to a fracture, and should prompt tests for leakage of cerebrospinal fluid into the nasal cavity.

*Olfactory auras* are a typical prodromal feature of uncinate epilepsy (see Panel 25.2).

---

Three efferent pathways link the olfactory cortical areas with the hypothalamus and brainstem: one is a dual pathway from the amygdala, one is the medial forebrain bundle, and the third is the stria medullaris thalami (for details, see under Limbic System). These pathways trigger autonomic responses such as salivation and gastric contraction, and arousal responses through the reticular formation (Chapter 18).

Points of clinical interest are mentioned in Panel 25.1.

## LIMBIC SYSTEM

### *Anatomy* (Figure 25.3)

The limbic system comprises the *limbic cortex* (so-called limbic lobe) and related subcortical nuclei. The term 'limbic' (Broca, 1878) originally referred to a limbus or rim of cortex immediately adjacent to the corpus callosum and diencephalon. The limbic cortex is now taken to include the three-layered allocortex of the hippocampal formation and septal region together with transitional, *mesocortex* in the parahippocampal gyrus, cingulate gyrus, and insula. The principal subcortical component of the limbic system is the subcortical amygdala. Cortical areas closely related to the limbic system are the orbitofrontal cortex and the temporal pole. Closely related subcortical areas are the hypothalamus and reticular formation, and the nucleus accumbens.

### *Parahippocampal gyrus*

The parahippocampal gyrus is a major junctional region between the cerebral isocortex and the

allocortex of the hippocampal formation. Its anterior part is the *entorhinal cortex* (area 28 of Brodmann), which is six-layered but has certain peculiar features. By way of the parahippocampal gyrus, the entorhinal cortex has two-way connections with all of the cortical association areas as well as with the hippocampal formation and piriform cortex.

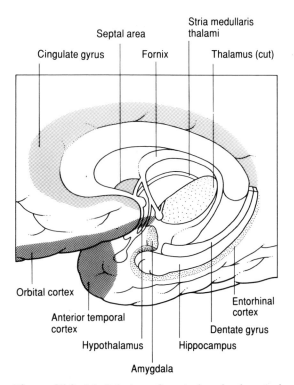

**Figure 25.3.** Medial view of cortical and subcortical limbic areas.

---

## CLINICAL PANEL 25.2 • SEIZURES

Next to vascular disorders, seizures (epileptic attacks) are the commonest group of problems encountered in clinical neurology. Some 3% of the population suffer two or more attacks during their lifetime.

Seizures are divided into two main categories. *Partial* seizures, the commoner form, begin in one hemisphere and may or may not spread to the other hemisphere. *Generalized* seizures begin with immediate involvement of both hemispheres. Seizures of either category may or may not be accompanied by loss of consciousness.

Partial seizures usually originate in the temporal lobe, most commonly in the hippocampus or amygdala. Premonitory 'auras' at the beginning of a temporal lobe attack include well-formed visual or auditory hallucinations (scenes, sound sequences), a sense of familiarity with the surrounding scene ('déjà vu'), a sense of strangeness ('jamais vu') or a sense of fear. Attacks originating in the uncus are ushered in by unpleasant olfactory or gustatory auras. A focus within the motor cortex produces *jacksonian attacks* (named after the British neurologist, Hughlings Jackson), characterized by a 'march' of contralateral motor activity from one part of the body to another (e.g., shoulder–arm–hand–face). A focus in the somatosensory cortex gives rise instead to a spreading sense of numbness. A focus in the occipital cortex may create unformed visual illusions (lights, patterns).

Generalized seizures take various forms but two varieties are especially common. *Primary tonic–clonic* seizures are characterized by sudden onset of unconsciousness with falling. The body stiffens for up to a minute (tonic stage) and then exhibits jerky movements of all four limbs and chewing movements of the mouth (often with frothing at the lips) for a second minute (clonic stage). A third minute is then spent in more relaxed unconsciousness. Where this picture is the result of spread from a unilateral ictal (attack) focus, it is described as a *secondary* tonic–clonic seizure.

The second common variety of generalized seizure takes the form of *absence attacks*, which usually begin during childhood and may recur frequently throughout the day. For up to 15 seconds, consciousness is interrupted, and the child stares vacantly, sometimes making small automatic movements. There is no warning and no later recall of the episode.

The term *symptomatic epilepsy* is used when seizures are brought on by a specific illness such as meningitis, brain tumor, or kidney failure with uremia. Where no organic cause can be found, the term *idiopathic* is used.

All seizures are caused by focal or generalized hyperexcitability of cortical cell columns. Biopsies of foci often show glial scarring and loss of inhibitory (GABA) neurons. In primary generalized epilepsy, there may be a genetic fault rendering glutamatergic cell membranes more easily depolarized, or GABAergic inhibition less effective.

Temporal lobe seizures often develop many years after seizures originating elsewhere. One interpretation (which has experimental support) is that the temporal allocortex (hippocampus, amygdala) has suffered damage from glutamatergic barrages from the entorhinal cortex, which itself has been bombarded from the association areas that feed into it. As a result, the temporal mesocortex could be in a permanently kindled state (for 'kindling,' see main text).

---

### Hippocampal formation *(Figure 25.4)*

Although the term 'hippocampus' is often used instead, in the context of memory, the *hippocampal formation* comprises the **subiculum,** the **hippocampus** proper, and the **dentate gyrus.** All three are composed of temporal lobe allocortex which has tucked itself into an S-shaped scroll along the floor of the lateral ventricle The band-like origin of the fornix from the subiculum and hippocampus is the **fimbria.**

The principal cells of the subiculum and hippocampus are spiny *pyramidal cells;* those of the dentate gyrus are spiny *stellate cells.* The hippocampus is also known as Ammon's horn (after an Egyptian deity with a ram's head); for research purposes it is divided into four CA *(cornu ammonis)* zones, of which CA1 and CA3 are the largest.

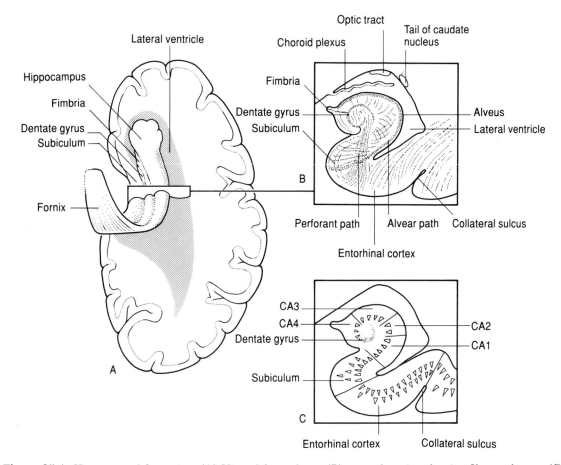

**Figure 25.4.** Hippocampal formation. (A) Viewed from above; (B) coronal section showing fiber pathways; (C) coronal section showing the four sectors of the hippocampus proper (cornu ammonis).

## Connections *(Figure 25.5)*

The largest *afferent* connection is the *perforant path,* which arises from the lateral part of the entorhinal cortex, perforates the subiculum, and synapses upon the dentate granule cells. The medial part of the entorhinal cortex gives rise to a second, *alvear path* which contributes to a sheet of fibers on the surface of the hippocampus, the alveus. Fibers of the alvear path synapse upon CA1 pyramidal cells. Both pathways from the entorhinal cortex are excitatory (glutamate).

The best known *intrinsic* connections are the *Schaffer collaterals* which run a recurrent course from CA3 to CA1. The hippocampus is also rich in inhibitory (GABA) internuncials.

The largest *efferent* connection is the **fornix** *(Figure 25.6).* The fornix is a direct continuation of the fimbria. The **crus** of the fornix arches up beneath the corpus callosum, where it joins its fellow to form the **trunk.** Anteriorly, a **pillar** descends on each side and divides above the anterior commissure. *Precommissural fibers* enter the septal area. *Postcommissural fibers* enter the anterior hypothalamus, the mammillary bodies, and the medial forebrain bundle.

In addition to the discrete connections mentioned above, the hippocampus is *diffusely* innervated from several sources, mainly by way of the fornix:

- A dense *cholinergic* innervation is received from the septal nucleus.
- A *noradrenergic* innervation is received from the locus ceruleus.
- A *serotonergic* innervation enters from the raphe

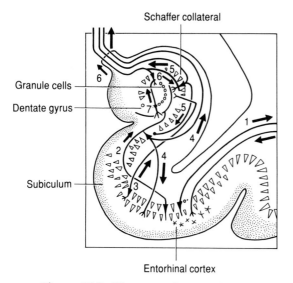

**Figure 25.5.** Hippocampal connections.

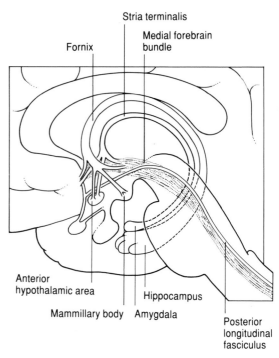

**Figure 25.6.** Limbic pathways.

nuclei of the midbrain. The possible linkage between serotonin and endogenous depression is mentioned in Chapter 18.

- A *dopaminergic* innervation enters from the ventral tegmental area of Tsai. The possible linkage between dopamine and schizophrenia is mentioned in Chapter 18.

## Mnemonic function of the hippocampal formation

Information from the sensory association areas is believed to be channeled through the entorhinal cortex, consolidated in the hippocampal formation, and returned to the association areas for long-term storage. The fornix is an alternative, circuitous pathway from the hippocampus to the cerebral isocortex.

The evidence for a mnemonic (memory) function in the hippocampal formation is discussed in psychology textbooks. Some insights are listed below:

- Bilateral damage or removal of the hippocampal formation is followed by *anterograde amnesia,* a term used to denote absence of conscious recall of newly acquired information for more than a few minutes. When asked to name a commonplace object the subject will have no difficulty because long-term memories are stored elsewhere, in association areas of the isocortex. However, when the same object is shown a few minutes later the subject will not remember having seen it. This is known as a loss of *declarative* (data-based) memory. *Procedural* (how-to-do) memory is preserved. If asked to assemble a jigsaw puzzle the subject will do it in the normal way. When asked to repeat the exercise the next day, the subject will do it faster although there will be no recollection of having seen the puzzle previously. There is some evidence that the cholinergic supply from the basal nucleus of Meynert to the isocortex of the frontal lobe may be relevant to procedural memory.

- Under experimental conditions, pyramidal cells and granule cells exhibit *long-term potentiation (LTP),* a phenomenon already noted in the cerebellar cortex (Chapter 19). A strong, brief (milliseconds) stimulus to the perforant or alveolar path induces long-lasting (hours) sensitivity to a fresh stimulus. LTP is associated with a cascade of biochemical events in the target neurons, following activation of appropriate glutamate receptors. In the hippocampus it is accompanied by the rapid (within minutes), transient appearance of new synaptic contacts and the expansion of old ones; this is especially true in the CA1 sector controlled by Schaffer collaterals. LTP is promoted by noradrenaline

## CLINICAL PANEL 25.3 • ALZHEIMER'S DISEASE

Alzheimer's disease (AD) is the commonest cause of dementia, *dementia* being defined as a severe loss of cognitive function without impairment of consciousness. The illness is ushered in by episodes of forgetfulness about names and faces, and progresses within weeks or months to amnesia for recent events (e.g., describing something within minutes of having already done so) and to general disorientation in time and space, inablity to manage personal affairs, etc. Later stages are characterized by disregard for personal hygiene and nutrition. The disease accounts for 20% of all patients in psychiatric institutions. It occurs in 4–5% of people over 60 years old, and in 20% of people over 80.

The great majority of cases are sporadic, but in some families it is an autosomal dominant aberration with a gene locus on the long arm of chromosome 21. In these families 50% of offspring are affected and the illness appears early, during the fourth or fifth decade.

MRI brain scans usually reveal severe atrophy of the cerebral cortex, with widening of the sulci and enlargement of the ventricular system. This can be confirmed at autopsy, and it is associated with loss of pyramidal neurons. Histological studies also reveal innumerable small (200–500 $\mu$m) *amyloid plaques* and *neurofibrillary tangles*, which are especially abundant in the hippocampus and amygdala. The plaques begin in the walls of small blood vessels and have not been explained except in terms of an enzyme defect resulting in abnormal protein production. The tangles are intraneuronal, and are made up of clumps of microtubules associated with an abnormal variant of a microtubule-associated *tau* protein. The tangles are progressively replaced by amyloid.

The hippocampus is shrunken, with considerable loss of pyramidal neurons. The most striking loss of neurons is not in the hippocampus but in the basal nucleus of Meynert. Up to 90% of the ACh neurons are lost from the basal nucleus, as are their projections to the cerebral isocortex and mesocortex. Indeed, degenerating ACh terminals seem to contribute to the neurofibrillary tangles.

As the relatives of Alzheimer victims know only too well, amnesia is the cardinal clinical feature. In view of the known relationship between the septohippocampal projection and learning, the main thrust of therapeutic research is being directed to the discovery of drugs capable of activating postsynaptic ACh receptors in the temporal lobe—not least because the receptors may survive for much longer than the presynaptic neurons.

---

and by dopamine, which may have a bearing on the attentional or motivational state at the time of learning.

• In both human and animal experiments, *cholinergic activity* in the hippocampus seems to be significant for learning. In human volunteers, central ACh blockade (by administration of scopolamine) severely impairs memory for lists of names or numbers whereas a cholinesterase inhibitor (physostigmine) gives above-normal results. Clinically, hippocampal cholinergic activity is severely reduced in *Alzheimer's disease*, which is particularly associated with amnesia (see Panel 25.3).

• *Kindling* ('lighting a fire') is a property unique to the hippocampal formation and amygdala, although its relationship to learning is not obvious. Kindling is the progressively increasing group response of neurons to a repetitive stimulus of uniform strength. In both humans and experimental animals, it can spread from mesocortex to isocortex and cause generalized convulsive seizures (see Panel 25.2).

Indirect evidence for a hippocampal function in relation to memory has been adduced from *diencephalic amnesia*, a state of anterograde amnesia following bilateral damage to the diencephalon. Such damage may interrupt the *Papez circuit* linking the fornix to the cingulate gyrus by way of the mammillary body and the anterior nucleus of the thalamus. Complete transection of the fornix may have the same effect, although amnesia is not an invariable result.

### Insula

Being completely covered by the frontal, parietal and temporal opercula, the insula is relatively inaccessible and its functions are poorly understood. The anterior insula is continuous with the orbitofrontal and anterior temporal cortex. In cases where the insula has been exposed at surgery, electrical stimulation has elicited olfactory and gustatory (flavor) hallucinations, as well as a variety of autonomic effects. The posterior insula is interconnected with the entorhinal cortex and the amygdala.

### Cingulate cortex

The cingulate cortex is part of the Papez circuit, receiving a projection from the anterior nucleus of the thalamus and becoming continuous with the parahippocampal gyrus behind the splenium of the corpus callosum.

The *anterior* cingulate cortex (area 24 of Brodmann) receives afferents from the intralaminar nuclei of the thalamus. It is one of three cortical areas that show a pronounced increase in metabolic activity in response to a painful stimulus applied to the body surface. The other two are the primary and secondary somatic sensory areas (*Figure 25.7*). Electrical stimulation of area 24 is not painful but it may elicit a *cry of pain*, and it is of interest that (in monkeys) the anterior cingulate projects to the nucleus ambiguus, which could produce the muscle contractions required. Undercutting area 24 *(anterior cingulotomy)* is a procedure sometimes performed for the relief of intractable pain. In successful cases the severity of the pain is not altered but the unpleasant, aversive quality is removed.

The *posterior* cingulate gyrus (area 23 of Brodmann) is richly interconnected with area 7 of the posterior parietal lobe, where visual and tactile information is integrated. The limbic connection may be responsible for the emotional 'tone' of what is seen or felt.

### Septal area

The septal area is the chief *pleasure center* of the brain. It comprises the **septal nucleus,** merged with the cortex directly in front of the anterior commissure, together with a few cells extending into the septum pellucidum.

*Afferents* are received from:

- The amygdala, via the diagonal band of Broca.
- The olfactory tract, via the medial olfactory stria.

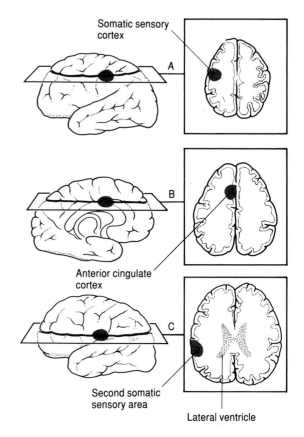

**Figure 25.7.** Cortical areas showing increased metabolic activity following application of noxious heat to the right volar forearm. (Adapted from Talbot *et al.* (1991) *Science* **251**: 1355–1358.)

- The hippocampus, via the fornix.
- Brainstem monoaminergic neurons, via the medial forebrain bundle.

*Efferent* projections run to the hypothalamus, brainstem, and hippocampus. The largest projection to the brainstem is by way of the **stria medullaris thalami** and the **habenular nucleus.** The habenular nuclei of the two sides are connected through the **habenular commissure** located close to the root of the pineal gland and often calcified (Chapter 2). The habenular nucleus sends the **fasciculus retroflexus** to synapse in an **interpeduncular nucleus** of the reticular formation in the midbrain. The interpeduncular nucleus is linked to autonomic nuclei in the brainstem and spinal cord.

The *septohippocampal pathway* runs to the hippocampus by way of the fornix.

The septal area appears to participate in several different functional activities:

- Electrical stimulation of the human septal nucleus produces a most agreeable sense of well-being. In animals, the nucleus is one of several 'reward areas' of the brain, as judged by eagerness to self-stimulate by means of a lever attached to an indwelling electrode. Rats may self-stimulate the septal nucleus to the exclusion of all other activities, even to the point of death from starvation. An electrolytic *lesion* of the nucleus has the opposite effect: the animal shows extreme displeasure (so-called 'septal rage').
- The nucleus provides the bulk of the cholinergic nerve supply to the hippocampus, with a probable mnemonic role.
- The septohippocampal projection is responsible for rhythmic, slow-wave activity (4–7 Hz) of hippocampal neurons. It is detectable as *theta rhythm* in the electroencephalogram. The functional significance of theta rhythm is unknown.

### Amygdala

The amygdala (Greek, almond; also called the amygdaloid body or amygdaloid complex) is a large group of nuclei blending with the mesocortex near the uncus of the temporal lobe. It consists of a *corticomedial group* of nuclei which merges with the piriform cortex, and a larger, *basolateral group*, which has a multiplicity of connections.

*Afferents* to the amygdala are as follows:

- Olfactory afferents (to the corticomedial group) from all areas of olfactory cortex.
- Visceral afferents from the nucleus solitarius (via the medial forebrain bundle).
- Septal afferents via the diagonal band.
- Afferents from the temporal neocortex containing visual, auditory, and even some tactile information.
- Hippocampal afferents.
- Monoaminergic afferents from the midbrain and pons (serotonin, dopamine, norepinephrine).

*Efferents* project widely, having target areas in the cerebral cortex, basal ganglia, thalamus, hypothalamus, and brainstem. Some of the efferents travel independently, others travel in the stria terminalis or in the ventral amygdalofugal pathway.

- *Independent* efferents reach the neocortex of the prefrontal and premotor areas, and the nucleus accumbens.
- The *stria terminalis* (*Figure 25.6*) follows the curve of the caudate nucleus and accompanies the thalamostriate vein along the upper surface of the thalamus. It sends fibers to the septum, to the hypothalamus, and, through the medial forebrain bundle, to the autonomic and respiratory nuclei of the brainstem.
- The *ventral amygdalofugal pathway* passes medially below the lentiform nucleus. It contains fibers going to the mediodorsal nucleus of the thalamus, and it provides an additional route to the septum, hypothalamus and brainstem.

The *functions* of the amygdala have yet to be clearly defined. This nuclear group is in a position to have *cognitive* effects through its linkages with the prefrontal cortex; to influence *movement* through its linkages with the ventral stiatum (nucleus accumbens); to influence *endocrine* and *feeding* functions through the hypothalamus; and to affect the *autonomic* functions of the brainstem.

The level of activity in the amygdala seems to be related to the general emotional state. In animals, weak electrical stimulation produces postural and autonomic adjustments indicative of *expectancy*. Strong electrical stimulation produces postural and autonomic changes associated with either *evasion* or *attack*. In humans, electrical stimulation most often produces an acute sense of *fear*, accompanied by intense sympathetic activity and sometimes by evasive movements.

Bilateral ablation of the amygdala has been carried out in humans for treatment of *rage attacks*, characterized by irritability, building up over several hours to dangerous aggressiveness. The operation has been successful in eliminating such attacks. In monkeys, bilateral ablation leads to placidity, together with a tendency to explore objects orally and a state of hypersexuality *(Kluver–Bucy syndrome)*. A comparable syndrome has occasionally been observed in humans.

### Basal forebrain (Figure 25.8)

The *basal forebrain* extends from the bifurcation of the olfactory tract as far back as the infundibulum, and from the midline to the amygdala. In its roof are the anterior commissure, the *ventral pallidum* (pierced by the commissure), and the *ventral stria-*

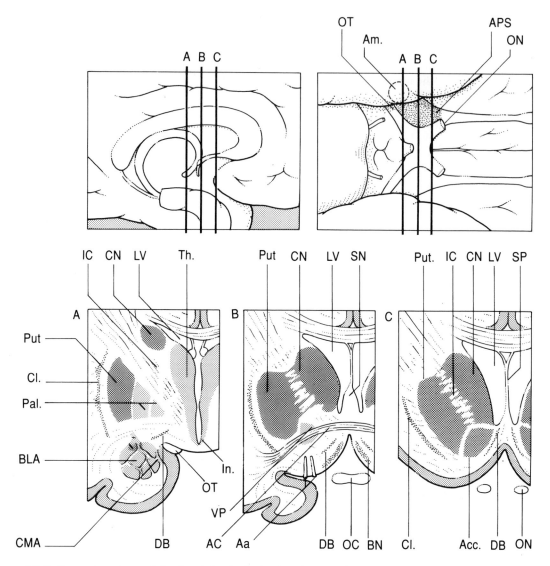

**Figure 25.8.** Coronal sections of the basal forebrain in the planes indicated. Aa, arteries piercing APS; Am., amygdala; Acc., nucleus accumbens; AC, anterior commissure; APS, anterior perforated substance; BLA, basolateral amygdala; BN, basal nucleus of Meynert; Cl., claustrum; CMA, corticomedial amygdala; CN, caudate nucleus; DB, diagonal band of Broca; IC internal capsule; In., infundibulum; LV, lateral ventricle; OC, optic chiasm; ON, optic nerve; OT, optic tract; Pal., pallidum; Put., putamen; SN, septal nucleus; SP, septum pellucidum; Th., thalamus; VP, ventral pallidum.

*tum* whose anterior end contains the **nucleus accumbens.** Above and medial to the nucleus accumbens is the **septal nucleus,** below the septum pellucidum. The septal nucleus has a two-way linkage with the amygdala through the diagonal band (of Broca), which contains a small nucleus of its own.

In the floor of the basal forebrain is the anterior perforated substance, pierced by central branches of the anterior and middle cerebral arteries. Here the cerebral cortex is replaced by scattered nuclear groups, of which the largest is the **nucleus basalis magnocellularis** of Meynert.

The *cholinergic neurons of the basal forebrain* have their somas mainly in the septal and basal nuclei (*Figure 25.9*). The septal nucleus gives rise to the

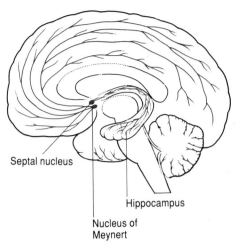

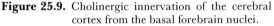

**Figure 25.9.** Cholinergic innervation of the cerebral cortex from the basal forebrain nuclei.

*septohippocampal pathway,* which reaches the hippocampus through the fornix. This projection is supplemented by cholinergic fibers from the nucleus of the diagonal band. The basal nucleus projects to all parts of the cerebral neocortex, which also contains scattered intrinsic cholinergic neurons.

The septal, basal and diagonal band nuclei are often called the *basal forebrain nuclei,* or 'the nucleus of Meynert' in the context of Alzheimer's disease. In the hippocampus, the cholinergic supply seems to be relevant to the consolidation of information into memory, as well as generating theta rhythm on EEG recordings. In the neocortex, the cholinergic supply is tonically active in the waking state, contributing to the 'awake' pattern on EEG recordings. In animals, activation of the basal nucleus potentiates and prolongs the responsiveness of cortical cell columns to inputs from the 'specific' sensory and motor thalamic nuclei.

## REFERENCES

Agranoff, B.W. (1989) Learning and memory. In *Basic Neurochemistry: Molecular, Cellular, and Medical Aspects,* 4th edn (Siegel, G.J. *et al.,* eds), pp. 915–927. New York: Raven Press.

Baudry, M. and Lynch, G. (1987) Properties and substrates of mammalian memory systems. In *Psychopharmacology: the Third Generation of Progress* (Meltzer, H.Y., ed.), pp. 449–462. New York: Raven Press.

Dekker, A.J.A.M., Connor, D.J. and Thal, L.J. (1991) The role of cholinergic projections from the nucleus basalis in memory. *Neurosci. Behav. Rev.* **15:** 299–317.

de Olmos, J. (1990) Amygdaloid nuclear gray complex. In *The Human Brain* (Paxinos, G., ed.), pp. 583–710. San Diego: Academic Press.

Macchi, G. (1989) Anatomical substrate of emotional reactions. In *Handbook of Neuropsychology, Vol. 3* (Boller, F. and Grafman, J., eds), pp. 283–303. Amsterdam: Elsevier.

Prah, J.D. and Benignus, V.A. (1985) Olfaction: anatomy, physiology, and behavior. In *Toxicology of the Eye, Ear, and other Special Senses* (Hayes, A.W., ed.), pp. 25–39. New York: Raven Press.

# 26

# Blood supply of the forebrain

Cerebrovascular disease is the third largest cause of death, after heart disease and cancer. Appreciation of the normal anatomy of the cerebrovascular arterial tree is quite fundamental to the interpretation of the effects of vascular occlusion or hemorrhage. Most of the better known syndromes arising from vascular occlusion are touched upon in the clinical panels.

As well as describing the arterial system, this chapter gives a brief account of the venous drainage of the brain, and of the blood–brain barrier.

The brain is absolutely dependent on a continuous supply of oxygenated blood. It controls the delivery of blood by sensing the momentary pressure changes in its main artery of supply, the internal carotid. It controls the arterial oxygen tension by monitoring respiratory gas levels in the the internal carotid artery and in the cerebrospinal fluid beside the medulla oblongata (Chapter 18). The control systems used by the brain are exquisitely sophisticated but they can be brought to nothing if a distributing artery ruptures spontaneously or is rammed shut by an embolus.

A *stroke* is defined as a sudden, nonconvulsive, focal neurological deficit lasting more than 24 hours. The most frequent deficit is a contralateral motor weakness or paralysis, but the possible variety of symptoms and symptom combinations is very large. The two chief underlying disorders are atherosclerosis and hypertension. *Atherosclerosis* is associated with development of fatty deposits in the intimal lining of the internal carotid artery. The deposits may cause *thrombotic* occlusion *in situ* or they may break away and cause *embolic* occlusion distally. Many cerebral emboli originate as

blood clots in the heart, in association with coronary or valvular disease. *Hypertension* is particularly associated with *cerebral hemorrhage*, which characteristically affects one of the lateral striate branches of the middle cerebral artery.

An area of brain destruction produced by vascular occlusion or hemorrhage is called an *infarct*. Cerebral infarcts become swollen after a few days, forming *space-occupying lesions* capable of causing subfalcal or tentorial herniation in the manner of a tumor (Chapter 5).

A separate form of stroke is unrelated to either atherosclerosis or hypertension. It is caused by spontaneous rupture of a berry-like *aneurysm* protruding from an artery at the base of the brain.

## ARTERIAL SUPPLY OF THE FOREBRAIN

The blood supply to the forebrain is derived from the two internal carotid arteries and from the basilar artery (*Figure 26.1*).

Each internal carotid artery enters the subarachnoid space by piercing the roof of the cavernous

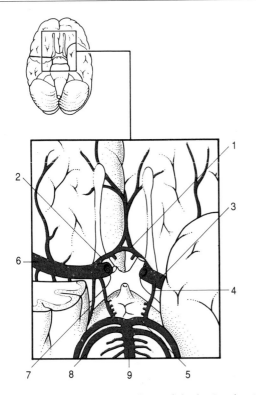

**Figure 26.1.** Arteries at the base of the brain. *Arteries forming the Circle of Willis:* 1, anterior communicating; 2, anterior cerebral; 3, internal carotid; 4, posterior communicating; 5, posterior cerebral. *Other arteries:* 6, middle cerebral; 7, anterior choroidal; 8, superior cerebellar; 9, basilar.

sinus. In the subarachnoid space it gives off **ophthalmic, posterior communicating** and **anterior choroidal arteries** before dividing into the **anterior** and **middle cerebral arteries**.

The basilar artery divides at the upper border of the pons into the two **posterior cerebral arteries.** The *arterial circle of Willis* is completed by a linkage of the posterior communicating artery with the posterior cerebral on each side, and by linkage of the two anterior cerebrals by the **anterior communicating artery**.

The choroid plexus of the lateral ventricle is supplied from the anterior choroidal branch of the anterior cerebral artery and by a posterior choroidal branch from the posterior cerebral artery.

Dozens of fine *central (perforating) branches* are given off by the constituent arteries of the circle of Willis. They enter the brain through the **anterior perforated substance** beside the optic chiasm and through the **posterior perforated substance**

behind the mammillary bodies. They have been classified in various ways but can be conveniently grouped into short and long branches. *Short* central branches arise from all of the constituent arteries and from the two choroidal arteries. They supply the optic nerve, chiasm and tract, and the hypothalamus. *Long* central branches arise from the three cerebral arteries. They supply the thalamus, corpus striatum and internal capsule. They include the striate branches of the anterior and middle cerebral arteries.

### Anterior cerebral artery (Figure 26.2)

The anterior cerebral artery passes above the optic chiasm to gain the medial surface of the cerebral hemisphere. It forms an arch around the genu of the corpus callosum. making it easy to identify in a carotid angiogram (*Figure 26.4*). Close to the anterior communicating artery it gives off a final central branch, *the recurrent artery of Heubner* (pron. 'Hoibner') which supplies the anterior half of the internal capsule immediately above the crus cerebri. Cortical branches of the anterior cerebral supply the medial surface of the hemisphere as far back as the parieto-occipital sulcus. The branches overlap onto the orbital and lateral surfaces of the hemisphere.

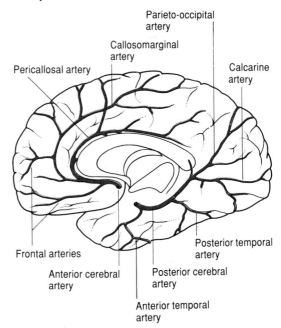

**Figure 26.2.** Cortical branches of the anterior and posterior cerebral arteries.

Named cortical branches* and their territories are as follows:

| | |
|---|---|
| Orbital | Orbital surface of frontal lobe |
| Frontopolar | Frontal pole |
| Callosomarginal | Cingulate and superior frontal gyri; paracentral lobule |
| Pericallosal | Corpus callosum |

*The term *cortical* is conventional. The official term *terminal* is better because these arteries supply the subjacent white matter as well.

Clinical syndromes involving the anterior cerebral artery are described in Panel 26.1. In this and later panels, the term 'occlusion' is used in a general sense, to signify infarction of arterial territories.

### Middle cerebral artery (Figure 26.3)

The middle cerebral artery is the main continuation of the internal carotid, receiving 80% of the carotid blood flow. It immediately gives off important central branches, then passes along the

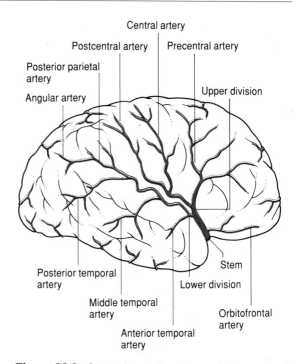

**Figure 26.3.** Cortical branches of the middle cerebral artery.

---

## CLINICAL PANEL 26.1 • ANTERIOR CEREBRAL ARTERY OCCLUSION

Complete interruption of flow in the anterior cerebral artery is very unusual because the opposite artery can nearly always perfuse its distal territory (through the anterior communicating) while continuing to supply its own side. However, central and cortical occlusions within the territory of the anterior cerebral are well recognized clinically:

- *Recurrent artery of Heubner:* the clinical picture resembles that of middle cerebral artery upper-division occlusion (see Panel 26.2), with motor weakness of the contralateral face and arm.
- *Callosomarginal:* the characteristic result is motor weakness and some cortical-type sensory loss in the contralateral lower limb, due to infarction within the paracentral lobule. Urinary incontinence may occur for some days owing to interference with the bilateral 'social' control of the pontine bladder center

(Chapter 18).* With dominant hemisphere lesions, initiation of speech may be difficult if the supplementary motor area is damaged.
- *Pericallosal:* infarction of the corpus callosum may produce 'split brain' effects (Chapter 23). In a right-handed patient a simple test is to ask the patient to feel an *unseen* object (e.g. a key) in the left hand and to name it. If the tactile information cannot be transferred from the right parietal lobe to the left, the object cannot be named ('tactile aphasia').

  If the premotor cortex has been compromised, the patient may not be able to reach out with the contralateral arm on command (so-called 'sympathetic apraxia').

*Urinary incontinence may accompany clouding of consciousness following any large infarct in the hemisphere. Recovery of bladder control can be assisted by means of general sensory and cognitive stimulation of the patient.

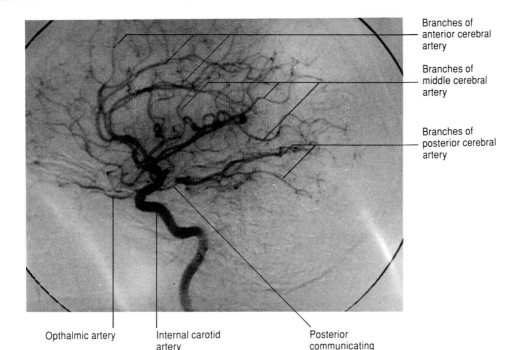

Opthalmic artery

Internal carotid artery

Posterior communicating artery

Branches of anterior cerebral artery

Branches of middle cerebral artery

Branches of posterior cerebral artery

**Figure 26.4.** Internal carotid angiogram, arterial phase. An embryonic pattern is apparent, with perfusion of the posterior cerebral artery via the posterior communicating branch of the internal carotid. (There is some filling of the contralateral anterior cerebral artery.) (Photograph kindly provided by Dr James Toland, Department of Radiology, Beaumont Hospital, Dublin.)

**Figure 26.5.** Distribution of perforating branches of the middle cerebral, anterior choroidal, and posterior cerebral arteries (schematic).

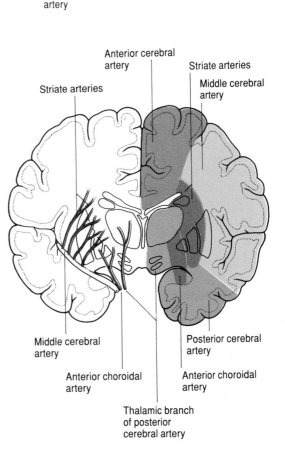

Anterior cerebral artery

Striate arteries

Striate arteries

Middle cerebral artery

Middle cerebral artery

Anterior choroidal artery

Posterior cerebral artery

Anterior choroidal artery

Thalamic branch of posterior cerebral artery

depth of the lateral fissure to reach the surface of the insula. There it usually breaks into upper and lower divisions. The upper division supplies the frontal and anterior parietal lobes, the lower division supplies the posterior parietal lobe, the temporal lobe, and the midregion of the optic radiation. (Named branches are shown in *Figure 26.4* and listed in Panel 26.2). Overall, the middle cerebral supplies two-thirds of the lateral surface of the brain.

The central branches of the middle cerebral are *medial* and *lateral striate arteries* (*Figure 26.5*). These arteries supply the corpus striatum, internal capsule, and thalamus. The lateral striate are especially prone to 'lacunar infarcts'—small pools

## CLINICAL PANEL 26.2 • MIDDLE CEREBRAL ARTERY OCCLUSION

Two forms of middle cerebral artery occlusion are frequent in late middle life and in the elderly. The first is an embolic event arising from detachment of a thrombus from the internal carotid artery or the heart. The second follows leakage of one of the striate branches of the middle cerebral artery, usually in association with hypertension.

### Embolism

An embolus may lodge in the *stem* of the artery, in the *upper division*, in the *lower division*, or in a *cortical branch* of either division.

### Stem

Occlusion of the stem affects the central as well as the cortical branches. The picture is one of contralateral hemiplegia with severe sensory loss, together with contralateral homonymous hemianopia. Left-sided lesions are usually accompanied by global aphasia, right-sided ones with contralateral sensory neglect. Prognosis for significant recovery is poor. Many patients die in coma following midbrain compression by a swollen infarct.

### Upper division

An embolus occluding the upper division gives rise to contralateral paresis (weakness) and cortical-type sensory loss in the face and arm, together with dysarthria arising from damage to supranuclear pathways involved in speech articulation. Left-sided lesions are usually accompanied by expressive aphasia, right-sided ones by contralateral hemineglect.

### Lower division

Embolism of the lower division produces contralateral homonymous hemianopia, and sometimes a confused, agitated state attributed to involvement of limbic pathways in the temporal lobe. Left-sided lesions are also accompanied by Wernicke's aphasia, alexia, and sometimes by bilateral ideomotor apraxia.

### Branch embolism

The following isolated deficits are attributable to an embolus lodged in one of the cortical branches:

- *Orbitofrontal:* elements of a dorsolateral prefrontal syndrome may be present (Chapter 23).
- *Precentral (prerolandic)* motor aphasia (left lesion); monotone speech (right lesion).
- *Central (rolandic):* contralateral loss of motor and/or sensory function in the face and arm.
- *Anterior parietal (postrolandic):* contralateral astereognosis.
- *Posterior parietal:* contralateral hemineglect (especially with right lesion).
- *Angular:* contralateral homonymous hemianopia; alexia with left lesion.
- *Posterior/middle temporal:* Wernicke's aphasia (left lesion); sensory aprosodia (right lesion).

### Hemorrhage

The commonest source of a cerebral hemorrhage is one of the lateral striate branches of the middle cerebral. The commonest location is the putamen, with spread into the anterior and posterior limbs of the internal capsule. The usual cause is a pre-existing systemic hypertension. The hematoma may be as small as a pea or as big as a golf ball. Large hemorrhages rupture into the lateral ventricle and are usually fatal within 24 hours.

A typical clinical case is one in which a sudden, severe headache is followed by unconsciousness within a few minutes. The eyes tend to drift toward the side of the lesion, as noted in Chapter 17. With recovery of consciousness there is a complete, flaccid hemiplegia (apart from the upper part of the face). Tendon reflexes are absent on the hemiplegic side and a Babinski sign is present. Conjugate movement of the eyes toward the hemiplegic side may be impossible initially.

Considerable return of function is possible during the ensuing weeks. The end result is often one of ambulatory spastic hemiparesis with hemihypesthesia (reduced sensation).

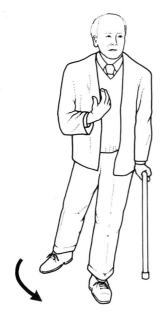

**Figure CP 26.2.1.** Hemiplegic gait. Patient's right side is affected.

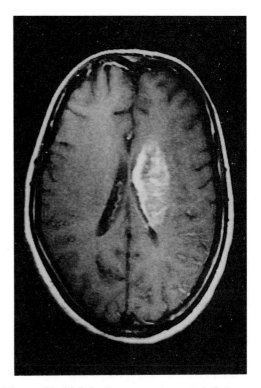

**Figure CP 26.2.2.** Contrast-enhanced MR image taken from a patient 11 days after an embolic stroke (see text). (Reproduced from Sato *et al.*, *Neuroradiology* (1991) **178:** 433–439 by kind permission of Dr. S. Takahashi, Department of Radiology, Tohoku University School of Medicine, Sendai, Japan, and the Editors.)

*Figure CP 26.2.1* shows the typical posture during walking: the elbow and fingers are flexed and the leg has to be *circumducted* during the swing phase (unless an ankle brace is worn) because of the antigravity tone of the musculature. During the early rehabilitation period an arm sling is required in order to protect the shoulder joint from downward subluxation; this is because the supraspinatus muscle is normally in continuous contraction when the body is upright, preventing slippage of the humeral head.

A small hemorrhage or embolus may select pyramidal tract fibers almost exclusively, giving rise to *pure motor hemiplegia*. A fascinating account of a personal case is that of the Norwegian neuroanatomist Alf Brodal (see Reference list). *Figure CP 26.2.2* is from an MR study of a patient who had suffered a right hemiplegia with sensory loss 11 days previously. The picture shows extensive infarction of the white matter on the left side, at the junctional region between the corona radiata and internal capsule, with compression of the lateral ventricle.

*(lacunes)* of vascular leakage into the upper part of the internal capsule, having a severe impact on the pyramidal tract.

### *Posterior cerebral artery* (Figure 26.2)

The two posterior cerebral arteries are the terminal branches of the basilar. However, in embryonic life they originated from the internal carotid, and in about 25% of individuals the internal carotid persists as the primary source of blood on one or both sides, by way of a large posterior communicating artery.

Close to its origin, each posterior cerebral gives branches to the midbrain and a **posterior choroidal artery** to the choroid plexus of the lateral ventricle. Additional, *central* branches are sent into the posterior perforated substance (*Figure 26.1*).

The main artery winds around the midbrain in company with the optic tract. It supplies the splenium of the corpus callosum and the cortex of the occipital and temporal lobes. Named cortical branches and their territories are as follows:

| | |
|---|---|
| Anterior temporal | Parahippocampal gyrus, hippocampal formation |
| Posterior temporal | Occipitotemporal gyri |
| Calcarine | Walls of calcarine sulcus |
| Parieto-occipital | Cuneus, precuneus |

The *central* branches, called *thalamoperforating* and *thalamogeniculate*, supply the thalamus, subthalamic nucleus, and optic radiation.

The effects of posterior cerebral artery occlusion are described in Panel 26.3.

### Internal carotid artery

As well as being a source of cerebral emboli, atheromatous plaques may cause partial or com-

---

## CLINICAL PANEL 26.3 • POSTERIOR CEREBRAL ARTERY OCCLUSION

A variety of effects may follow occlusion of branches of the posterior cerebral artery. Usually the occlusion is limited to a branch to the midbrain, *or* to the thalamus, *or* to the subthalamic nucleus, *or* to the cerebral cortex.

### Midbrain

The classical picture of a unilateral infarct of the midbrain is that of a *crossed third nerve palsy*, i.e. a complete oculomotor paralysis (Chapter 17) on one side with a hemiplegia on the other side (Weber's syndrome). The hemiplegia is due to infarction of the crus cerebri, which contains corticospinal and corticonuclear fibers in its mid-portion.

### Thalamus

Occlusion of a thalamogeniculate branch may cause infarction of the ventral posterior nucleus of the thalamus (resulting in contralateral sensory loss) and of the lateral geniculate nucleus (resulting in homonymous hemianopia). The rare, *thalamic syndrome* (Chapter 21) seems to result from damage to the white matter lateral to the thalamus, in the territory of the *middle* cerebral artery.

### Subthalamic nucleus

Occlusion of a thalamoperforating branch may destroy the small subthalamic nucleus and give rise to *ballism* on the contralateral side, usually affecting the arm (Chapter 24).

### Corpus callosum

Infarction of the splenium of the corpus callosum blocks transfer of written information from the right visual association cortex to the left. The result of infarction is alexia for written material presented to the left visual field.

### Cortex

Occlusion of the posterior cerebral artery behind the midbrain gives rise to a homonymous hemianopia in the contralateral field. Macular vision may be spared. One view of 'macular sparing' is that it signifies bilateral representation of the fovea in the primary visual cortex. Another view is that the occipital pole is supplied by a long branch from the middle cerebral artery supplying the angular gyrus.

Occlusion of the *left* artery also produces alexia for written material, the left visual field being the only area detectable by the patient.

A pure alexia, without agraphia, may follow a lesion of the left lingual gyrus.

BILATERAL OCCLUSION
Partial or complete *cortical blindness* may result from a 'riding thrombus' arrested astride the basilar bifurcation, with consequent blockage of both posterior cerebral arteries. It has also been recorded following cardiac arrest with resuscitation.

Temporary cessation of flow in both posterior cerebral arteries sometimes affects the anterior territories alone. If damage is confined to the occipitotemporal junctions, *prosopagnosia* (inability to identify faces) may occur alone. If the entorhinal cortex/hippocampus is compromised, anterograde amnesia may follow.

---

### CLINICAL PANEL 26.4 • INTERNAL CAROTID ARTERY OCCLUSION

The lumen of the internal carotid artery may become progressively obstructed by atheromatous deposits. Common sites of obstruction are the point of commencement in the neck, and the cavernous sinus. A slowly progressive obstruction may be compensated for by the opposite internal carotid artery, through the circle of Willis. Substantial additional blood may be provided by anastomotic branches of the external carotid artery; for example, carotid angiography may show significant retrograde flow through the ophthalmic artery from the facial artery. At the other extreme, sudden occlusion may cause death from infarction of the entire anterior and middle cerebral territories, and sometimes the posterior cerebral as well.

*Warning signs* of carotid occlusion take the form of *transient ischemic attacks* lasting for a few minutes (sometimes for a few hours). The territory of the middle cerebral artery is most often affected. Individual symptoms tend to occur in isolation and include any of the following: unilateral motor weakness, unilateral 'pins and needles' or numbness, aphasia, or hemianopia. Disturbance of flow in the ophthalmic artery may cause dimness of vision or monocular blindness (one eye may be filled with 'white steam').

---

plete occlusion of the internal carotid artery itself (see Panel 26.4).

### *Anterior versus posterior circulatory occlusion*

Clinicians refer to the internal carotid artery and its branches as the *anterior circulation* of the brain, and the vertebrobasilar system as the *posterior circulation*. About 25% of CVAs (cerebrovascular accidents) originate in the posterior circulation, notably in the brainstem.

Some of the clinical features of brainstem lesions have been mentioned in chapters dealing with cranial nerves. In more general terms, the following features are suggestive of a lesion within the posterior circulation:

- *Crossed hemiplegia:* lower motor neuron lesion(s) on the side contralateral to the hemiplegia.
- Ataxia in the presence of long-tract motor or sensory impairment.
- Horner's syndrome in the presence of long tract impairment.
- Dissociated sensory loss on one side, indicating damage to *either* the medial or the spinal lemniscus.
- Facial analgesia to pin-prick with or without loss of the corneal reflex.
- Bilateral long-tract signs (motor and/or sensory) without visual impairment could be suggestive of spinal cord damage but could be caused by blockage of the pontine artery with continued perfusion of the posterior cerebrals through the circle of Willis.
- Early and prolonged coma.

It is not always possible to distinguish between supratentorial and infratentorial lesions by clinical examination alone. For example, a pure motor hemiparesis may be produced by a lacune *either* in the upper part of the pons *or* in the upper part of the internal capsule.

### *Aneurysms*

In addition to the hazards of embolic, thrombotic and hemorrhagic strokes, the cerebral circulation poses a further threat. *Subarachnoid hemorrhage* may occur without warning, from a ruptured aneurysm at the base of the brain. About 25 000 cases occur annually in the United States. See Panel 26.5 for details.

### VENOUS DRAINAGE OF THE BRAIN

The venous drainage of the brain is of great importance in relation to neurosurgical procedures. It is also important to the professional neurologist because a variety of clinical syndromes can be produced by venous obstruction, venous thrombosis, and congenital arteriovenous communications. In general medical practice, however, problems caused by cerebral veins are rare in comparison with arterial disease.

---

### CLINICAL PANEL 26.5 • SUBARACHNOID HEMORRHAGE

Blister-like *berry aneurysms* 5–10 mm in diameter are a routine autopsy finding in 2% of adults. Most are in the anterior half of the circle of Willis. *Spontaneous rupture* of an aneurysm into the interpeduncular cistern usually occurs in early or late middle age. The characteristic presentation is a sudden blinding headache, with collapse into semiconsciousness or coma within a few seconds. On physical examination, the only characteristic feature is *neck rigidity;* this is caused by movement of blood into the posterior cranial fossa, where the dura mater is supplied by the upper cervical nerves (Chapter 16).

The massive rise in intracranial pressure may be fatal within a few hours or days. Recovery may be impeded by a secondary elevation of intracranial pressure caused by obstruction of cerebrospinal fluid circulation through the tentorial notch or even within the arachnoid granulations.

About a quarter of all cases develop a neurological deficit 4–12 days after the initial attack. The deficit is fatal in a quarter of those who get it. The immediate cause is *vasospasm* of the main, conducting segments of the cerebral arteries. The amount of spasm is proportionate to the size of the blood clot that collects in the interpeduncular cistern containing the circle of Willis.

It is usual practice to define the aneurysm by means of carotid angiography, and to ligate it surgically. Without operation, most aneurysms will leak again at some future date.

---

The cerebral hemispheres are drained by superficial and deep cerebral veins. Like the intracranial venous sinuses, they are devoid of valves.

### Superficial veins

The *superficial cerebral veins* lie in the subarachnoid space overlying the hemispheres. They drain the

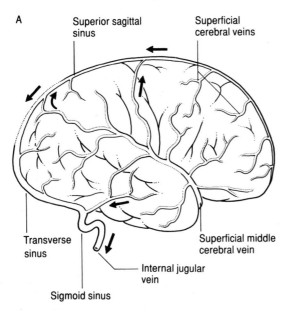

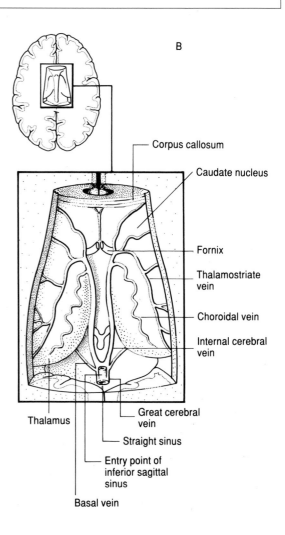

**Figure 26.6.** Cerebral veins. (A) Superficial veins viewed from the right side; arrows indicate direction of blood flow. (B) Deep veins viewed from above.

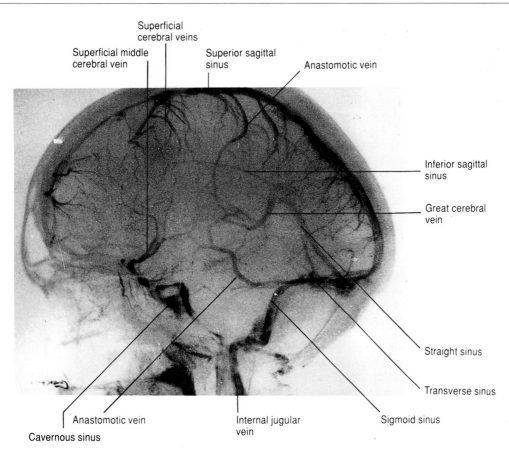

**Figure 26.7.** Internal carotid angiogram, venous phase. The dye is draining into the dural venous sinuses. (Photograph kindly provided by Dr James Toland, Department of Radiology, Beaumont Hospital, Dublin.)

cerebral cortex and underlying white matter and empty into intracranial venous sinuses (*Figures 26.6A* and *26.7*).

The upper part of each hemisphere drains into the superior sagittal sinus. The middle part drains into the cavernous sinus (as a rule) by way of the **superficial middle cerebral vein.** The lower part drains into the transverse sinus.

### Deep veins *(Figure 26.6B)*

The deep cerebral veins drain the corpus striatum, thalamus, and choroid plexuses.

A **thalamostriate vein** drains the thalamus and caudate nucleus. Together with a **choroidal vein** it forms the **internal cerebral vein.** The two internal cerebral veins unite beneath the corpus callosum to form the **great cerebral vein** (of Galen).

A **basal vein** is formed beneath the anterior

perforated substance by the union of **anterior** and **deep middle cerebral veins.** The basal vein runs around the crus cerebri and empties into the great cerebral vein.

Finally, the great cerebral vein enters the midpoint of the tentorium cerebelli. As it does so, it unites with the inferior sagittal sinus to form the straight sinus. The straight sinus empties in turn into the left transverse sinus.

### *Regulation of blood flow*

Blood flow in the cerebral vessels is primarily controlled by *autoregulation*, which is defined as the capacity of a tissue to regulate its own blood supply.

The most powerful source of autoregulation in the CNS is the $H^+$ *ion concentration* in the extracellular fluid surrounding the arterioles within the brain parenchyma. Generalized relaxation of arteriolar smooth muscle tone is produced by hypercapnia (excess plasma $PCO_2$) On the other hand, hypocapnia causes arteriolar vasoconstriction.

A second powerful source of autoregulation is the *intraluminal pressure* within the arterioles. Any increase in pressure elicits a direct, myogenic response. When other factors are controlled (in animal experiments), the myogenic response is sufficient to maintain steady-state perfusion of the brain within a systemic blood pressure range of 80–180 mmHg (11–24 kPa).

*Focal* blood flow increases within cortical foci and deep nuclei involved in particular motor, sensory or cognitive tasks. The local arteriolar relaxation can be accounted for by a rise in $K^+$ levels caused by propagation of action potentials, and by a rise in $H^+$ caused by increased cell metabolism. At precapillary level neuronal peptides and amines may be significant, the most promising candidate being VIP (vasoactive intestinal polypeptide).

A large number of vasoactive substances have been identified in neural networks surrounding the cerebral conducting arteries and the arterioles. A specific role is difficult to assign to any of them, within the physiological range of blood flow.

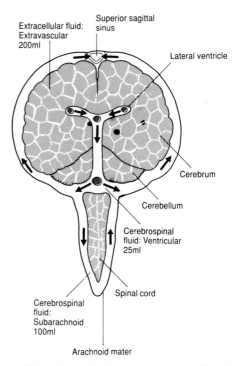

**Figure 26.8.** Extracellular compartments of the brain. Arrows indicate circulation of cerebrospinal fluid (CSF).

## THE BLOOD–BRAIN BARRIER

The nervous system is isolated from the blood by a barrier system that provides a stable and chemically optimal environment for neuronal function. The neurons and neuroglia are bathed in *brain extracellular fluid* (ECF) which accounts for 15% of total brain volume.

The extracellular compartments of the CNS are shown diagrammatically in *Figure 26.8*. As previously described (Chapter 4), cerebrospinal fluid (CSF) secreted by the choroid plexuses circulates through the ventricular system and the subarachnoid space before passing through the arachnoid villi into the dural venous sinuses. *In addition*, CSF diffuses passively through the ependyma–glial membrane lining the ventricles and enters the brain extracellular spaces. It adds to the ECF produced by the capillary bed and by cell metabolism, and it diffuses through the pia–glial membrane into the subarachnoid space. This 'sink' movement of fluid compensates for the absence of lymphatics from the CNS.

Metabolic water is the only component of the

CSF which does not pass through the blood–brain barrier. It carries with it any neurotransmitter substances that have not been recaptured following liberation by neurons, and it accounts for the presence in the subarachnoid space of transmitters and transmitter metabolites that could not penetrate the blood–brain barrier.

Relative contributions to the CSF obtained from a spinal tap are approximately as follows:

| | |
|---|---|
| Choroid plexuses | 60% |
| Capillary bed | 30% |
| Metabolic water | 10% |

The blood–brain barrier has two components. One is at the level of the choroid plexus, the other resides in the CNS capillary bed.

### Blood–CSF barrier

The blood–CSF barrier occupies the specialized ependymal lining of the choroid plexuses. This *choroidal epithelium* differs from the general ependymal epithelium in three ways:

1. Cilia are almost completely replaced by microvilli.

## CLINICAL PANEL 26.6 ● BLOOD–BRAIN BARRIER PATHOLOGY

The following five conditions are associated with breakdown of the blood–brain barrier:

1. Patients suffering from hypertension are liable to attacks of *hypertensive encephalopathy* should the blood pressure exceed the power of the arterioles to control it. The pressure may then open the tight junctions of the brain capillary endothelium. Rapid exudation of plasma causes *cerebral edema* with severe headache and vomiting, sometimes progressing to convulsions and coma.

2. In patients with severe *hypercapnia* brought about by reduced ventilation of the lungs (as in pulmonary or heart disease, or after surgery), relaxation of arteriolar muscle may be sufficient to induce cerebral edema even if the blood pressure is normal. In this case the edema may be expressed by mental confusion and drowsiness progressing to coma.

3. *Brain injury*, whether from trauma or spontaneous hemorrhage, leads to edema due to the osmotic effects of tissue damage (and other factors).

4. *Infections* of the brain or meninges are accompanied by breakdown of the blood–brain barrier, perhaps because of the large scale emigration of leucocytes through the brain capillary bed. The breakdown can be exploited because the porous capillary walls will permit the passage of non-lipid-soluble antibiotics.

5. The capillary bed of *brain tumors* is fenestrated. As a result, radioactive tracers too large to penetrate healthy brain capillaries can be detected within tumors.

---

2. The cells are bonded by tight junctions. These pericellular belts of membrane fusion are the actual site of the blood–CSF barrier.

3. The epithelium contains numerous enzymes specifically involved in transport of ions and metabolites.

### Blood–ECF barrier

The blood–ECF barrier resides in the CNS capillary bed, which differs from that of other tissues in three ways:

1. The endothelial cells are bonded by tight junctions.
2. Pinocytotic vesicles are rare, and fenestrations are absent.
3. The cells contain the same transport systems as those of the choroidal epithelium.

The surface area of the brain capillary bed is about the size of a tennis court. This huge area accounts for the brain's consumption of 20% of basal oxygen intake by the lungs.

### Functions of the blood–brain barrier

● Modulation of the entry of metabolic substrates. *Glucose*, in particular, is a fundamental source of energy for neurons. The level of glucose in the brain ECF is more stable than that of the blood because the specific carrier becomes saturated when blood glucose rises and becomes hyperactive when it falls.

● Control of ion movements. $Na^+$–$K^+$ ATPase in the barrier cells pumps sodium into the CSF and pumps potassium out of the CSF into the blood.

● Prevention of access to the CNS by toxins and by peripheral neurotransmitters escaping into the blood stream from autonomic nerve endings.

For some clinical notes concerning the blood–brain barrier, see Panel 26.6.

### EXERCISES

Indicate the most likely anatomical site of a lesion (e.g. infarct/hemorrhage, patch of demyelination, tumor) responsible for each of the following deficits.

**1** *(a)* Slow, laborious speech
  *(b)* Paralysis of the right arm and lower face.

**2** *(a)* Difficulty with speech initiation
  *(b)* Spastic weakness of the right leg.

**3** *(a)* Inability to name an unseen object placed in the left hand.

**4** Bitemporal hemianopia.

**5** Central blind spot in the visual field of the right eye.

**6** *(a)* Homonymous lower quadrant anopia on the left side
   *(b)* Neglect of the left side of the body.

**7** Right hemiplegia with reduced sensation in the paralyzed limbs.

**8** *(a)* Fluent but largely unintelligible speech
   *(b)* Right homonymous upper quadrant anopia.

**9** Flaccid left hemiplegia with paralysis of contraversive gaze.

**10** Epileptic aura consisting of flashes of light in the right visual field.

## REFERENCES

Adams, R.D. and Victor, M. (1989) *Principles of Neurology*, 4th edn. New York: McGraw-Hill.

Betz, A.L., Goldstein, G.W. and Katzman, R. (1989) Blood-brain-cerebrospinal fluid barriers. In *Basic Neurochemistry: Molecular, Cellular, and Medical Aspects*, 4th edn (Siegel, G.J. *et al.*, eds), pp. 591–605. New York: Raven Press.

Brodal, A.(1973) Self-observations and neuro-anatomical considerations after a stroke. *Brain* **96:** 675–694.

Brust, J.C.M. (1989) Cerebral infarction. In *Merritt's Textbook of Neurology*, 8th edn (Rowland, L.P., ed.), pp. 206–214. Philadelphia: Lea & Febiger.

Duus, P. (1983) *Topical Diagnosis in Neurology*. New York: Thieme-Stratton, Inc.

Toole, J.F. (1990) *Cerebrovascular Disorders*, 4th edn. New York: Raven Press.

# Index